Orthostatic Disorders of the Circulation

MECHANISMS, MANIFESTATIONS, AND TREATMENT

Orthostatic Disorders of the Circulation

MECHANISMS, MANIFESTATIONS, AND TREATMENT

David H. P. Streeten, M.B., B.Ch., D.Phi., F.R.C.P., F.A.C.P.
Professor of Medicine
and Chief of Endocrine Section
State University of New York Health Science Center
Syracuse, New York

PLENUM MEDICAL BOOK COMPANY
New York and London

Library of Congress Cataloging in Publication Data

Streeten, David H. P., 1921-
Orthostatic disorders of the circulation.

Bibliography: p.
Includes index.
1. Hypotension, Orthostatic—Complications and sequelae. 2. Edema. 3. Blood pressure—Regulation. I. Title. [DNLM: 1. Blood Circulation. 2. Edema—physiopathology. 3. Hypotension, Orthostatic—physiopathology. 4. Posture. QZ 170 S915o]
RC685.078S87 1986 616.1 86-18748
ISBN 978-1-4684-8964-4 ISBN 978-1-4684-8962-0 (eBook)
DOI 10.1007/978-1-4684-8962-0

Softcover reprint of the hardcover 1st edition 1987
233 Spring Street, New York, N.Y. 10013

Plenum Medical Book Company is an imprint of Plenum Publishing Corporation

This book is dedicated to my wife, Barbara, who encouraged me to prepare the manuscript, and to clinical investigators in all lands, who seek to alleviate illness and suffering by studying the underlying derangements of physiological processes.

Preface

Most of us spend at least two-thirds of our lives either sitting or standing. It is somewhat surprising, therefore, to find not a single book devoted to disorders caused by derangements of the normal physiological adjustments to changes in posture. In fact, until very recently, medical students have not even been advised to measure the blood pressure and heart rate in the upright posture as part of the routine physical examination. Although Bradbury and Eggleston first described orthostatic hypotension as a consequence of autonomic insufficiency in 1925, interest in orthostatic disorders has been slow to develop in the subsequent years.

It is well known that the change from recumbency to the standing posture stimulates neurological, endocrine, and cardiovascular adjustments that ensure maintenance of a normal circulation despite the effects of gravitational forces. The mechanisms of these physiological responses to orthostasis have been studied by many investigators. Some of the defects to which antigravitational compensatory mechanisms are subject, such as postural hypotension resulting from autonomic failure, have been studied intensively and have become part of the general knowledge of most medical practitioners. Other orthostatic disorders—such as various other postural abnormalities of blood pressure control, and orthostatic edema—have received far less attention and have been unable to compete with the more dramatic and life-threatening ailments of humankind for a place in our standard medical texts. These disorders often give rise to distressing symptoms and may lead to severe impairment of health. Since they do not appear to have been described and discussed systematically before, I have attempted in the present volume to collate our own studies performed over the past 30 years, as well as those reported by others, on the pathogenesis, clinical manifestations, and treatment of these and other postural disorders of the circulation.

ACKNOWLEDGMENTS

In this endeavor, I have enjoyed the constant stimulation of colleagues in the Endocrine Section of the Department of Medicine, especially Dr. Arnold

Moses, Dr. Gunnar Anderson, Jr., Dr. Stanley Blumenthal, and Dr. Myron Miller, as well as participants in our interdepartmental Endocrine Study Group at the State University of New York Health Science Center at Syracuse, particularly Drs. Jay and Helen Tepperman and Dr. Robert Richman. Dr. Howland Auchincloss, Jr., Dr. Harold Smulyan, Dr. Anis Obeid, Dr. Robert Eich, Dr. Deaver Thomas, and Dr. Robert Richardson have made valuable contributions to the investigations. The studies have been performed in collaboration with a series of research fellows, particularly Dr. Philip Speller, Dr. Theodore Dalakos, Dr. Gunnar Anderson, Jr., Dr. Michael Freiberg, and Dr. Timothy Howland, to all of whom it is a pleasure to acknowledge my profound indebtedness.

A succession of keen and inquisitive medical students has participated in the performance and discussion of the clinical experiments. The studies could not have been undertaken without the devoted and careful assistance of the nurses and dietitians at our Clinical Research Center or the skillful biochemical analyses performed by our technicians in the Endocrine Research Laboratory: Mary Kearney, Thomas Scullard, Carol Jones, and Suzanne Brennan. Suzanne Brennan and David Peppi were responsible for preparing most of the diagrams and the photographs were taken by the Photography Department of the SUNY Health Science Center. To all these collaborators I offer my sincere thanks.

The United States Public Health Service supported a large number of the investigations on which much of this book is based, with grants RR 229, A 3795, AM 04488, AM 07793, HL 14076, and HL 22051.

Last but not least, I am very grateful to the patients who have cheerfully endured the discomfort involved in so many of the studies described in this book.
I believe they have understood that virtually no advance in alleviating human disorders can be achieved without studies on some of the sufferers themselves, and I sincerely hope that most have derived some therapeutic benefit from the results of these investigations.

David H. P. Streeten

Syracuse, New York

Contents

1

Physiology of the Microcirculation

Functional integrity of the blood vessels is an essential ingredient of a normal circulatory system. In its simplest terms, physiological "normality" of the microcirculation includes the capacity to bring about dynamic changes in the function of the arterioles, the precapillary sphincters, the muscular venules, and the veins, so as to ensure appropriate perfusion of the relatively passive capillaries under the variable conditions of daily life. Arteriolar contraction and relaxation serve both to maintain an adequate diastolic blood pressure for the organism as a whole and to redistribute blood flow to different vascular beds as metabolic requirements dictate. In most circumstances requiring increased tissue perfusion—say, to the muscles during vigorous exercise—dilatation of arterioles and precapillary sphincters increases the flow of blood into an expanded capillary bed. After perfusion of the tissues, the return of blood to the heart is enhanced by tonic contraction of the muscular venules. Venous return is further facilitated by the negative intrathoracic pressure and by the massaging action of skeletal muscular contraction on venous flow directed centrally by venous valves.

1.1. CONTROL OF THE PERIPHERAL VASCULATURE

The sympathetic nervous system and the circulating and locally released humoral agents control the peripheral vasculature.

1.1.1. Sympathetic Innervation

Figure 1 shows the variable density of sympathetic innervation of the vascular system, which is sparse in the large elastic arteries, increasing as the arteries become smaller, and reaching a peak in the arterioles. The precapillary sphincters are noninnervated in many vascular beds (Altura, 1978*b;* Chambers and Zweifach, 1944; Furness, 1973), such as the mesenteric circulation, but are

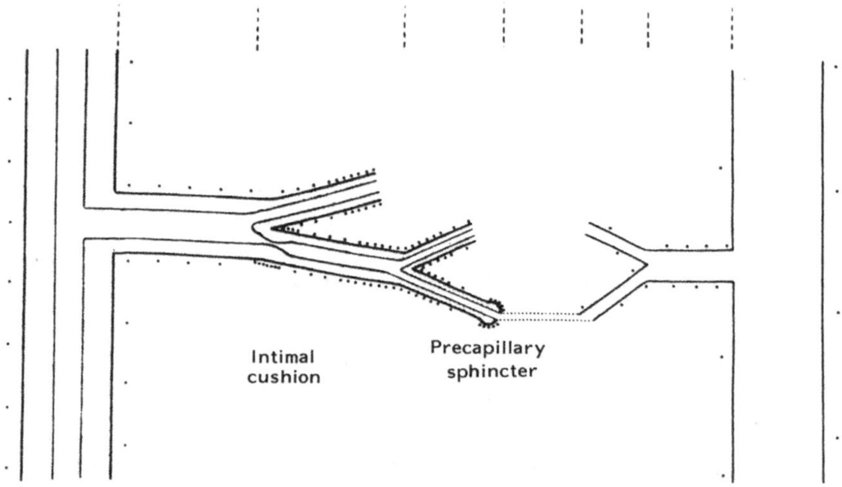

FIGURE 1. Diagrammatic representation of innervation density in different regions of the vascular system. (From Burnstock, 1975.)

richly supplied with adrenergic innervation in other parts of the vascular tree, such as the coronary circulation (Burnstock *et al.*, 1981). The capillaries and the collecting venules are generally thought not to be innervated (Burnstock *et al.*, 1981; Altura, 1978*b*). Most of the muscular venules are sparsely supplied with sympathetic nerve endings and are unresponsive to drugs that (1) stimulate norepinephrine release, e.g., ephedrine; (2) inhibit neuronal uptake of norepinephrine, e.g., guanethidine; or (3) block α-adrenergic receptors, e.g., phenoxybenzamine (Altura, 1978*a*). Muscular venules have a preponderance of β- over α-receptors, which might imply that they are normally dilated by the action of circulating epinephrine on their receptors (Altura, 1978*a*). Some of the large muscular veins, however, including the saphenous veins of man, have heavy adrenergic innervation (Ehinger *et al.*, 1967). The sympathetic nerve supply of the large veins probably mediates sympathetic increases in venous tone (Furness, 1973), since norepinephrine is known to induce venous constriction *in vivo* (Wood and Eckstein, 1958).

There are variations in the nerve supply of the blood vessels to different organ systems in the body. The sympathetic nerves supplying the vasculature of skeletal muscle, for instance, contain cholinergic vasodilator fibers. Adrenergic nerves supply mainly the adventitial side of the media of blood vessels, thus providing for dual control of vascular contraction by the transmitter (norepinephrine) released from these nerve endings and by circulating catecholamines and other vasoactive humoral agents. In view of the many species differences that have been described, it is unfortunate that our knowledge of vascular innervation in the human subject is incomplete.

1.1.2. Humoral Agents and Local Tissue Metabolites

In the precapillary sphincters, the venules, and perhaps the capillaries themselves, it seems likely that control of luminal diameter depends to a large extent on circulating hormones and local tissue metabolites (Devine, 1978). The large variety of these vasoactive agents includes circulating norepinephrine, epinephrine, and perhaps dopamine, angiotensin II, and vasopressin, as well as (predominantly) locally released histamine, bradykinin, serotonin, acetylcholine (ACh), and various prostaglandins.

Vascular contractility may also be affected by the vascular uptake of renin and by the local synthesis of renin as well as angiotensin I and II within the vascular endothelium or the smooth muscle cells (Dzau, 1984*a,b;* Oliver and Sciacca, 1984). In addition to its intrinsic actions on contractility of the vascular muscle, angiotensin II in the vascular walls may indirectly increase contractility by facilitating the local release of norepinephrine from sympathetic nerve endings (Zimmerman, 1978). On many vascular structures, including the mesenteric arterioles, metarterioles, precapillary sphincters, and muscular venules of the rat, the potency of epinephrine is about 10 times that of norepinephrine and five or six orders of magnitude greater than that of dopamine (Altura, 1978*b*). Moreover, precapillary sphincters are 500–10,000 times more sensitive to the constrictive actions of epinephrine and norepinephrine than are the arterioles and venules (Altura, 1971); therefore, they are probably largely controlled by circulating rather than by locally released catecholamines. Since circulating concentrations of epinephrine are seldom less and sometimes more than one-tenth those of norepinephrine in man, it follows that, quantitatively, epinephrine may be as important as norepinephrine in its role as a circulating vasoconstrictor of the microvasculature, at least beyond the arterioles. Epinephrine also has qualitatively different effects from norepinephrine, including its vasodilatory and cardioacceleratory actions on arteriolar and cardiac β-adrenergic receptors, respectively.

Dilatation of most reactive components of the microcirculation, including that of the liver, results from the action of histamine, bradykinin, prostacyclin, vasoactive intestinal peptide (VIP), ACh, serotonin, and some substances from functioning tissues, such as potassium and inorganic phosphate (McCuskey, 1966; Haddy and Scott, 1978). However, the actions of some of these agents are not the same at all vascular sites; e.g., serotonin and histamine both dilate arterioles and constrict venules (Vanhoutte, 1978). Some prostaglandins, such as prostacyclin, are predominantly vasodilators, whereas others, such as prostaglandin F (PGF), are predominantly vasoconstrictors (Kaley, 1978); also PGE_2

dilates many vascular beds but contracts the aorta in rabbits and the coronary arteries in dogs (Strong and Bohr, 1967; Kaley, 1978). Species and site differences are apparent in the actions of PGF (Kaley, 1978) and in those of bradykinin, which contracts unbilical vessels, most large arteries, and veins but dilates the entire microvasculature (Vanhoutte, 1978; Altura, 1967, 1978*a*). Angiotensin II exerts a potent vasoconstrictor action on the arterioles but is far weaker than norepinephrine in its constrictor activity on the veins (Rose *et al.*, 1962; Haddy *et al.*, 1962).

Thus, in determining whether an observed vascular phenomenon in man might have resulted from adrenergic nervous changes or from circulating or locally produced vasoactive agents, it is necessary to know whether the reaction in the specific vessels of interest could have resulted from the agent in question, in the human subject. Unfortunately, this information is frequently unavailable.

There is evidence that changes in the availability of free calcium ions (Ca^{2+}) in the intracellular fluid (ICF) may be the "final common path" of the actions of many vasoconstrictor and vasodilator agents. Increases in free, ionized calcium concentration promote contraction of the smooth muscle, while reductions in intracellular Ca^{2+} concentration lead to muscular relaxation (Bohr *et al.*, 1978).

1.2. PHYSIOLOGICAL REQUIREMENTS IMPOSED BY ORTHOSTASIS

Assumption of the upright posture imposes gravitational forces that raise the intravascular pressures in the parts of the body below the "hydrostatically indifferent point" (E. Wagner, 1886), which is close to the diaphragm (Gauer and Thron, 1965), and cause pooling of blood in the vessels below this level. This orthostatic pooling, which is known to be absent during space flight (Kirsch *et al.*, 1984), would produce a profound fall in blood pressure in the absence of rapid and sustained adjustments in the circulation. The necessity of maintaining blood flow to the brain and other vital organs requires circulatory changes that obviously become more critical as the vertical distance between the heart and the head is increased. To satisfy this need, orthostasis is associated with immediate and sustained constriction of the arterioles and probably of the precapillary sphincters, the venules, and the large veins (Wood, 1958), where the changes are relatively small and transient (Gauer and Thron, 1962, 1965). These changes restrict the magnitude of gravitational pooling, which would otherwise cause profound hypotension and, if sufficiently long lasting, edema. The gravitational pooling of blood in the legs during orthostasis is also reduced by contractions of the calf muscles. By compressing the deep veins of the calf, this "muscle pump" accelerates the return of blood toward the heart during standing, and particularly during exercise (Gauer and Thron, 1965). Absence of this muscular action on venous return is responsible for the pronounced effects of orthostasis and often for troublesome symptoms (i.e., a fall in cardiac output, progressive narrowing of pulse pressure, a drop in mean blood pressure, and syncope) when normal subjects are passively tilted, head up, or during motionless standing, as in a military parade. These changes are aggravated by a warm environment (Robinson, 1949), long-distance running (Allen *et al.*, 1945), previous hemorrhage (Barcroft and Swan, 1953; Gullbring *et al.*, 1960), and prolonged bed rest (Deitrick and Whedon, 1946).

In some animals, the tight hide that binds the tissues of the lower limbs provides added protection from the effects of gravity by physically preventing peripheral vascular overdistention and significant edema formation in the upright posture (Goetz *et al.*, 1960). This protective mechanism enables such animals to remain on their feet and even to sleep in this position for many hours at a time without developing peripheral edema. The need to raise blood a long distance from the heart to the brain has been satisfied in the giraffe by the maintenance of extremely high mean arterial blood pressure levels—in the vicinity of 250 mm Hg (Folkow, 1978).

1.3. ORTHOSTATIC CIRCULATORY ADJUSTMENTS: NEUROHUMORAL MECHANISMS

1.3.1. Catecholamine Responses

When human beings assume the erect posture, immediate vagal inhibition accelerates the heartbeat, and increased sympathetic activity results in contraction of the microvessels in the dependent limbs. Almost instantaneously upon rising from recumbency, the baroreceptor reflex is initiated in receptors located in the major arteries, the atria, and the cardiopulmonary circulation. The reflex, operating through the nucleus tracti solitarii in the medulla, results in stimulation of a sympathetic discharge, directed predominantly toward the cardiac nerves, ending in the sinoatrial node, and toward the nerves supplying the peripheral arterioles. Release of norepinephrine at these neuronal terminals (Rosenthal *et al.*, 1978; Sever, 1983) brings about an immediate increase in heart rate and arteriolar constriction. So rapid is this response that leakage of norepinephrine from the neuronal synaptic clefts into the circulation results in a striking elevation of the plasma norepinephrine concentration, measurable in blood from an antecubital vein within 2 min, and rising to more than double the reclining concentration within 5 min of standing (Fig. 2). A more gradual, slight, but progressive further increase in plasma norepinephrine concentration indicates continued sympathetic discharge (since plasma norepinephrine half-life is less than 2 min in man), as long as the individual remains on his feet, or at least for 9

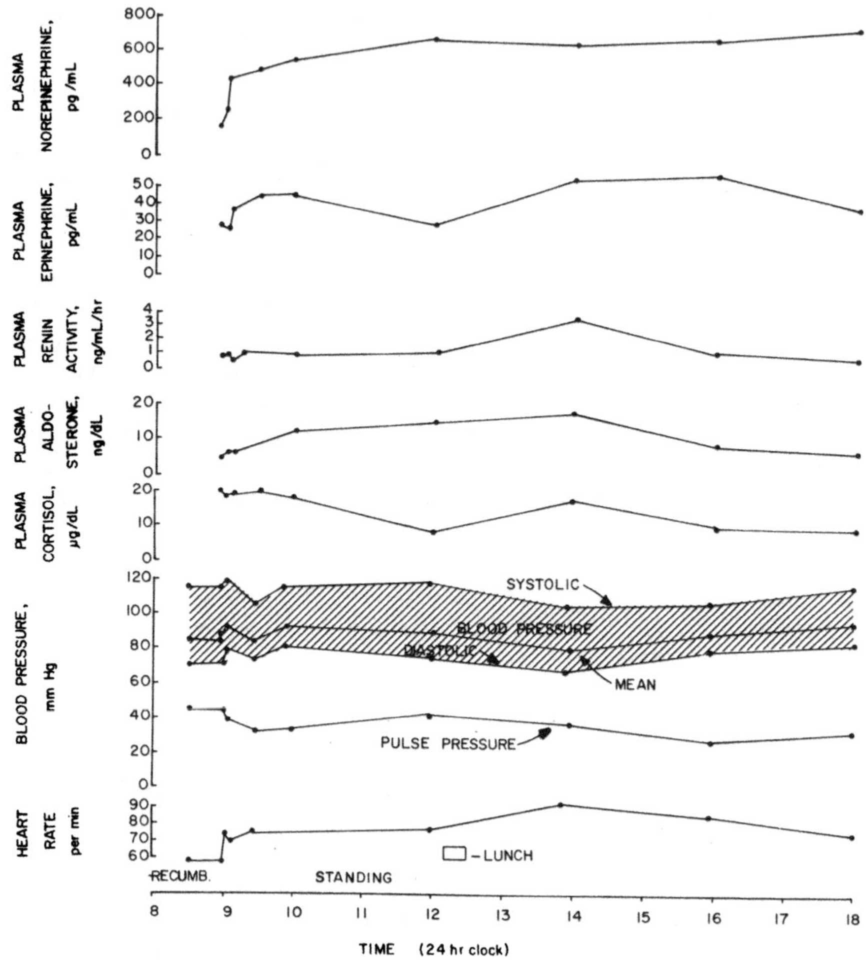

FIGURE 2. Humoral changes in a normal male upon assumption and during maintenance of the upright posture for several hours. Note the slight, inconsistent increases in plasma renin activity and plasma aldosterone and epinephrine concentrations, which contrast with the immediate, striking, and uninterrupted rise in plasma norepinephrine concentration.

hr, as shown in Figure 2. This sympathetic discharge in the upright posture appears to involve the adrenal medullae to a lesser extent—whereas plasma norepinephrine concentration was found to rise in this normal subject from 162 to 709 pg/ml, plasma epinephrine concentration, resulting mainly from adrenal medullary secretion (von Euler *et al.*, 1954), rose only from 28 to 56 pg/ml and eventually declined to 37 pg/ml at 9 hr. Similar increases in plasma catecholamine concentrations and in urinary output of norepinephrine and epinephrine occur in other normal subjects (Fig. 3) and have been reported by several investigators (Sundin, 1956; Molzahn *et al.*, 1972; Eide *et al.*, 1978; Robertson *et al.*, 1979; Hjemdahl and Eliasson, 1979; Campese *et al.*, 1980). Significant positive correlations have been reported (Eide *et al.*, 1978) between the recumbent plasma norepinephrine concentration and the orthostatic changes in systolic blood pressure and pulse pressure. It is evident from Figure 4 that the mean plasma norepinephrine concentration rose by 62% after 5 min of standing and by 97–100% after standing for 10, 15, and 30 min to above 400 pg/ml, while the mean rise in plasma epinephrine concentration was smaller and not statistically or (probably) biologically significant.

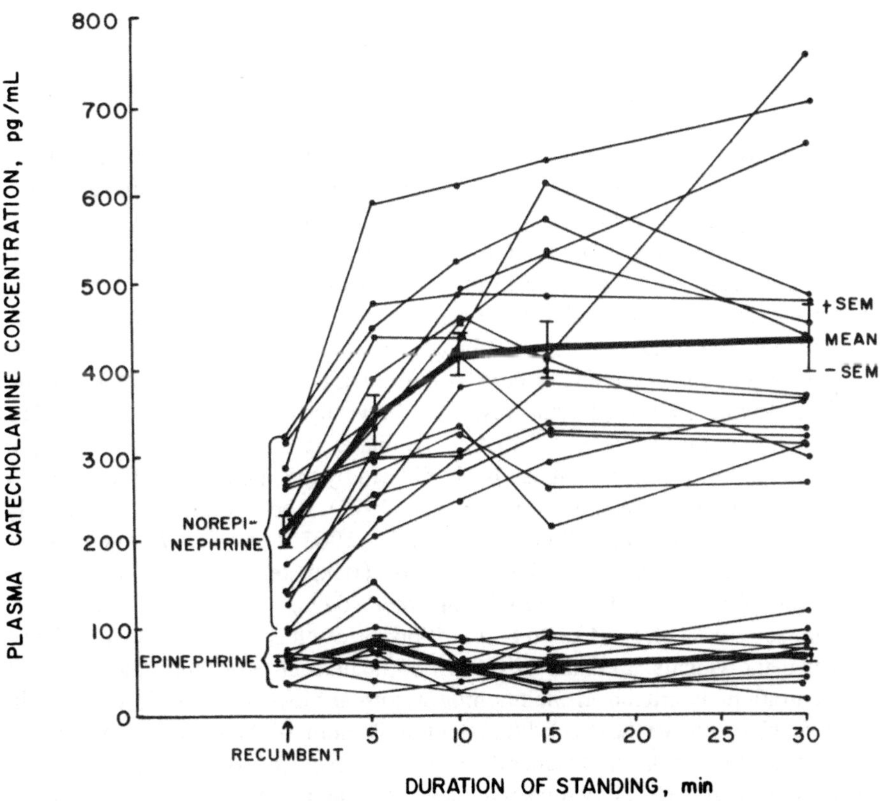

FIGURE 3. Concentrations of norepinephrine and epinephrine in the plasma of normal subjects after recumbency for 45–60 min and while standing for 30 min. Heavy lines indicate mean concentrations.

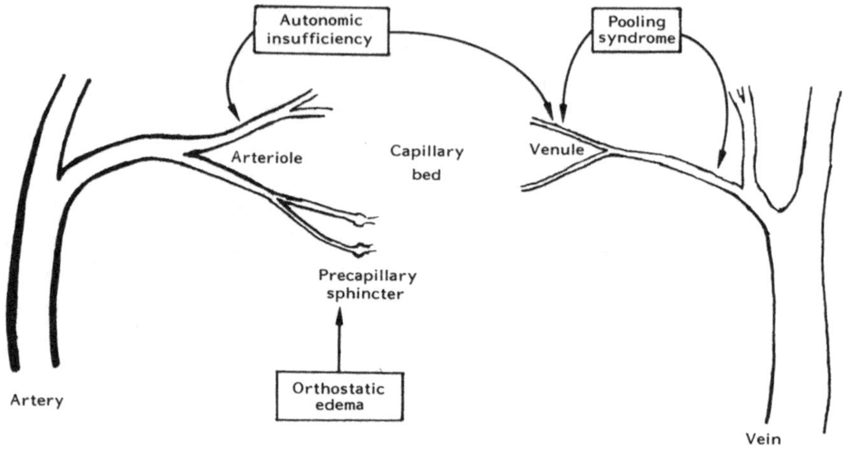

FIGURE 4. Defects responsible for orthostatic disorders. Known and postulated sites.

1.3.2. Changes in the Renin-Angiotensin-Aldosterone System

The orthostatic rise in plasma renin activity (PRA), first described by Gordon *et al.* (1966), has been amply confirmed (Cohen *et al.*, 1966; Streeten *et al.*, 1969*a*). In the normal subject, whose data are shown in Figure 2, the rise in PRA was smaller and more delayed than the increase in plasma norepinephrine concentration. Thus, the PRA rose from a recumbent level of 0.6 ng/ml-hr to 0.9 ng/ml-hr after 3 hr, and 3.7 ng/ml-hr after 5 hr, declining to recumbent values, despite continued standing, after 9 hr (see Fig. 2). The fall in PRA in the late afternoon and early evening occurs in the recumbent as well as in the upright posture despite continued orthostasis, as shown by Gordon *et al.* (1966). The orthostatic increase in PRA is probably stimulated by the gravitational pooling of blood in the lower limbs, as it can be duplicated by the application of lower body negative body pressure (Fasola and Martz, 1972). The rise in PRA is partially dependent on sympathetic stimulation (Vander, 1965; Tobian *et al.*, 1965) and is usually (Gordon *et al.*, 1966), but not always (Bannister *et al.*, 1977), absent in autonomic failure. It is far more striking when sodium deprivation or natriuresis accompanies orthostasis (Cohen *et al.*, 1966; Streeten *et al.*, 1969*a*). In sodium-depleted individuals, too, the postural rise in plasma renin and angiotensin II concentrations is crucial in maintaining a normal blood pressure in the upright posture, since, under these conditions, administration of the angiotensin II receptor antagonist, saralasin, frequently causes hypotension (Gavras *et al.*, 1976; Anderson *et al.*, 1977), which may lead to syncope despite continuing catecholamine release. Even in the absence of sodium depletion, however, the angiotensin II formed by the orthostatic rise in PRA interacts with the sympathetic nervous system to facilitate maintenance of the blood pressure (Hatton *et al.*, 1982).

Aldosterone secretion and excretion rates are increased when normal subjects assume and maintain the upright posture, as was first clearly documented by Muller *et al.* (1958*a,b*) and was confirmed by many studies (Gowenlock *et al.*, 1959; Wolfe *et al.*, 1966; Williams *et al.*, 1972; Streeten *et al.*, 1973). The stimulus to orthostatic elevation in the production and plasma concentration of aldosterone appears to result from the pooling of blood in the dependent parts of the body, since it can be almost completely suppressed by immersion in a water bath up to the neck (Gowenlock *et al.*, 1959; M. Epstein and Saruta, 1971). That the orthostatic rise in plasma aldosterone concentration results mainly from a large increase in aldosterone secretion rate, and only minimally from the small concomitant fall in metabolic clearance rate of aldosterone in the upright posture, was clearly demonstrated by Balikian *et al.* (1968). There is little doubt that the primary mechanism whereby orthostasis increases aldosterone secretion is the orthostatic increase in renin release and the consequent rise in plasma angiotensin II concentration (Laragh *et al.*, 1960; Davis *et al.*, 1961), although increased aldosterone production occasionally occurs without a rise in plasma renin or angiotensin II concentration (Best *et al.*, 1971). Plasma aldosterone concentration remains elevated for at least 9 hr of continued orthostasis. Despite continued standing, however, it then begins to fall to levels that, by 15 hr, are even below reclining concentrations of the steroid. This reduction in plasma aldosterone concentration in the face of continued orthostasis does not occur if the orthostatic stimulus is augmented by severe volume depletion, induced by the combination of a restricted sodium intake and the administration of a potent diuretic (Williams *et al.*, 1972).

1.3.3. Other Physiological Changes in the Erect Posture

Orthostatic increases in aldosterone secretion augment the effects of orthostatic reduction in the glomerular filtration rate (GFR) (Gowenlock *et al.*, 1959) to cause sodium and water retention, probably contributing to maintenance of blood pressure during prolonged orthostasis, although certainly not acutely. Normal cortisol production is certainly essential for the prevention of orthostatic hypotension (see Chapter 6). Although the normal circadian fluctuations in plasma cortisol concentrations may be blunted by prolonged orthostasis (see Fig. 2), we do not know whether orthostasis-induced attenuation of the normal circadian decreases and the consequent small increases in plasma cortisol concentration are important in maintaining the blood pressure during standing.

It is evident from Figure 2 that assumption of the erect posture was associated with an immediate slight rise in heart rate that persisted as long as orthostasis continued. This almost certainly reflected β-receptor action of norepinephrine released at the sinoatrial node, since β-blocking drugs consistently prevent this response. Standing caused an immediate slight rise in diastolic blood pressure, which was sustained for 9 hr, associated with a more variable slight drop in systolic blood pressure, so that mean blood pressure was consistently slightly higher and pulse pressure consistently slightly narrowed (from a mean value of 44.5 mm Hg to 27–39 mm Hg) in the upright position.

1.3.3.1. Changes in Blood Bradykinin Concentration

Blood bradykinin concentration increases in the upright posture (Streeten *et al.*, 1972; Wong *et al.*, 1975). This small change might reflect a more important local phenomenon at the sites of release of kinins in the tissues, but is not likely to have much effect on blood pressure control in the standing position under normal conditions, since simultaneously released norepinephrine would almost certainly overcome any hypotensive action of these low levels of bradykinin in normal subjects (Adamski *et al.*, 1983).

1.3.3.2. Changes in Plasma Vasopressin Concentration

Plasma vasopressin concentration rises in the upright posture in most patients with orthostatic hypotension (Zerbe *et al.*, 1983) and vasopressin excretion in the standing position is excessive in many patients with orthostatic edema (Thibonnier *et al.*, 1979; GH Anderson, Jr. and DHP Streeten, unpublished results). Whether orthostasis increases vasopressin release in normal subjects is unknown.

1.4. DISORDERS OF THE PERIPHERAL CIRCULATION

Functional abnormalities of the peripheral circulation may be caused by subnormal contractility of the arterioles, the precapillary sphincters, or the venules, as well as by deranged capillary permeability, venous obstruction, and malfunction of the venous valves or of the venous musculature. One would expect—and, in general, the expectation is realized—that excessive arteriolar tone would lead to arterial hypertension, while reduction or loss of arteriolar contractility would produce hypotension. Subnormal orthostatic contraction of the precapillary sphincters would be expected to result in excessive capillary perfusion. In the absence of compensatory changes in other parts of the vasculature, overperfusion of the capillaries might increase transudation beyond the capacity of the veins and the lymphatics to return the transudate to the heart, thus causing edema. By contrast, subnormal dilatation of the precapillary sphincters in response to heat or during reactive hyperemia has been shown to occur in diabetic patients (Tooke, 1980; K. Alexander *et al.*, 1967) and might be expected to restrict the flow of blood-borne nutrients to the tissues, in this disease. Subnormal venular tone would be expected to cause excessive pooling of blood within the peripheral capacitance vessels, while excessive tone in the venules, by increasing intracapillary pressure, could cause or aggravate edema. Impaired flow of blood in the veins has long been thought to cause edema and stasis changes due to inadequate oxygenation of the tissues.

1.5. ORTHOSTATIC DISORDERS OF THE CIRCULATION

Circulatory disorders that are evident exclusively in the upright posture in man have many etiologies, but most appear to result from faulty or inadequate adjustments of the peripheral circulation to the effects of gravity. Impaired arteriolar constriction causes orthostatic hypotension, often, paradoxically, associated with recumbent hypertension (Appenzeller, 1982). Subnormal constriction of the precapillary sphincters in the erect posture is the most likely mechanism of orthostatic edema in many patients (Streeten, 1978). It has been postulated that inadequate constriction of the capacitance vessels during maintenance of the upright posture initiates the series of physiological responses that result in orthostatic hypertension (Streeten *et al.*, 1985) and other disorders of blood pressure control in the upright position—the *pooling syndrome*. The mechanisms of these orthostatic derangements of the circulation, their clinical manifestations, and their most satisfactory treatment are discussed in Chapters 7–10. The known and postulated sites of origin of these orthostatic disorders are shown schematically in Figure 4.

1.6. SUMMARY

Among the many physiological influences on the peripheral vasculature, norepinephrine released from the sympathetic nerve endings, circulating catecholamines, and angiotensin II, as well as locally released vasodilators (histamine, bradykinin, prostaglandins) may all be involved in the orthostatic disorders of the circulation discussed in this book: edema and abnormalities of blood pressure control.

The normal sympathetic nervous system response to orthostasis is known to start almost instantaneously and to be sustained for several hours. This is evident in the obvious rise in plasma norepinephrine concentration demonstrable after standing for 1 or 2 minutes and maintained as long as orthostasis continues. Increases in PRA and plasma aldosterone concentration follow and serve a particularly important physiological role in the presence of sodium depletion and hypovolemia. Orthostatic disorders of the circulation may arise from inadequate arteriolar contraction (orthostatic hypotension), from subnormal contraction of the capacitance vessels (in the variety of blood pressure and heart rate abnormalities seen in the "venous pooling syndrome"), or probably from lack of precapillary sphincter tone (in orthostatic edema).

2

ORTHOSTATIC EDEMA

Definition and Pathogenesis

2.1. DEFINITION OF ORTHOSTATIC EDEMA

Orthostatic edema is defined as a disorder characterized by edema that becomes detectable after a period of time (no more than 12 hr) in the sitting or standing posture and that disappears spontaneously in recumbency. Its occurrence does not depend on intrinsic cardiac, renal, hepatic, or obstructive venous disorders, nor is it associated with an abnormal tendency to retain fluids in recumbency. A specific maximal duration of orthostasis required for the development of manifest edema has to be included in the definition, as ankle edema may develop in individuals in robust health after more prolonged periods of sitting or standing. Thus, pitting edema was readily demonstrable at the ankles of six healthy passengers (three of them males) that I was able to examine at the end of a flight from various American cities to Copenhagen, *via* Amsterdam, which lasted 15–16 hr, in 1960. In unusually hot weather, too, it is common for persons in apparently good health to note some puffiness at the ankles after being on their feet all day. For this reason, orthostatic edema should be considered present when edema is evident after what might be considered a "normal" day's activity, under "normal" environmental conditions.

The syndrome of idiopathic edema was actively studied by Dr. George W. Thorn, at the Peter Bent Brigham Hospital in Boston from about 1949 and was first described as being associated with hyperaldosteronism by Mach *et al.* (1955*a*,*b*). Among a group of 169 of these patients on whom we have performed metabolic balance studies over the course of the past 31 years, it has been determined that in at least 80% of cases (patients #1–135 in Appendix I), orthostasis was the most important factor in the pathogenesis of the edema. Since the effect of the upright posture has generally not been described in the literature related to idiopathic edema, one cannot be sure that the data recorded here will always be in accord with some of the published findings on patients with idiopathic edema of undescribed types. It seems likely, however, that in the data described in the literature as having been obtained from patients with idiopathic edema, a similar, overwhelming preponderance of the patients actually had *orthostatic edema.*

2.2. GENERAL MECHANISMS OF EDEMA FORMATION

Edema occurs when there is either imbalance between Starling's forces acting on fluid exchange between the capillary blood and the interstitial fluid or an abnormally leaky capillary. Transudation of fluid from the capillary is enhanced by increased hydrostatic pressure within the capillary, which may result from excessive inflow into the capillary or from retarded outflow at the venous end of the capillary. Edema may also result from reduction of the oncotic pressure of the capillary blood plasma due to a fall in plasma protein concentration. Abnormalities of the oncotic or hydrostatic pressures of the interstitial fluid may also have a role in the genesis but are seldom the prime cause of edema. Lymphedema occurs when return of lymph to the venous system is retarded or prevented. As fluid accumulates in the extracellular compartment, the pressure of the tissue fluid rises rapidly and by so doing reduces further capillary filtration (Landis and Gibbon, 1933).

Each of the major factors in the pathogenesis of edema may have several causes. These are shown in Figure 5 and include the following:

2.2.1. Increased Capillary Hydrostatic Pressure

Most commonly, this reflects venous hypertension resulting from reduction of outflow from the venous end of the capillary. It may be caused by heart failure, associated with increased peripheral venous tone (Sharpey-Schafer, 1963); venous obstruction; venous stasis in varicose veins or veins with incompetent valves (Cooper, 1981); prolonged orthostasis; anemia or beriberi, in which arteriolar dilatation is associated with venous constriction (Sharpey-Schafer, 1961); or cirrhosis, resulting in portal vein hypertension and ascites. Elevation of the capillary hydrostatic pressure may follow plasma hypervolemia, itself the consequence of renal retention of fluid in patients taking sodium-retaining drugs or suffering from renal insufficiency or mineralocorticoid excess with failure of the *escape phenomenon* (August *et al.*, 1958). Capillary blood volume is probably also increased when humoral agents (bradykinin, prostaglandins, histamine) released in response to infections, burns, trauma, or drugs dilate the precapillary sphincter and expand the capillary bed. Orthostatic elevation of the hydrostatic pressure within such an expanded capillary bed is the probable mechanism of some types of orthostatic edema.

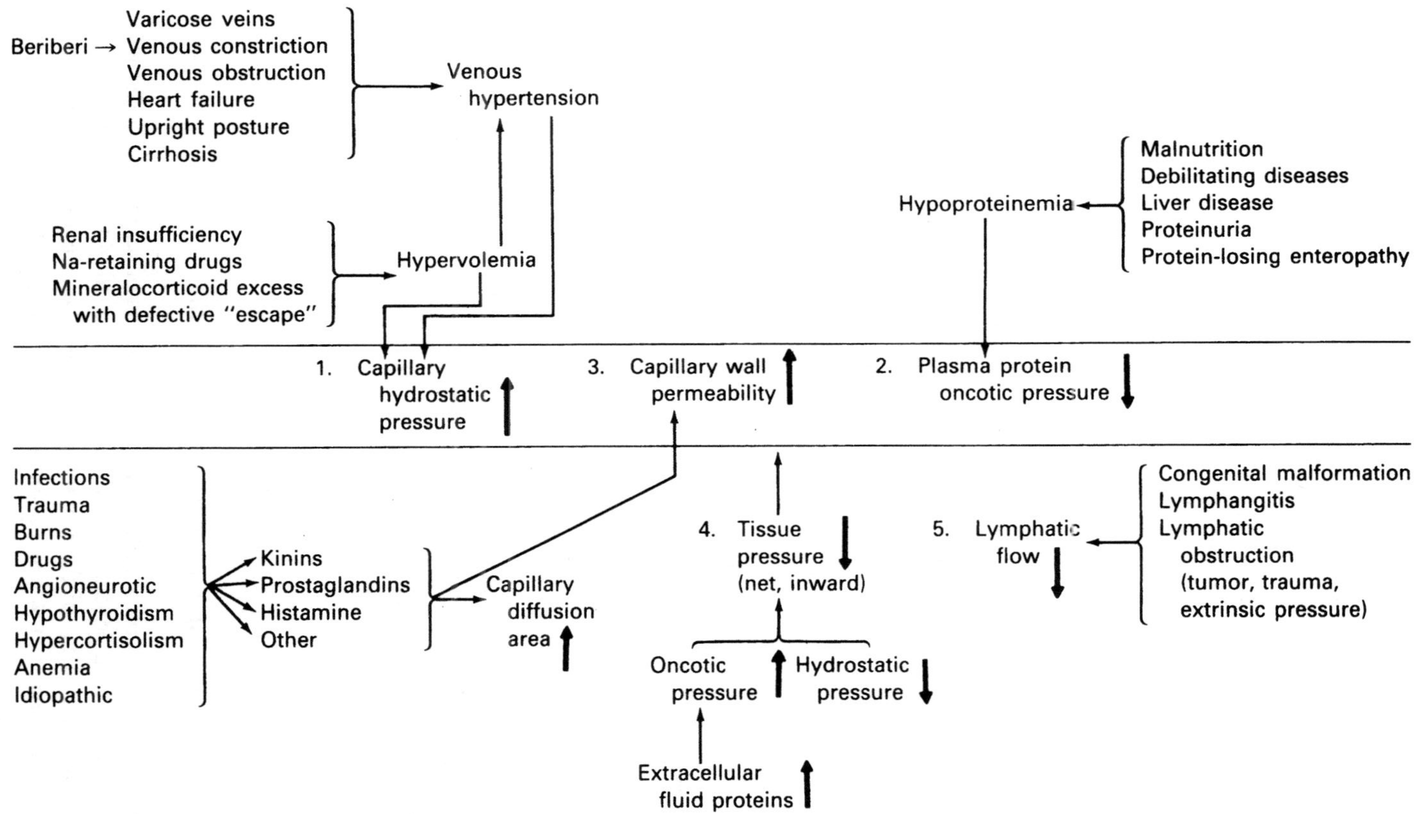

FIGURE 5. Primary mechanisms in the pathogenesis of edema. Since almost all mechanisms cause increased leakage of fluid from the vascular into the extravascular space, the extent of edema would be limited by the fall in blood pressure that would occur with increasing hypovolemia, were it not for secondary mechanisms (not depicted) that result in renal retention of Na and water: secondary aldosteronism, possible vasopressin release and intrinsic renal changes (e.g., fall in GFR).

2.2.2. Reduced Plasma Protein Oncotic Pressure

This is a consequence of *hypoproteinemia,* which may result from inadequate protein intake, subnormal hepatic synthesis of plasma proteins in various intrinsic liver diseases or general, debilitating diseases, and abnormal excretion of protein in the urine (in nephrosis) or the stool (in diarrheal states or protein-losing enteropathy).

2.2.3. Pathologically Leaky Capillaries

This condition is thought to cause a rare form of episodic or sustained edema, occasionally associated with profound hypotensive crises which may be fatal (Emerson *et al.*, 1955; Clarkson *et al.*, 1960; Horwith *et al.*, 1967; Atkinson *et al.*, 1977). It is possible that milder degrees of the same excessive leakiness of the capillaries to protein might occur in other patients with less acute and less dramatic forms of edema. *Hypothyroid edema* might depend on such a mechanism, since it is associated with acceleration of the loss of labeled protein from the plasma compartment (Parving *et al.*, 1979).

2.2.4. Tissue Pressure Changes

Tissue pressure may become altered by abnormal accumulations of protein in the extravascular space, which through an increase in oncotic pressure within the tissues might increase subcutaneous fluid content and cause edema.

2.2.5. Lymphatic Obstruction

The normal runoff of transuded fluid into the lymphatics is decreased in lymphatic edema, caused by congenital malformation of the lymphatics or by obstruction of the lymphatics attributable to lymphatic spread of malignant neoplasms, surgical transsection of lymphatics (Porter, 1972), or recurrent bouts of (usually) streptococcal lymphangitis.

2.3. PATHOGENESIS OF ORTHOSTATIC EDEMA

2.3.1. Role of Posture in the Pathogenesis of Edema

The importance of orthostasis in the pathogenesis of idiopathic edema was first suggested when a patient with severe edema was admitted for study to the Metabolic Research Unit of the University of Michigan, in 1955. Much to my embarrassment, the edema had disappeared completely when the patient was presented at ward rounds the next day. Several months later, when the possible role of orthostasis had occurred to me, the patient was readmitted and found to show the development of pitting edema of both legs when she remained upright all day, with complete loss of the retained fluid after recumbency for 24 hr. During the next 5 years, metabolic balance studies, with strictly controlled posture, disclosed the reproducible occurrence of orthostatic fluid retention in several of these patients. Subnormal ability to dilute the urine and to excrete a water load (20 ml/kg) during 4 hr in the upright posture was observed in a small group of these patients in whom normal orthostatic water excretion could be restored by ethanol (Streeten and Conn, 1959, 1960), a known inhibitor of vasopressin release (Rubini *et al.*, 1955). A systematic study of the role of posture was performed between 1960 and 1968 at the Upstate Medical Center in Syracuse. Parts of this study were reported (Speller and Streeten, 1964; Streeten and Speller, 1966) before the complete results were published (Streeten *et al.*, 1973). Thirty-one females with idiopathic edema were compared with six healthy female controls in their responses to standing from 8:00 a.m. to 8:00 p.m. on three successive days, preceded by 2 days in recumbency, after coming into balance on a constant, weighed, metabolic diet, containing 200 mEq sodium, 65–90 mEq potassium, 3 liters of fluid, and maintenance calories daily. The patients had been on no diuretic or other treatment for at least 10 days before the definitive observations were made during the second 3-day period, when they remained upright for 12 hr/day. Of the 31 patients, 26 were found to have a cumulative weight gain greater than that of any of the normal subjects, from 8 o'clock on the morning of the first day in the upright posture, to 8 o'clock on the morning after the third day of standing, and/or a greater loss of weight during 2 days of recumbency than in any of the control subjects (Fig. 6). These patients were all devoid of detectable edema after 2 days of recumbency, and all developed obvious pitting edema at the end of each day spent in the upright posture. Since their weight gain associated with the development of edema was apparently attributable entirely to maintenance of the erect posture, they were considered to have *orthostatic edema*. The five other patients whose posturally induced changes in body weight fell within the range of changes found in the normal controls, were considered to have *nonorthostatic edema* (Streeten *et al.*, 1973).

2.3.1.1. Sodium Excretion in the Upright Posture: Differentiation of Orthostatic Sodium and Water Retainers

Urinary sodium excretion on the second day of recumbency and on the subsequent first day of standing for 12 hr, is shown in Figure 7. It is evident that most of the patients excreted more sodium in recumbency, while their edema was disappearing, than did the normal (nonedematous) subjects on this day. When the patients remained standing for 12 hr (except for mealtimes), sodium excretion fell below that of the normal controls in 16 of the patients said to have *edema with orthostatic sodium retention,* while sodium excretion was within the normal range in the remaining 10 patients with orthostatic water retention and in the patients with nonorthostatic edema.

2.3.1.2. Posture Test

On a separate occasion, during the continued intake of the constant 200-mEq sodium diet, the effects of orthostasis on sodium excretion were compared by an independent procedure called a *posture test.* In this procedure, the individuals received 12 mEq sodium in the form of 150 ml of a dilute saline solution (0.14% NaCl solution) by mouth, every 30 min for 6 hr, while they remained recumbent for the first 4 of these hours, and then walked about at their leisure for the remaining 2 hr. Urinary sodium excretion during the 2 hr of orthostasis was expressed as a percentage of the urinary sodium excretion during the last 2 hr in recumbency. This ratio was between 33 and 100% in 26 normal subjects. The upright/recumbent urinary sodium ratio fell within this normal range in all the

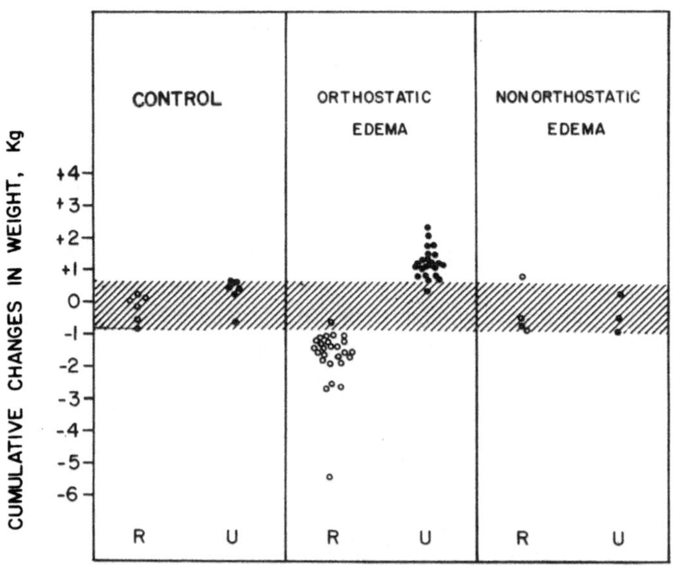

FIGURE 6. Differentiation of orthostatic and nonorthostatic edema states by measurement of cumulative changes in body weight (on a 200-mEq Na diet) during 2 days in recumbency (R) and 3 days in the upright posture from 8:00 a.m. to 8:00 p.m. (U). Weight changes depicted were from 8:00 a.m. on the first day of the recumbent and standing periods, to 8:00 p.m. the day after the respective periods. The ranges of weight decreases in the recumbent periods and of weight increases in the upright periods in the control subjects are shaded. (From Streeten *et al.*, 1973.)

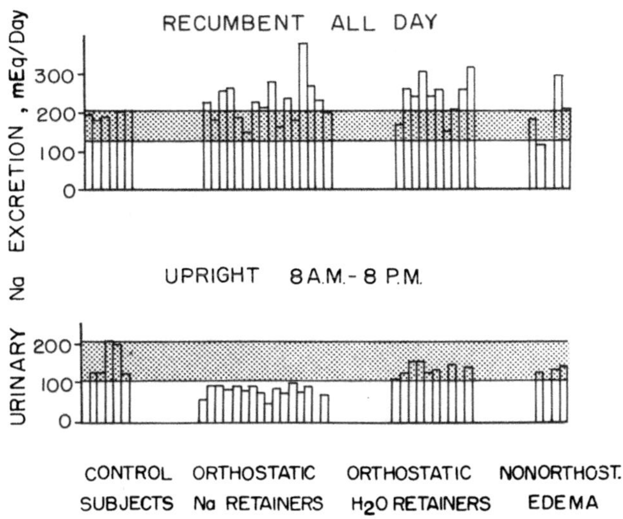

FIGURE 7. Differentiation of patients with orthostatic sodium retention from those with orthostatic water retention and others with nonorthostatic edema, by measurements of urinary sodium excretion on the second day of recumbency all day and the first day of standing for 12 hr, during intake of a constant high-sodium (200 mEq/day) diet. It is evident that Na excretion was below the range of values found in the control subjects (shown by cross-hatching) in one group of patients who were therefore considered to have edema with orthostatic Na retention, but not in the other edematous patients. (From Streeten, 1978.)

eight patients who had been found by the more laborious balance technique to have orthostatic water but not sodium retention, and fell below 33% in 15 of 16 patients who were found by the balance technique to be orthostatic sodium retainers (Streeten, 1978; see Fig. 8). Thus, in these two independent procedures, the findings concurred in 96% of patients, and the presence of orthostatic sodium or water retention in the two groups of patients was strongly confirmed by this simpler method.

2.3.1.3. Leg Volume Measurements

Further confirmation of the role of orthostasis in the genesis of edema in these patients was derived from an additional independent measurement—that of changes in leg volume. The volume of the legs, from the soles to 33.5 cm above the soles, was measured by a simple water displacement technique (see Streeten *et al.*, 1973, for details), at 8:30 a.m. and 8:30 p.m. daily, during the balance studies. In control healthy subjects on the 200-mEq sodium diet, leg volume changed very little from morning to evening when the individuals were reclining

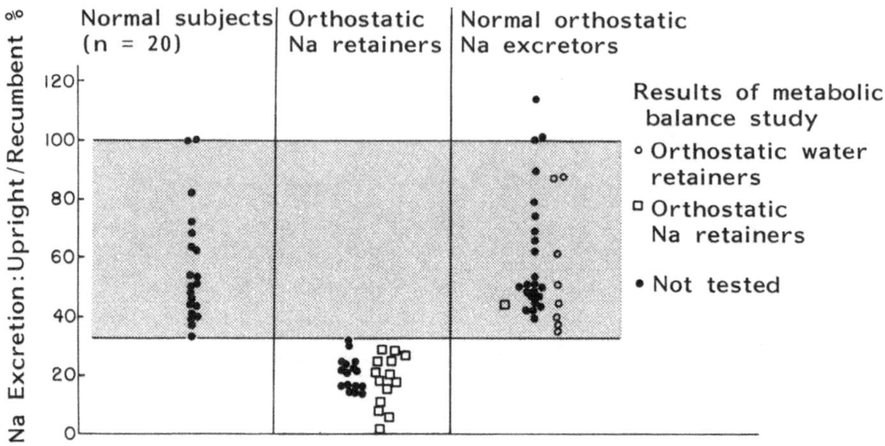

FIGURE 8. Differentiation of edematous patients with orthostatic sodium retention from those without abnormal orthostatic sodium retention, by a 6-hr posture test. The ratio, Na excretion while standing 2 hr/Na excretion while lying 2 hr, was >33% in normal subjects and in all edematous patients except those with orthostatic sodium retention. Good agreement between the results of this procedure and the results of the more prolonged metabolic balance study is evident, with only one patient found to have had orthostatic Na retention (designated by open squares) by the balance study but not according to the 6-hr posture test. (From Streeten, 1978.)

all day (mean change: −16 ml), and changed by −60 to +270 ml (mean ±129 ml) during orthostasis for 12 consecutive hours (from 8:00 a.m. to 8:00 p.m.). These findings confirmed the old observations made by Asmussen (1943) that the volume of the feet increases while standing, such as during a day of work in the laboratory, in normal subjects. In patients with orthostatic edema, leg volume usually declined strikingly on the first day of recumbency (mean reduction 134 ± 31 ml), in parallel with a decline in body weight; these changes reflected the clinically evident rapid reduction of edema. When the patients with orthostatic edema remained upright for 12 hr, their leg volumes invariably increased by more than the greatest mean increment (+177 ml) and almost always more than the greatest individual increase in leg volume (+270 ml) in any of the normal subjects. Simultaneously, body weight increased excessively, and edema became obvious by the end of the day in the patients' legs. Thus, the mean increase in leg volume during 12 hr of the upright posture, in the 57 patients with orthostatic edema whose leg volume changes are shown in Appendix I, was 481 ± 63 ml, or almost four times the mean increase observed in normal subjects. Moreover, maintaining the upright posture for 12 hr each day, for three successive days, resulted in cumulative increases of leg volume over the 72-hr period, of +280 ± 34 (SEM) ml in the orthostatic sodium retainers, and +218 ±

34 ml in the orthostatic water retainers, both values being significantly greater ($p < 0.005$) than the cumulative change of $+20 \pm 31$ ml in the normal controls, or $+75 \pm 13$ ml in patients who were characterized by their weight changes as having nonorthostatic edema (Fig. 9). By contrast, 2 days of recumbency caused a significantly greater cumulative decline in leg volume, in both the orthostatic sodium retainers (-231 ± 28 ml, $p < 0.001$) and the orthostatic water retainers (-215 ± 44 ml, $p < 0.005$), compared with normal subjects (-33 ± 22 ml). Thus, the excessive cumulative reduction in leg volume during 2 days of recumbency, and the excessive cumulative increases in leg volume during 3 days of standing, closely paralleled the corresponding changes in body weight in these patients. The observations provided further evidence that orthostasis not only causes excessive leg swelling during the hours spent in the upright posture but also results in excessive accumulation of leg edema over a period of at least 3 days.

It is of interest to recall that prolonged standing has been known for many years to cause an initially rapid and a later slow increase in leg volume in normal subjects. The rapid increase in leg volume is demonstrable by plethysmography within a few minutes of standing (Atzler and Herbst, 1923; Looke, 1937) and must certainly be largely the result of blood pooling within the venous system. We have found that intravascular blood content increases to 230% of recumbent values after 5–10 min of standing in normal subjects but changes only slightly with more prolonged orthostasis (Streeten *et al.*, 1985). The slower increase in

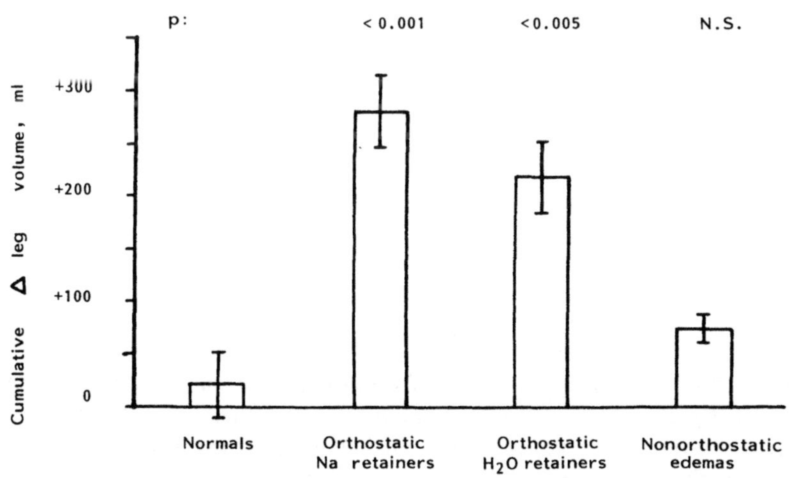

FIGURE 9. Cumulative changes in leg volume from beginning to end of a 3-day period of standing for 12 hr/day, showing the excessive increase in leg volume in the patients with orthostatic sodium and orthostatic water retention, but not in the patients with nonorthostatic edema.

leg volume that continues for at least 2 hr in normal subjects (Atzler and Herbst, 1923; Looke, 1937) has been attributed mainly to extravasation of plasma transudate in the legs (Gauer and Thron, 1965; Atzler and Herbst, 1923; Waterfield, 1931*a;* Youmans *et al.*, 1935; Grill, 1937; Looke, 1937; Wells *et al.*, 1938). Grill (1937) recognized that leg volume changes in the upright posture were excessive in some and minimal in other patients with edema.

2.3.1.4. Weight Measurements

Upon the conclusion of the balance studies, our patients were asked to record their body weights over the course of at least 2 weeks, at home, in the nude, each morning after arising and each evening before retiring, immediately after emptying the bladder on each occasion. These weights showed a mean change of 0.455 kg (range +0.31 to +0.58 kg) from morning to evening (i.e., intra diem), in eight normal subjects (Streeten *et al.*, 1960), while every patient diagnosed by the balance technique or the "posture test" as having "orthostatic edema" experienced a mean weight gain, over 2 weeks, of more than 0.6 kg, intra diem (Fig. 10). Thus, evidence was obtained from four entirely different and independent measurements (the balance studies, the "posture tests," the leg volumes and the weight changes intra diem) to show that the upright posture induced excessive fluid retention and excessive leg swelling in the patients characterized as having orthostatic edema. Moreover, in the recumbent posture, under identical conditions of food intake, fluid intake, environment, and attending staff, pitting edema always disappeared, and there was no evidence of excessive retention of sodium or water, in these patients. There appeared to be good reasons for believing, therefore, that orthostasis was the proximate cause both of fluid retention and of the development of edema in these patients.

2.3.2. *Mechanisms of Orthostasis-Induced Fluid Retention*

2.3.2.1. Findings in Normal Subjects

a. *Water Excretion.* It has long been known that normal subjects show reductions in urinary excretion of water and electrolytes in the upright posture (Erlanger and Hooker, 1905). These postural effects are greater when individuals are tilted to 60° (head-up) (Brun *et al.*, 1945; Pearce and Newman, 1954) or stand still (Epstein *et al.*, 1951; Surtshin *et al.*, 1956; Thomas, 1957)—circumstances that often reduce venous return sufficiently to cause syncope—than when muscular activity, such as walking about slowly, is encouraged (Streeten and Speller, 1966). We have confirmed the reports of Pearce and Newman (1954) by finding that ethanol will reduce the usual fall in urine flow rate and in free water

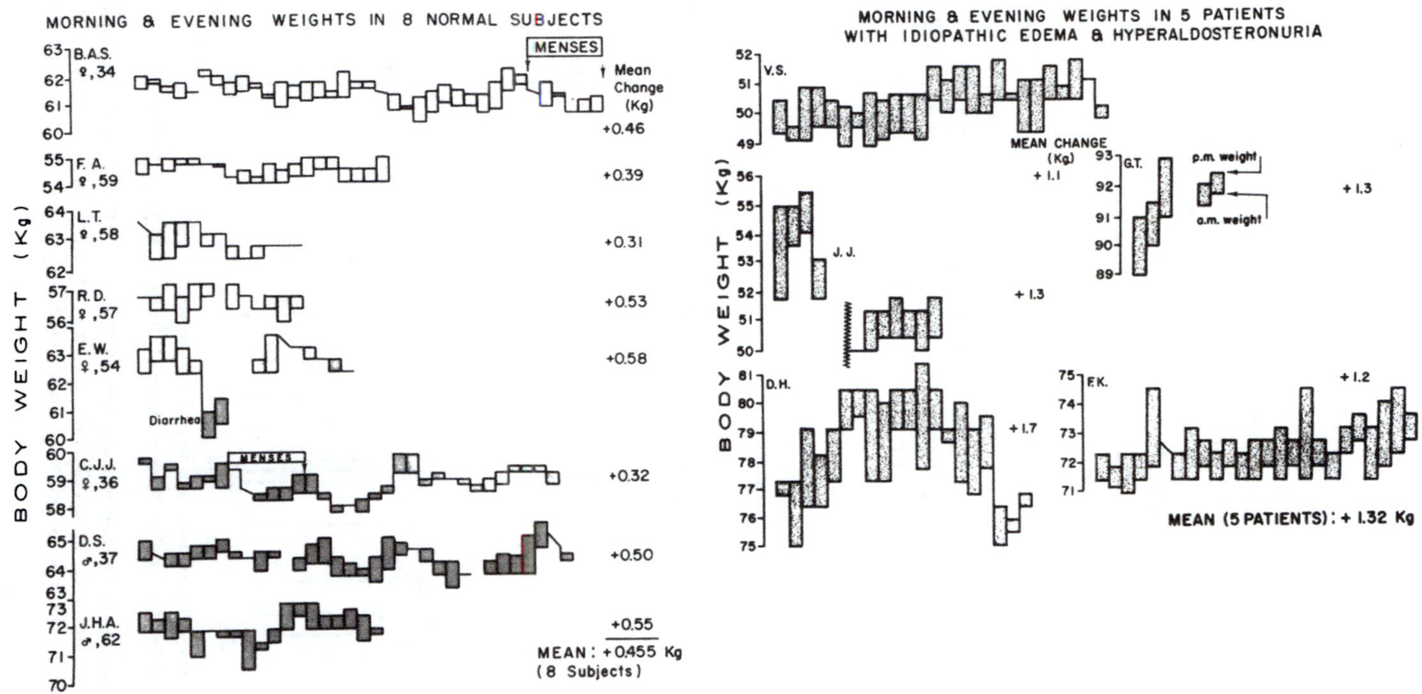

FIGURE 10. Body weight changes from morning to evening over a period of more than a week, in normal subjects and patients with orthostatic edema. In each instance, morning weight is depicted by the lower border, whereas evening weight is shown as the upper border of each rectangle, so that the vertical height of the rectangle represents weight gain intra diem. (From Streeten *et al.* 1960.)

clearance during the first 30 min of slow ambulation to values very similar to those found under the same conditions in patients with diabetes insipidus (Streeten and Speller, 1966). These findings are illustrated in Figure 11. During the oral intake of 0.14% NaCl solution, 150 ml every half-hour, both urine flow rate and free water clearance fell when normal subjects changed from recumbency (period A) to the upright posture (periods B and C) for 2 hr. When these normal subjects were given 95% ethanol, 25 ml, 30 min before standing, the falls in urine volume and free water clearance were significantly reduced in the first half-hour of standing only. In patients with diabetes insipidus, the falls in urine flow rate and free water clearance were significantly less than in normal subjects during the first half-hour of standing, and were virtually identical with those seen in normal subjects who had been given ethanol. Since ethanol is known to inhibit vasopressin release (Rubini *et al.*, 1955), these findings strongly suggest that increased release of antidiuretic hormone is the major mechanism of the reduced urine flow rate during at least the first half-hour of orthostasis. However, in their

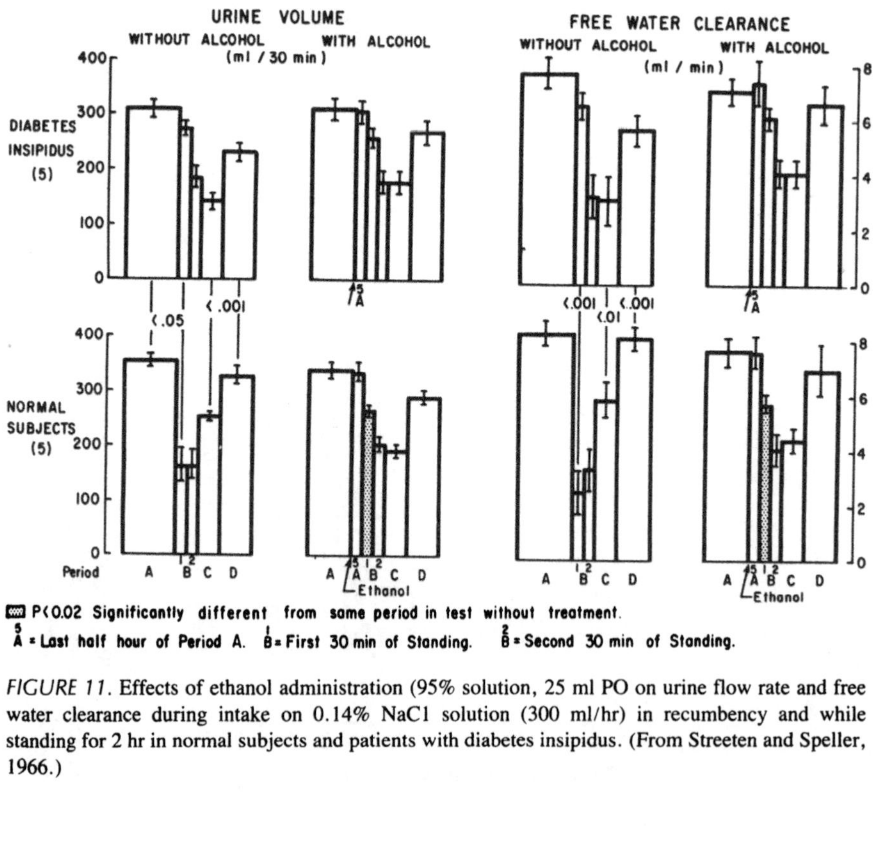

FIGURE 11. Effects of ethanol administration (95% solution, 25 ml PO on urine flow rate and free water clearance during intake on 0.14% NaCl solution (300 ml/hr) in recumbency and while standing for 2 hr in normal subjects and patients with diabetes insipidus. (From Streeten and Speller, 1966.)

later responses to the upright posture, too, patients with diabetes insipidus responded similarly to normal subjects treated with ethanol, in manifesting large (~50%) reductions in the rate of urine flow during the third and fourth half-hours of orthostasis. In fact, this delayed oliguric response to orthostasis is actually more severe in patients with diabetes insipidus than in untreated normal subjects (Streeten and Speller, 1966). Therefore, orthostatic release of vasopressin probably causes the immediate oliguric response to standing but is certainly not the only mechanism of the more prolonged orthostatic fall in urine flow rate in healthy subjects.

b. Sodium Excretion. Tilt-table experiments showed the existence of an orthostatic fall in the excretion of sodium as well as of water (Pearce and Newman, 1954). Bandaging the legs of the subjects with wide elastic bandages was found to reduce the orthostatic fall in sodium excretion from 38.4–62.9% of the recumbent rate, while it reduced the orthostatic fall in water excretion less effectively, from 34.7–44.2% of the recumbent rate. Like the fall in flow rate, the reduction in sodium excretion starts within the first 30 min of standing. The secretion of aldosterone is known to be stimulated in the upright posture (Muller *et al.*, 1958*a,b*, Streeten *et al.*, 1973). However, increased aldosterone production probably has no role in the sodium retention that occurs during the first 1 or 2 hr of orthostasis in normal subjects, because (1) measurable effects of aldosterone on sodium transport in the toad bladder are not evident during the first hour (Barger *et al.*, 1958; Crabbé, 1961), and (2) the orthostatic fall in sodium excretion was unaffected by the aldosterone receptor antagonist, spironolactone, and was just as evident in hydrocortisone-treated adrenalectomized patients as in normal subjects (Streeten and Speller, 1966) (see Fig. 12).

c. Role of Dopamine. The renal excretion of sodium has been shown to be affected by increases in sympathetic nervous system activity and by the administration of sympathomimetic amines (Speller and Streeten, 1964; Gill, 1969). There is undoubtedly increased sympathetic activity in the upright posture; Cuche *et al.* (1972) reported that normal subjects excrete in their urine more norepinephrine and epinephrine but less dopamine in the upright than in the recumbent posture. These workers also reported a correlation between the urinary excretion of dopamine and sodium, on a low-sodium diet, as well as during normal sodium intake. The observations suggested that orthostatic reduction in dopamine release might be involved in the decrease in sodium excretion in the upright posture. This is a plausible hypothesis, since dopamine administration certainly causes natriuresis, associated with increases in the renal blood flow and GFR in man (McDonald *et al.*, 1964; Burns *et al.*, 1967). Adjustment from a low- to a high-salt intake and the more acute response to a saline infusion in normal humans is associated with an increase in dopamine and a decrease in

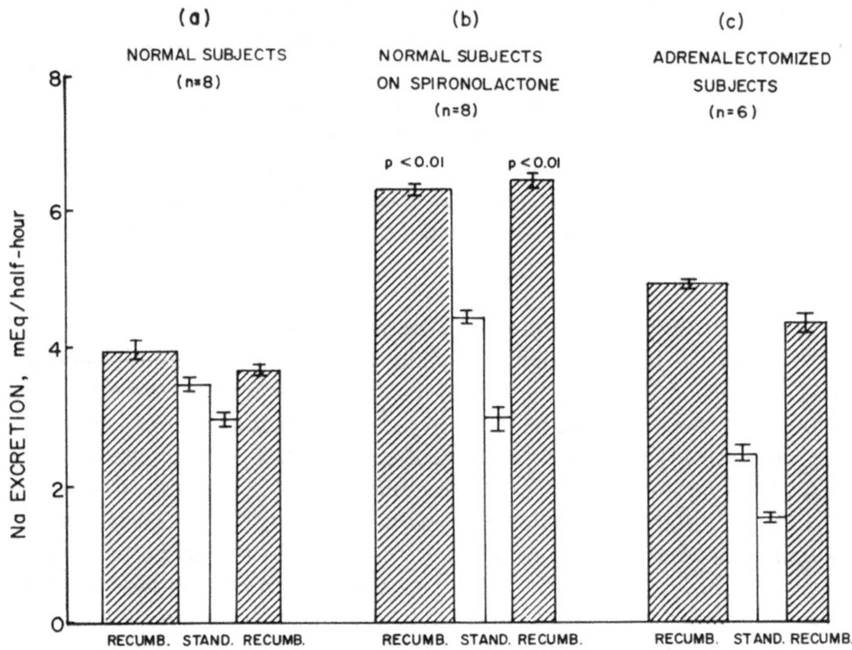

FIGURE 12. Comparison of recumbent and standing excretion during the "posture test" in (a) untreated normal subjects, (b) normal subjects pretreated with the aldosterone antagonist, spironolactone, and (c) patients who were aldosterone deficient because of previous bilateral adrenalectomy for Cushing's syndrome, and receiving maintenance doses (25–30 mg) of hydrocortisone alone. Note that reduced aldosterone action increased recumbent Na excretion but did not abolish the orthostatic reduction of Na excretion.

norepinephrine excretion (Alexander *et al.*, 1974). All these potentially important findings suggest that renal dopamine may have a physiological role as a natriuretic hormone in man that could be of special significance in the normal and abnormal changes in sodium excretion in the upright posture.

2.3.2.2. Findings in Patients with Edema and Orthostatic Sodium Retention

Patients with edema associated with orthostatic sodium retention show reduction of renal sodium excretion in the upright posture, which is qualitatively similar to but quantitatively greater than that found in normal subjects (Fig. 12). The mechanisms of the excessive orthostatic responses of patients with orthostatic edema are as follows:

a. Aldosterone Excretion and Secretion Rates. The balance studies alluded to in Chapter 1 measured these rates, which were found to be consistently excessive in the upright posture only, in 7 of the 15 patients who had edema with orthostatic sodium retention, and in none of the other patients with orthostatic or nonorthostatic edema (Streeten *et al.*, 1973), as shown in Figure 13. Many investigators have described hyperaldosteronism in patients with idiopathic

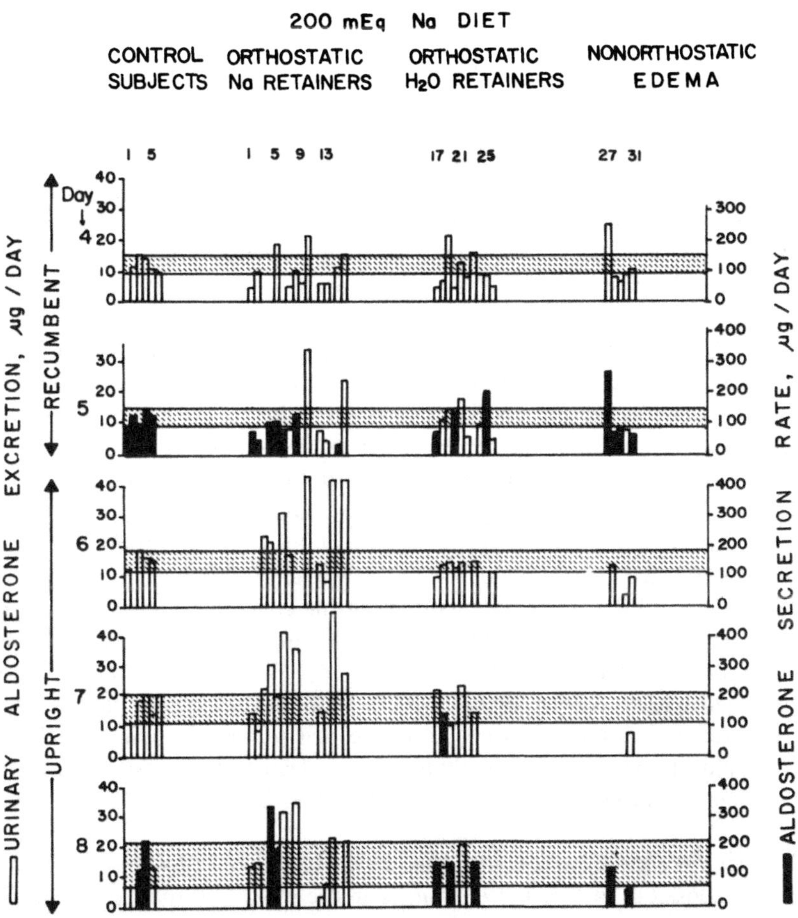

FIGURE 13. Aldosterone excretion (open columns) and secretion rates (solid columns) during 200 mEg Na intake daily, in normal control subjects and in patients with orthostatic sodium retention, orthostatic water retention, and nonorthostatic edema during recumbency for 24 hr (days 4 and 5) and on 3 days (days 6, 7, and 8) when the subjects remained standing from 8:00 a.m. to 8:00 p.m. It is evident that excessive aldosterone excretion or secretion occurred consistently only in most of the patients with orthostatic sodium retention. (From Streeten *et al.*, 1973.)

edema (Mach *et al.*, 1955*a,b;* Luetscher *et al.*, 1957, 1964; Streeten and Conn, 1960; Thorn, 1957, 1968; Hill *et al.*, 1960; Kuchel *et al.*, 1970; Oelkers *et al.*, 1975, 1977), but its occurrence exclusively in the upright posture was a new finding (Streeten *et al.*, 1973). Since it occurred only in persons with excessive orthostatic sodium retention, and since aldosterone is a potent endogenous mediator of sodium retention, the conclusion that orthostatic hyperaldosteronism played some part in the excessive sodium retention in the upright posture in these patients certainly appears reasonable. However, neither constant daily administration of aldosterone (August *et al.*, 1958) nor its consistently excessive secretion in patients with primary aldosteronism causes edema, since the sodium-retaining action of the steroid is overcome in a few days, by the "escape phenomenon," in normal circumstances. Intermittent exclusively orthostatic hypersecretion of aldosterone might aggravate renal retention of sodium and might not be subject to relief by the "escape phenomenon." Evidence on this possibility is conflicting, however, since mineralocorticoid escape has been reported to be normal in most patients with idiopathic edema (Gill *et al.*, 1972*a,b;* Edwards and Bayliss, 1976) but abnormal in others (Jones, 1973).

b. Changes in Plasma Renin Activity. The predominant physiological stimulus to aldosterone secretion is renin release and increased angiotensin II formation. For this reason, and because orthostasis is known to stimulate renin release, it was anticipated that the excessive orthostatic rise in aldosterone secretion in orthostatic sodium retainers resulted from excessive renin release. Our own data (Streeten *et al.*, 1973), obtained by bioassay (Boucher *et al.*, 1964), failed to demonstrate excessive elevations in PRA in any of the edematous patients. Evidence published by other investigators has been conflicting, an excessive rise in PRA in patients with idiopathic edema being reported by some (Veyrat *et al.*, 1968; Kuchel *et al.*, 1970), but being found only exceptionally or never by others (Werning *et al.*, 1969; Oelkers *et al.*, 1975; Katz, 1977; MacGregor *et al.*, 1979; Sowers *et al.*, 1982*b*). More studies are required to remove this uncertainty, as there is some evidence that restricted sodium intake may increase aldosterone secretion without raising plasma angiotensin II concentrations in man (Catt *et al.*, 1971; Best *et al.*, 1971; Boyd *et al.*, 1972).

c. Orthostatic Changes in Renal Blood Flow and Glomerular Filtration Rate. The possible role of these changes in the excessive fluid retention manifested in the upright posture by patients with orthostatic edema has been explored by measurements of inulin and *p*-aminohippurate (PAH) clearances. Wesson (1957) and Gauer and Henry (1963) measured the small orthostatic reductions in glomerular filtration in normal subjects. In our studies of 10 normal females, after recumbency for 90 min, orthostasis for 120 min was associated with a fall in RBF of 7.6 ± 4.1% (SEM) and a fall in GFR of 5.2 ± 3.5% (Fig.

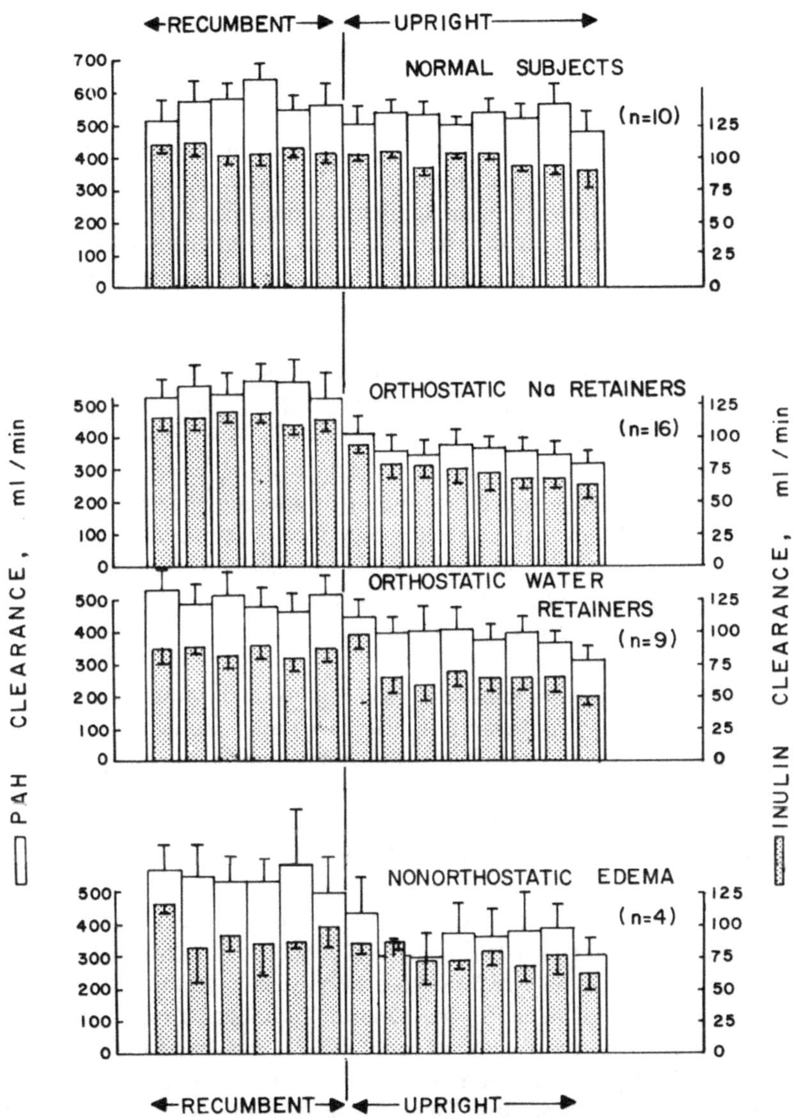

FIGURE 14. Effect of changing from recumbent to upright posture for 2 hr, on glomerular filtration rate (inulin clearance, open columns) and renal blood flow (PAH clearance, stippled columns) in 10 control and 34 edematous subjects on a 200-mEq Na diet. Means and SEM for each of the six 15-min periods in recumbency and the eight 15-min periods in the upright posture are shown. Note the orthostatic fall in both clearances, which was statistically significant only in the orthostatic sodium retainers. (From Streeten *et al.*, 1973.)

14). In patients who had edema with orthostatic sodium retention, RBF and GFR were normal while they were lying down, but there were far greater orthostatic reductions in RBF (32.7 + 5.6%, $p < 0.005$) and in GFR (34.7 + 5.2%, $p < 0.001$). In four of 15 patients, the orthostatic reduction in RBF exceeded 50%. Because of these findings, one patient whose RBF fell by 55% when she stood was subsequently studied by renal angiography at another hospital. Constriction of the major renal arteries was strikingly evident when renal angiograms were repeated after a few minutes in the upright posture (Fig. 15).

Among nine patients with orthostatic water retention, four had subnormal levels of RBF and/or GFR in recumbency; although these values fell excessively in the upright posture in one-half of the patients, the mean orthostatic reductions in RBF and GFR were not significantly greater than corresponding changes measured in the control subjects. The patients with nonorthostatic edema showed no consistent or significant changes in RBF or GFR either in recumbency or in the upright posture (Fig. 14). It is evident from these studies that a strikingly excessive drop in RBF, causing a concomitant excessive reduction in GFR, must have reduced the filtered load of sodium by an average of one-third in patients with orthostatic sodium retention while they were standing for 2 hr. Since the orthostatic changes were clearly more severe in the second than in the first hour of standing (Streeten *et al.*, 1973), it is possible that considerably greater reduction in the renal filtered load of sodium might have occurred during 12 hr of standing.

Patients with edema associated with orthostatic sodium retention also showed a statistically significant fall in urinary creatinine excretion during the 12-hr periods in the upright posture. Although serum creatinine concentrations were not measured daily in these studies, it is likely that this change, which did not occur in either the other groups of edematous patients or the normal control subjects, was a reflection of the severe fall in GFR documented by inulin clearance measurements in the same patients. Moreover, measurements of creatinine excretion in the posture tests of renal function demonstrated a highly significant drop in creatinine excretion in 54% of 48 patients with excessive orthostatic sodium retention but in only 18% of those with excessive orthostatic retention of water and in 12.5% of patients with nonorthostatic edema (Fig. 16). In 19 of these posture tests, serum creatinine concentration was found to show an insignificant mean change (2.8%) from the end of the recumbent period to the end of the period in the upright posture. Thus, the changes in urinary creatinine excretion closely reflected changes in endogenous creatinine clearance and confirm the previous evidence of a profound fall in glomerular filtration rate in the upright posture in patients with orthostatic sodium retention.

d. Conclusions. The combination of a severe fall in the filtered load of sodium and (frequently) excessive aldosterone-induced tubular reabsorption of

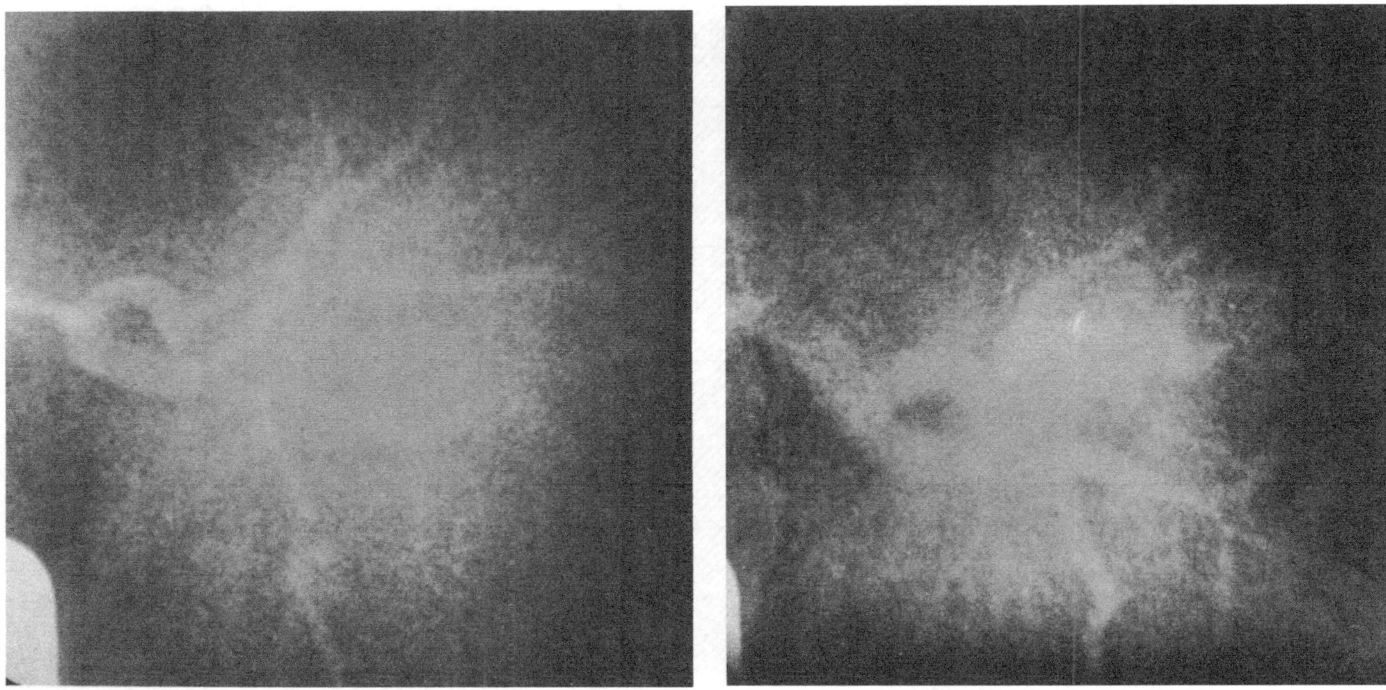

FIGURE 15. Dramatic orthostatic change in the caliber of the renal artery (reduction by more than one-third), in a patient with severe orthostatic sodium retention, when she changed from recumbency (left) to the standing posture (right). Renal blood flow (PAH clearance) fell by 55% in the upright posture in this patient.

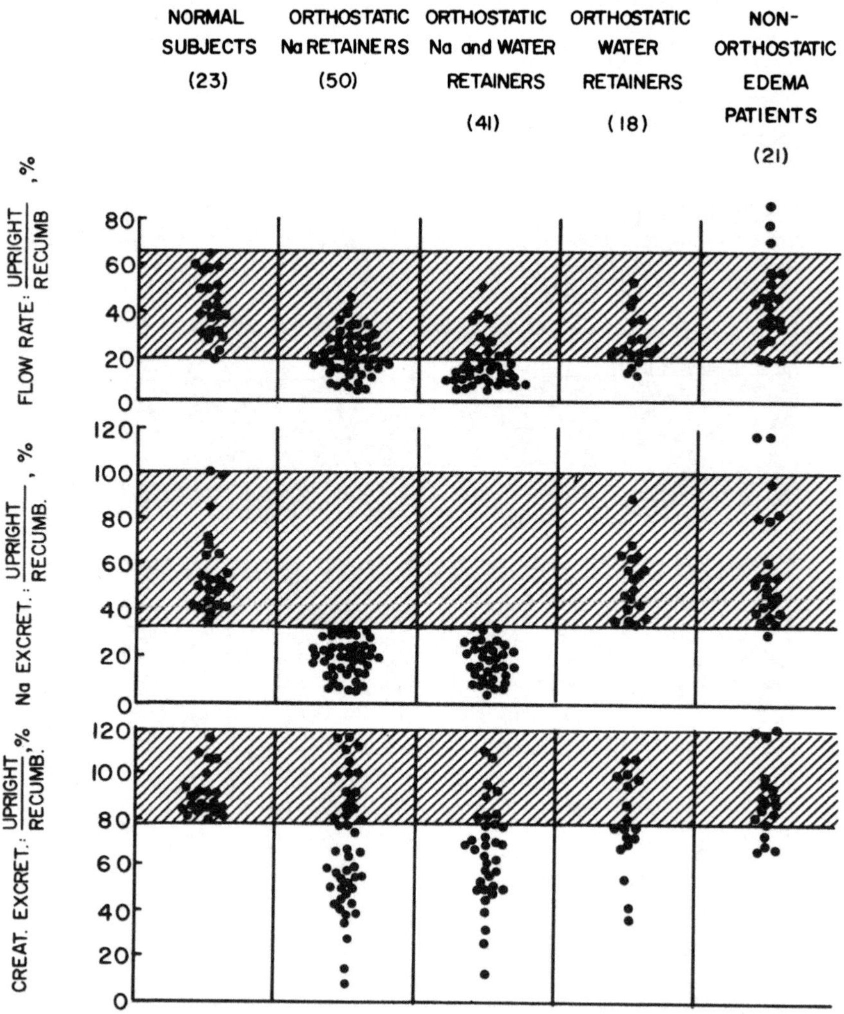

FIGURE 16. Upright/recumbent ratios of urinary flow rate, sodium excretion, and creatinine excretion during posture tests in 23 normal subjects and 130 patients with orthostatic and nonorthostatic edema. The excessive orthostatic reductions in urinary flow rate and creatinine excretion in the orthostatic sodium retainers are evident.

sodium is the mechanism whereby sodium excretion is excessively reduced in the upright posture in patients who have edema with orthostatic sodium retention. Neither of these postural abnormalities can be invoked to explain the edema of patients with orthostatic water retention or nonorthostatic edema.

2.3.2.3. Findings in Orthostatic Water Retainers

a. *Water Excretion Test.* Patients who were considered to have edema with orthostatic water retention were initially so designated because they gained weight excessively yet did not retain sodium excessively during 3-day periods of standing for 12 hr. Since diet was constant, these increments in weight could not have resulted from changes in caloric intake and must have been attributable to water retention without excessive sodium retention. This conclusion was tested more directly by measuring the renal response to a standard water load. Patients and normal control subjects were asked to drink 20 ml tap water per kg of ideal body weight (up to a maximum of 1500 ml) for a 15–20-min period, at about 8:00 a.m., after an overnight fast. They then remained on their feet, walking or standing at their leisure for 4 hr, and the bladder was emptied by voluntary voiding every hour for measurements of volume, osmolality, sodium and creatinine output, and vasopressin excretion, measured by radioimmunoassay (RIA). The same test was repeated with the patient recumbent for 4 hr, and the sequence of the tests was varied. A few subjects experienced nausea, vomiting, or diarrhea shortly after drinking the large volume of water. When this happened, the results of the test were disregarded in view of the known antidiuretic effects of nausea and vomiting. The reproducibility of responses to the standard water load test was found to be reasonably good, with a mean difference of 14.4% between percentage water excretion in two tests on the same individual, and a coefficient of variation of 16.7%.

Findings in Recumbency. In the recumbent posture, 11 of 16 normal persons excreted more water in 4 hr than they had imbibed at 8:00 a.m. Water excretion in 4 hr averaged 106 ± 4% (SEM) and always exceeded 65% (range 66–138%) of the water load administered. Urinary osmolality always fell below 112 (usually below 90) mOsm/kg. Maximal rates of urine flow and greatest urinary dilution generally occurred during the second hour after the water load had been given (Fig. 17). Urinary excretion of vasopressin fell below 0.7 μU/ml in seven of eight normal subjects, and to 1.0 μU/ml in the eighth individual, usually during the second but sometimes in the third hour after the water load. A similar fall in vasopressin excretion after a water load in recumbent normal subjects has long been suspected and was first measured by RIA and reported by Thibonnier *et al.* (1979, 1981). Among 59 of our patients with orthostatic and nonorthostatic edema who were tested in recumbency, every patient excreted the administered water entirely normally and with normal suppression of urinary

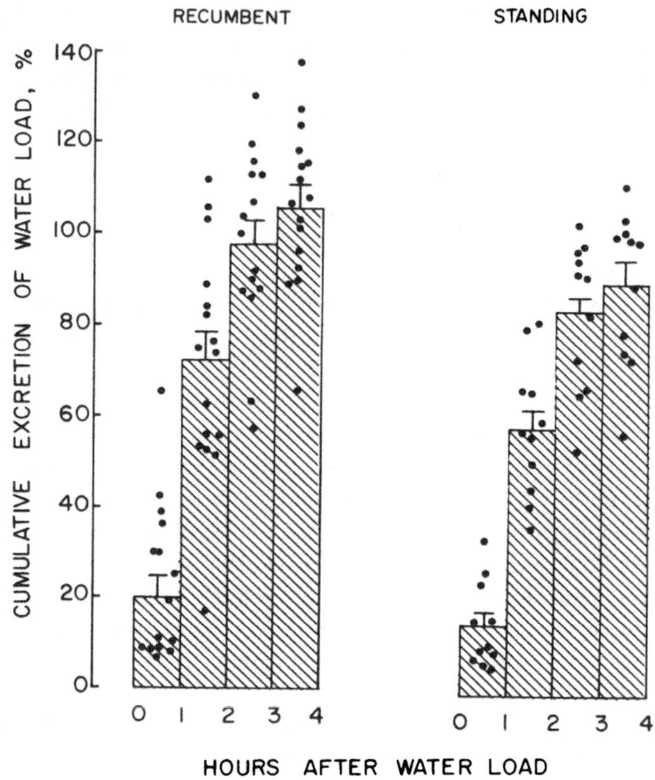

FIGURE 17. Cumulative hourly urine volumes (mean ± SEM) after a 20-ml/kg water load in normal subjects during recumbency and while in the upright posture. Slight orthostatic reduction in excretion is evident during each hour of the test.

vasopressin concentration below 1.0 μU/ml, confirming other evidence of the normality of renal function in recumbency, in these patients.

Findings in Standing Posture. In the upright posture, normal subjects almost invariably excreted less of the water load than in recumbency (Streeten and Conn, 1960; Kuchel *et al.*, 1970), water excretion in 4 hr varying from 55 to 120% of the water load administered, in 45 of 46 normal subjects tested [mean 87 ± 3% (SEM)] (Streeten, 1978). Among the patients with edema who were given water load tests (see Appendix I) less than 55% of the load was excreted in 4 hr, in the upright posture, in (1) all the 26 patients tested considered to have orthostatic water retention (patients #105–135 in Appendix I), confirming previous reports (Streeten and Conn, 1960; Kuchel *et al.*, 1970; Streeten, 1978; Thorn, 1968; Thibonnier *et al.*, 1979, 1981); (2) one of 13 nonorthostatic edema patients (patient #151); and (3) 26 of 46 patients tested who were orthostatic sodium retainers (Streeten, 1978). Thus, of the patients with orthostatic sodium retention, approximately one-half (51 of 104 patients in Appendix I) have evidence of excessive orthostatic retention both of sodium and of water and are referred to as orthostatic sodium and water retainers (patients #52–104, Appendix I). Minimal hourly urine osmolality was less than 100 mOsm/kg in all normal subjects. However, urinary osmolality failed to drop below 100 mOsm/kg in 33% of patients with orthostatic sodium retention, 16% of the patients with nonorthostatic edema, and 100% of those with orthostatic water retention (Fig. 18). The inadequate urinary dilution and subnormal decline in free water clearance after a water load in the upright posture have been confirmed by Thibonnier *et al.* (1979, 1981).

Urinary Sodium Excretion. It has been reported that after water loading sodium excretion in the upright posture is far less in patients with idiopathic edema than in control subjects (Kuchel *et al.*, 1970; Thibonnier *et al.*, 1979, 1981). In our experience, orthostatic sodium excretion after a water load showed no significant or consistent differences between normal subjects and patients with orthostatic edema of any type, as is clearly evident in Figure 36.

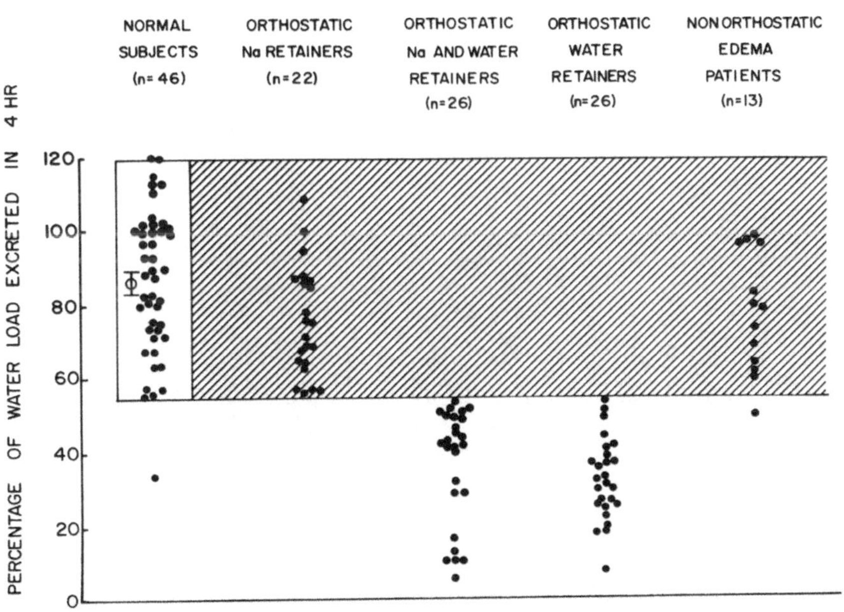

FIGURE 18. Percentage excretion of a water load during 4 hr in the upright posture in normal subjects and patients with orthostatic and nonorthostatic edema. Of the 48 orthostatic sodium retainers tested, 22 excreted water normally and 26 had combined orthostatic sodium and water retention.

Effects of Ethanol on Water Excretion. Patients who failed to excrete more than 55% of the water load in the upright posture were given a third water load test in which 95% ethanol, 25 ml, flavored with orange juice, was imbibed with the water. Ethanol increased water excretion into the normal range (>55% in 4 hr) in 19 of 20 patients with orthostatic water retention and was even followed by excretion of more than 100% of the load in five of these patients (Fig. 19). In two patients with orthostatic sodium retention and in two patients with nonorthostatic edema, the effect of ethanol was less dramatic, while in six of 14 patients with the combined defect (i.e., orthostatic sodium and water retention) ethanol restored water excretion in the upright posture to normal levels (Fig. 19). Ethanol is thought to promote water excretion mainly by inhibition of vasopressin release (Rubini *et al.*, 1955) and certainly exhibits little or no diuretic action in patients with diabetes insipidus (Streeten and Speller, 1966). The ethanol responses clearly suggest that excessive orthostatic release and action of vasopressin are the major mechanisms of the water retention in orthostatic water retainers.

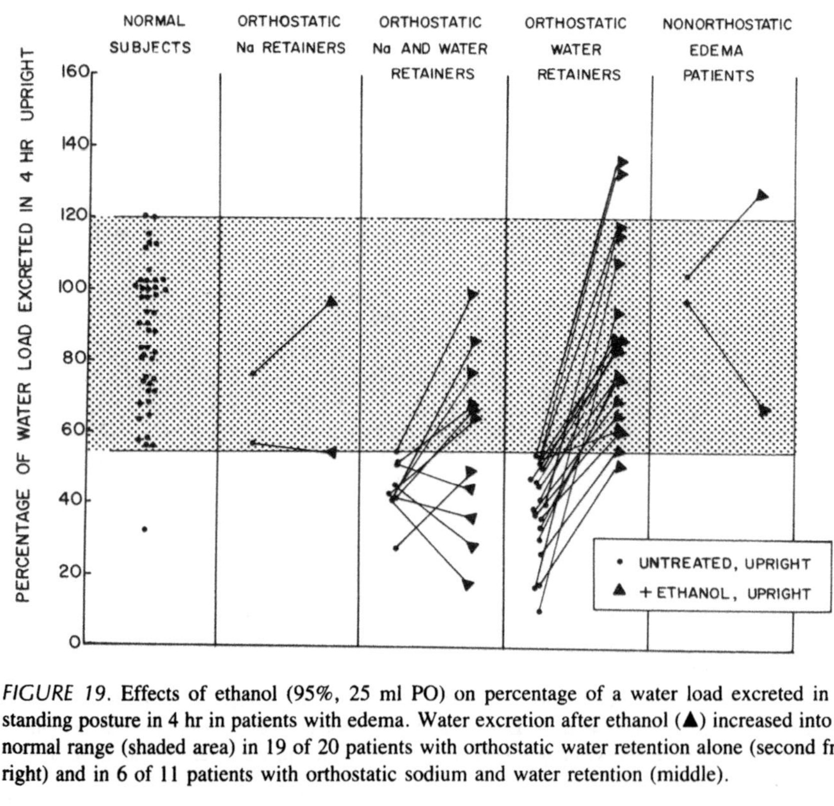

FIGURE 19. Effects of ethanol (95%, 25 ml PO) on percentage of a water load excreted in the standing posture in 4 hr in patients with edema. Water excretion after ethanol (▲) increased into the normal range (shaded area) in 19 of 20 patients with orthostatic water retention alone (second from right) and in 6 of 11 patients with orthostatic sodium and water retention (middle).

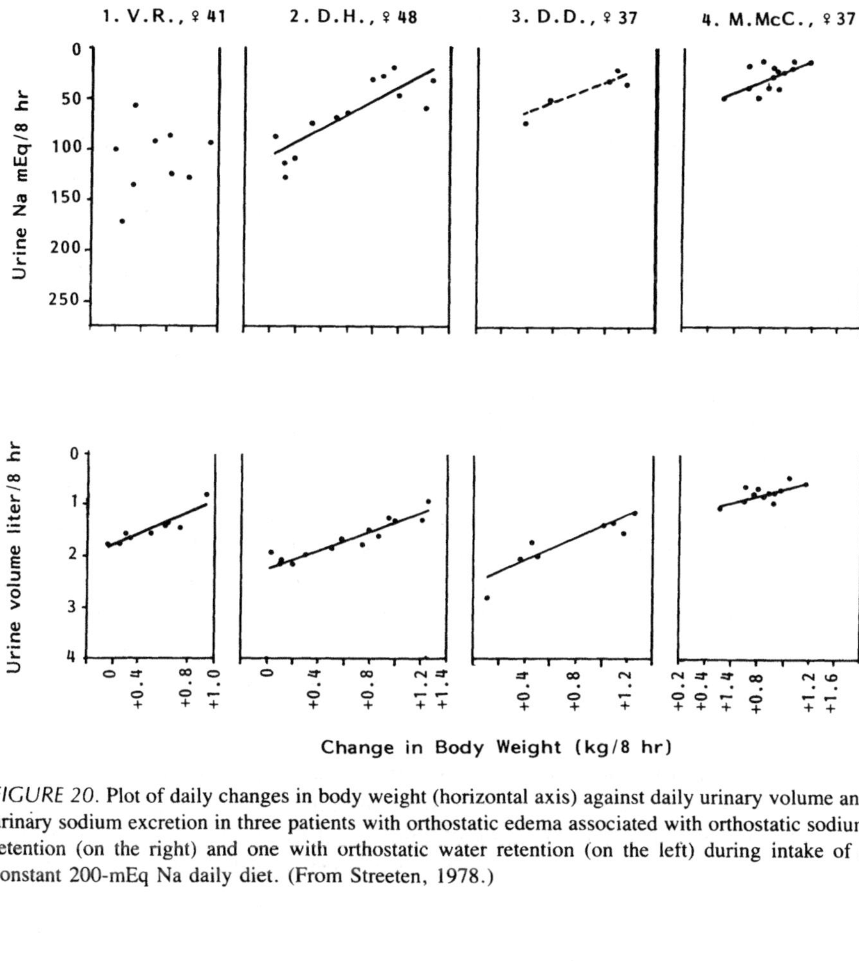

FIGURE 20. Plot of daily changes in body weight (horizontal axis) against daily urinary volume and urinary sodium excretion in three patients with orthostatic edema associated with orthostatic sodium retention (on the right) and one with orthostatic water retention (on the left) during intake of a constant 200-mEq Na daily diet. (From Streeten, 1978.)

b. Metabolic Balance Data. Additional evidence that orthostatic water retainers actually retain water in excess of sodium when they are upright was adduced in the balance studies described in Chapter 1. In all patients with orthostatic edema, there was an excellent correlation between 24-hr changes in body weight and 24-hr urine volumes in response to orthostasis (Fig. 20), confirming the assumption that the body weight changes reflected changes in fluid balance. An equally impressive significant correlation was found between 24-hr changes in body weight and 24-hr urinary sodium excretion in the three orthostatic sodium retainers for whom the data are depicted, but not in the one patient in whom we had previous independent evidence of orthostatic water retention. In this patient (see Fig. 13), the large orthostatic increases in body weight were clearly unrelated to changes in sodium excretion, and resulted from water retention without concomitant sodium retention.

c. Urinary Vasopressin Measurements. The role of excessive vasopressin release in the upright posture, implied by the effects of ethanol in the orthostatic water retainers (Streeten and Conn, 1960) was first shown by vasopressin measurements when Thibonnier *et al.* (1979) reported that excretion of urinary vasopressin was not normally suppressed by a water load in a group of 10 patients with idiopathic edema, most of whom probably had orthostatic edema. Our studies showed that after the standard water load in the upright posture, urinary vasopressin concentration fell below 1.0 μU/ml in 10 normal subjects (Fig. 21), lowest urinary vasopressin concentrations again being reached during the second hour in all subjects. In patients with edema, urinary vasopressin concentration fell normally, to below 1.0 μU/ml in 11 of 12 patients with orthostatic sodium retention (mean 0.69 ± SEM 0.35 μU/ml), and in all 12 patients with nonorthostatic edema (mean 0.28 ± 0.08 μU/ml). However, in four of six patients with orthostatic water retention, and in eight of 17 with orthostatic sodium and water retention, urinary vasopressin excretion failed to fall below 1.0 μU/ml, mean ± SEM being 1.0 ± 0.22 and 2.81 ± 0.77 μU/ml, respectively, in these two groups. In the patients with orthostatic water retention and in those with the combined orthostatic retention of sodium and water, but in none of the other groups, the lowest vasopressin concentrations in the urine after the water load in the upright posture were highly significantly greater than the mean values in all patients studied in the recumbent posture ($p < 0.001$) (Fig. 21).

In six of the patients with orthostatic water (± Na) retention, in whom the water load test was restored to normal by ethanol administration, lowest urinary vasopressin concentration fell after ethanol by 0.87 ± 0.36 (mean ± SEM) μU/ml. This reduction was of borderline statistical significance ($p = 0.05$).

d. Role of Vasopressin Excess. From the evidence described, it appears likely that excessive vasopressin, or antidiuretic hormone (ADH) production in the upright posture (which can be corrected by ethanol) is an important component of the mechanism of excessive water retention in the upright posture. This is true in patients with edema and orthostatic water retention, whether concomitant orthostatic sodium retention is present or not. Since ethanol corrected the orthostatic defect in water excretion in 95% of orthostatic water retainers, but only in six of 13 patients with orthostatic sodium and water retention, it follows that excessive vasopressin (ADH) secretion in the upright posture may be considered the mechanism of orthostatic water retention in virtually all patients with orthostatic water retention alone, but only in about one-half of the patients with orthostatic sodium and water retention.

The postulated role of an orthostatic excess of vasopressin release in the

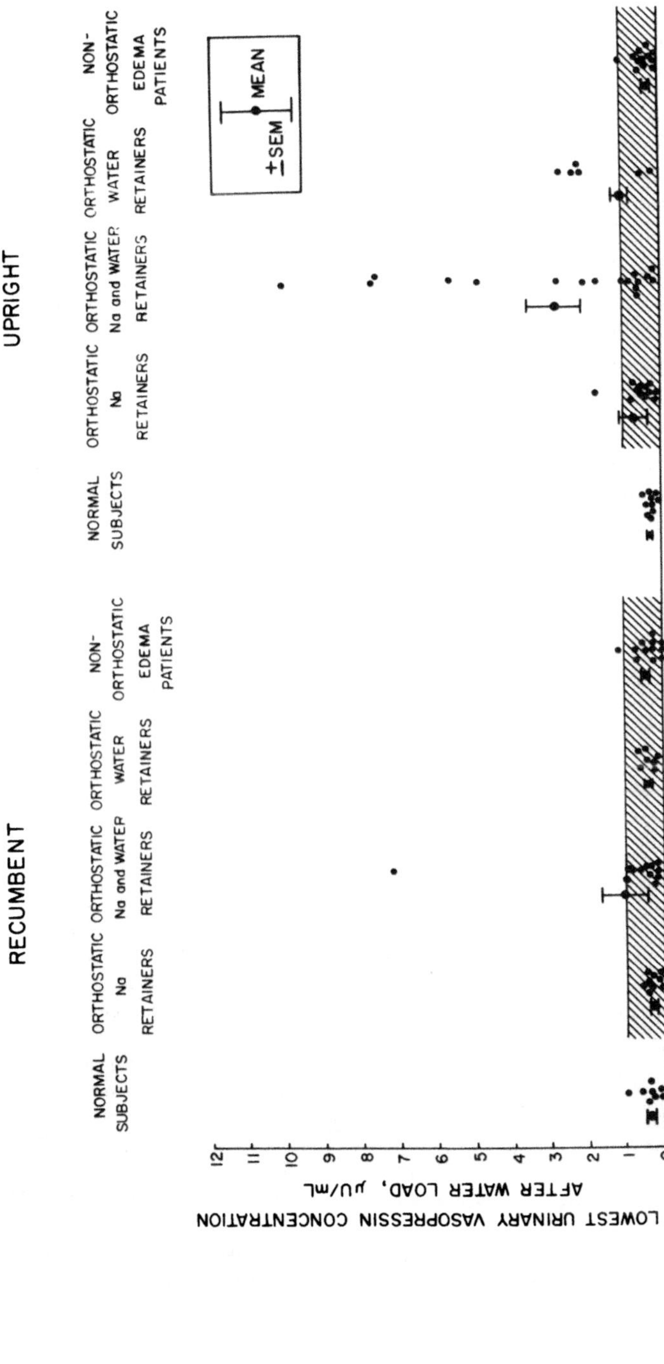

FIGURE 21. Urinary excretion of vasopressin (lowest hourly vasopressin concentration) after a 20-ml/kg water load in recumbency and in the upright posture, in normal subjects and in patients with nonorthostatic and various types of orthostatic edema.

pathogenesis of the edema of patients with orthostatic water retention has been contested in the past on two grounds:

Absence of Edema in SIADH. Edema is characteristically absent in the syndrome of inappropriate secretion of antidiuretic hormone (SIADH) (Bartter and Schwartz, 1967) and

Hyponatremia in SIADH. This typical manifestation of SIADH is seldom seen in orthostatic edema (Thorn, 1968; Werning *et al.*, 1969). Whether these arguments are valid is unclear; if ADH is involved in the pathogenesis of orthostatic water retention, as the above data imply, it is only through the action of an intermittent excess present during orthostasis and absent during sleep at night. The effects of such an intermittent ADH excess might well be different from those of persistent hypersecretion of the hormone, as in SIADH. Furthermore, one would expect that hyponatremia would be most severe in the evening in patients with orthostatic water retention.

We know of no reports of evening measurements of serum sodium concentration in patients with orthostatic water retention, except for observations in a single patient (Streeten, 1978). During a 2-day admission, this patient had serial measurements made of serum sodium concentration, body weight, and water balance, during orthostasis and recumbency. This patient, previously found to excrete 14% of a water load for 4 hr in the upright posture and 127% in recumbency, was found to have hyponatremia on the morning of admission (Fig. 22). While she remained on her feet from 8:00 a.m. to 8:00 p.m. on the first day of balance studies, she retained 1.3 liter water, gained 1.35 kg in weight, and experienced a fall in serum sodium concentration from 123 to 115 mEq/l. On the second day, when she lay in bed all day, despite the same intake of water, she

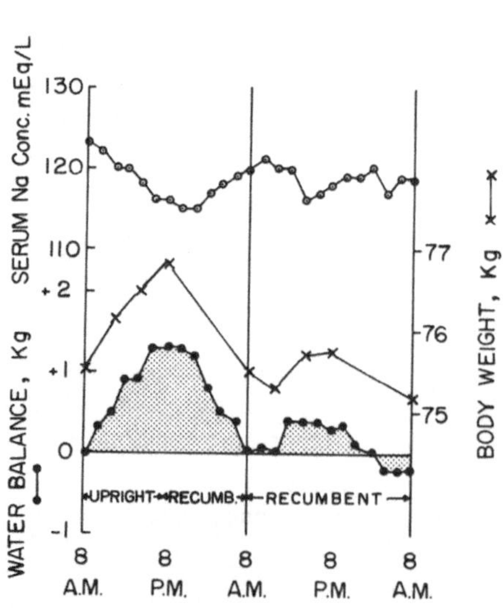

FIGURE 22. Effects of posture on serum sodium concentration, body weight, and water balance in a patient with orthostatic water retention. When she remained upright from 8:00 a.m. to 8:00 p.m. body weight increased by 1.35 kg, resulting mainly from retention of 1.30 kg water (estimated from measurement every 2 hr of intake and output and correction for insensible loss at 100 ml/2 hr), and serum Na fell from 123 to 115 mEq/liter. These changes were reversed in recumbency from 8:00 p.m. to 8:00 a.m. During recumbency the next day, all changes were reduced. (From Streeten, 1978.)

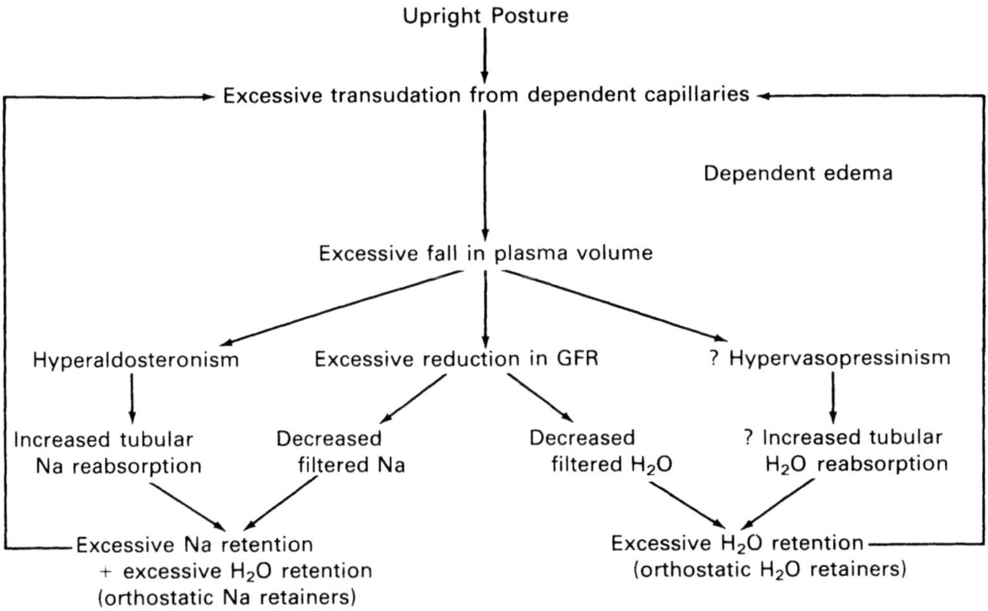

FIGURE 23. Summary of pathogenetic events leading to orthostatic edema.

retained only 300 ml fluid, gained 0.2 kg, and experienced a smaller fall in serum sodium concentration, from 120 to 116 mEq/l. Thus, hyponatremia can be aggravated by water retention when patients with orthostatic water retention remain on their feet. This patient actually displayed an element of compulsive water drinking, superimposed on her demonstrated orthostatic defect in water excretion, which might well have been responsible for her unusual morning hyponatremia. Evidence for this conclusion is that hyponatremia disappeared when the patient was able to accept our advice to restrict water intake voluntarily to volumes that might be considered normal, less than 1 liter/day. We have seen this unfortunate combination of disorders in two other patients with orthostatic water retention, both of whom also showed a good response to water restriction.

2.3.3. *Summary of Pathogenesis*

2.3.3.1. Orthostatic Sodium Retainers

Volume receptors, probably in the atria, sensing the excessive orthostatic fall in plasma volume, appear to stimulate aldosterone production, as shown in Figure 23. The consequent renal retention of sodium serves to replenish the reduced plasma volume and to potentiate continuation of further edema formation. Thus, hyperaldosteronism, when present, is not a primary component of the pathogenesis of orthostatic sodium retention but a secondary event that serves to protect the individual from progressive plasma volume depletion, thereby sustaining the capillary transudation that causes the edema.

2.3.3.2. Orthostatic Water Retainers

In patients with orthostatic water retention, orthostasis appears to stimulate excessive vasopressin release by a mechanism that might involve a milder (not statistically significant) fall in plasma volume and/or reduced distention of the left atrium, activating increased vasopressin release through the volume receptors in the atrium (Johnson *et al.*, 1969; Brennan *et al.*, 1971). The sequence of pathogenetic events leading to edema with orthostatic sodium and/or water retention is shown schematically in Figure 23.

2.3.4. How Does Orthostasis Trigger the Abnormal Responses in Patients with Orthostatic Sodium Retention?

2.3.4.1. Evidence from Plasma Volume Measurements

a. Plasma Volume in Recumbency. Measurements of changes in plasma volume during the development of orthostatic edema should throw light on the role of the upright posture in the pathogenesis of the disorder. Plasma volume is influenced by sodium intake (Streeten *et al.*, 1969*a*), posture (Streeten *et al.*, 1969*a*), relationship to meals, environmental temperature, and other factors. It is therefore important that plasma volume be measured under strictly standardized conditions. Expressed in terms of body weight, plasma volume falls with increasing obesity. For this reason, in our studies the basal plasma volumes of fasting recumbent subjects who were in electrolyte balance on a known standardized daily intake of salt and water, at 8:30 a.m., were found to vary widely, from values as low as 31.7 ml/kg in an obese (109.5-kg) patient to some as high as 52.0 ml/kg in a lean (62.8-kg) patient with apparently similar types of edema resulting from orthostatic sodium retention (Streeten *et al.*, 1973). These findings may explain some of the discrepancies in the literature reported by investigators who have described basal plasma volumes in idiopathic edema as being subnormal (Veyrat *et al.*, 1968; Gill *et al.*,1972*a,b*) and those who have found them to be normal (Fisher, 1965; Streeten *et al.*, 1973; Edwards and Bayliss, 1976). These basal plasma volume measurements also appear to rule out the theoretical possibility that hypervolemia and consequent elevation of capillary hydrostatic pressure might be part of the primary mechanism of edema formation in most patients with orthostatic edema.

b. Orthostatic Changes in Plasma Volume. The finding of a fall in plasma volume in the upright posture, in normal subjects, was described many years ago (Thompson *et al.*, 1928; Waterfield, 1931*b;* Youmans *et al.*, 1935; Asmussen *et al.*, 1939; Brun *et al.*, 1945; Aull *et al.*, 1957; Fawcett and Wynn, 1960). Our initial studies (Streeten *et al.*, 1973) showed that orthostasis for 1 hr in the fasting state was associated with a fall in plasma volume (measured directly with labeled serum albumin injections) of 3.5 ± 2.13% in five normal control subjects, 9.94 ± 1.55% in 10 orthostatic sodium retainers ($p < 0.05$), 6.44 ± 2.35% in five orthostatic water retainers (NS), and 4.00 ± 1.80% in three patients with non-orthostatic edema. Whether the lack of statistical significance of the changes in orthostatic water retainers was caused by the small number of patients studied is unknown. From measurements of hematocrit (Hct) in the standing and recumbent postures, Edwards and Bayliss (1975) found, in general agreement with our data, that patients with idiopathic edema showed a greater orthostatic fall in plasma volume than did normal females, during the luteal phase of the menstrual cycle. In their studies, Hct rose, indicating a fall in plasma volume, by 10.3 ± 0.6%, while the change in normal subjects was 7.9 ± 0.7% ($p < 0.025$) within 10 min of standing. Thibonnier *et al.* (1979) reported similar results. These findings suggested rapid excessive transudation of fluid from the capillaries in the upright posture in patients with orthostatic edema. It should be recognized that an excessive fall in plasma volume upon changing from recumbency to standing is not pathognomonic for patients with orthostatic edema, since it has also been described in patients with glomerulonephritis, nephrosis, cirrhosis, and nutritional edema (Fawcett and Wynn, 1960).

2.3.4.2. Capillary Leak Syndrome

In very rare instances (Clarkson *et al.*, 1960; Preston *et al.*, 1962; Weinbren, 1963; Horwith *et al.*, 1967; Jacox *et al.*, 1973; Atkinson *et al.*, 1977), patients have been found to experience repeated dramatic episodes of acutely developing edema, associated with rapid increases in Hct and plasma protein concentration, a precipitous fall in blood pressure to shock levels, and eventually, death during one of the episodes. Rapid disappearance of Evans Blue dye from the circulation (32% in 1 hr) during one episode of shock and a profound fall in measured plasma volume by as much as 50% in another episode showed unequivocally that this disorder is indeed, as it has been described, a "capillary leak syndrome." Elevations of plasma IgG concentrations have occurred in some of these patients (Atkinson *et al.*, 1977), but the cause of this striking syndrome is unknown. This disorder is probably unrelated. A possible exception might be some similarities of its mechanism to orthostatic edema, since edema is absent even in the upright posture, as we have had the opportunity to confirm, in one of these patients, between episodes of rapid plasma leak from the capillaries. However, evidence of excessive permeability of the capillaries to protein was found by Behar *et al.* (1976) in patients with idiopathic edema. Extravasation of labeled protein after inflation of a cuff around the forearm at 80 mm Hg for 12 min was below 10% in 30 normal control subjects and in all patients with cardiac or renal edema, but exceeded 10% in all 15 patients with idiopathic edema, in a few patients with cirrhosis, and in others with lymphedema.

2.3.4.3. Effects of Leg Wrapping and Pressure Suit

In an attempt to determine whether excessive orthostatic pooling of blood occurs in the capacitance vessels of patients with typical orthostatic edema, we compared the effects of posture on excretory responses to administered 0.14%

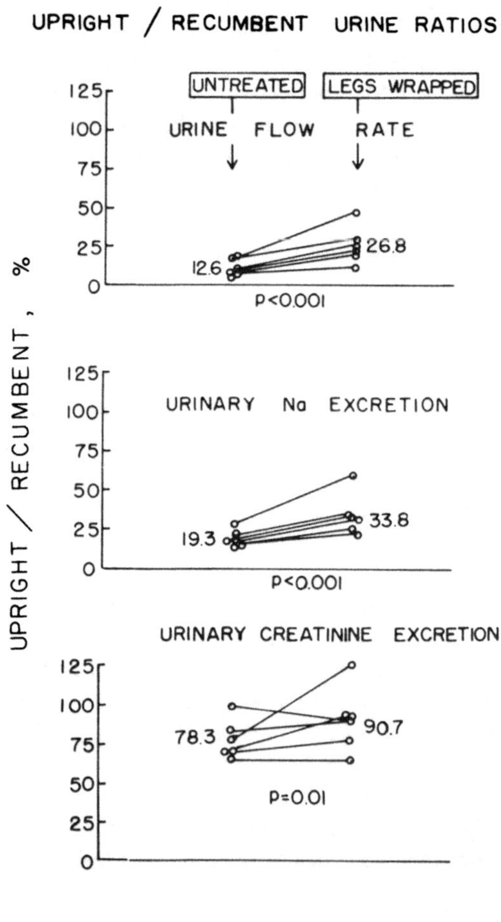

FIGURE 24. Effects of wrapping the legs (with Ace bandages) in six patients with orthostatic sodium retention. Changes are seen in their upright/recumbent ratios of urine flow rate, urinary Na excretion, and urinary creatinine excretion during salt loading (150 ml 0.14% NaCl solution each half-hour) in a posture test. Slight but significant improvement in all parameters resulted from bandaging the legs. (From Streeten, 1978.)

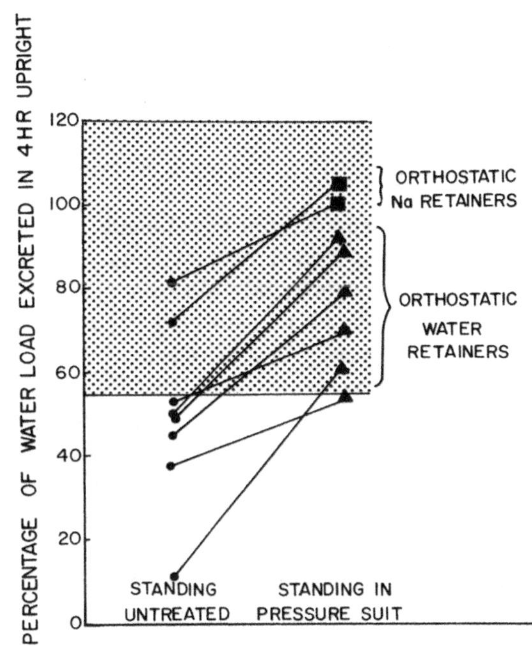

FIGURE 25. Effects of antigravity suit on excretion of water load in eight patients with orthostatic edema. Water excretion in the upright posture was improved in all patients, being restored virtually into the normal range in all of six patients with orthostatic water retention.

NaCl solution (the posture test) with and without wrapping the legs of six patients with orthostatic sodium retention. Leg wrapping produced modest but significant increases in the excretion of water, sodium, and creatinine in the patients studied (Fig. 24). These findings supported the concept that excessive orthostatic pooling of blood in the capacitance vessels of the legs led to excessive transudation from the capillaries, with consequent edema formation and reduction of renal function in these patients. Kuchel *et al.* (1970) reported that the subnormal excretion of a 1200-ml water load, in the upright posture, in six patients with orthostatic edema, was completely corrected by tightly bandaging the lower limbs and the abdomen during the test. Figure 25 shows that inflation of a pressure suit increased the excretion of a water load from subnormal to normal or very close to normal in six patients with orthostatic water retention and increased excretion within the normal range in two patients with orthostatic sodium retention. The effects of the pressure suit were highly significant statistically ($p < 0.001$).

2.3.4.4. Effects of Vasodilatation on Changes in Leg Volume

Youmans *et al.* (1935) studied the effects of orthostasis on leg volume in normal subjects by measuring the amount of water displaced from a rigid metal boot reaching 48.5 cm up the leg to about the knee. These workers found the orthostatic increase in leg volume to be exaggerated by vasodilatation in the legs, which was induced by immersing the hands and forearms in warm water.

2.3.4.5. Effects of Environmental Heat

Some patients with orthostatic edema report that high environmental temperatures greatly aggravate their edema. This phenomenon was studied in one of our patients who complained of severe heat sensitivity (Streeten, 1960*b*), and has been reported also by Edwards and Bayliss (1976). Our patient was shown (Fig. 26) to have oliguria, low sodium excretion, and excessive weight gain associated with the development of pedal edema, when she remained standing for 7 hr in a hot room (temperature 33–35°C). In striking contrast with these findings, the patient excreted more sodium and water, experienced a loss of weight, developed no pitting edema, and felt considerably more comfortable when she stood for the same length of time and ingested the same food in a walk-in refrigerator (temperature 4°C). A plot of the daily temperatures in her home against evening body weights over a 5-month period (see Streeten, 1960*b*) revealed a significant correlation ($r = +0.41$, $p < 0.001$), as shown in Figure 27. It seems likely that these effects of heat resulted from vasodilatation that aggravated the underlying excessive pooling of blood in the capacitance vessels and the consequently excessive transudation of fluid in this patient with orthostatic edema. This conclusion is supported by the observation (Streeten *et al.*, 1960*b*) that when the patient stood in the hot room for 7 hr in an inflated antigravity suit, her urinary

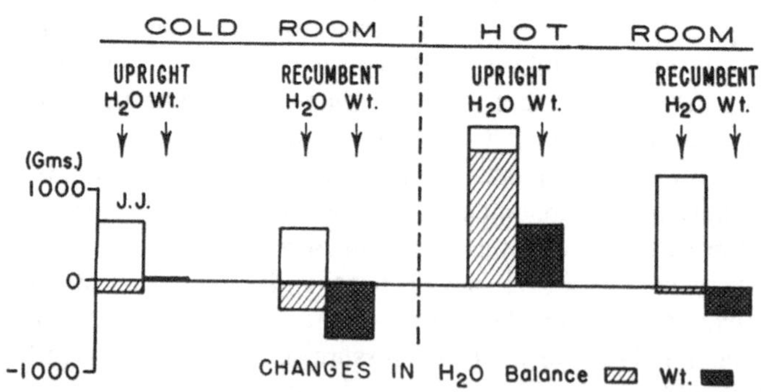

FIGURE 26. Predominant effect of heat on orthostatic fluid retention and weight gain in a euthyroid patient with orthostatic sodium retention and severe heat intolerance. During 7-hr days in recumbency or standing, either in a hot room (33–35°C) or a cold room (1–7°C), water retention (cross-hatched area above horizontal line) and weight gain (plotted above baseline) occurred only when she was standing in the hot room. Water intake is plotted from the baseline upward, urine output from the top of intake downwards. (From Streeten, 1960*b*.)

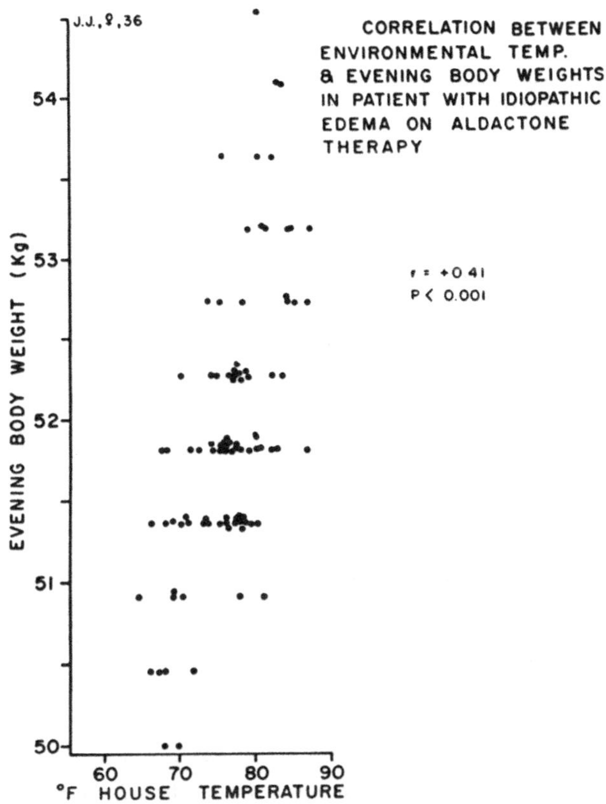

FIGURE 27. Correlation between house temperatures and evening body weights in patient with orthostatic sodium retention and heat intolerance whose other data are shown in Figure 26. The correlation ($r = +0.41$) was significant ($p < 0.001$). (From Streeten, 1960*b*.)

sodium output was increased from 17 to 50 mEq, urine volume was increased from 467 to 1510 ml, and weight gain (0.56 kg) was converted into a loss of 0.04 kg in the 7-hr period of orthostasis (Fig. 28).

2.3.4.6. Effects of Orthostasis on Leg Volume During Restricted Sodium Intake

In the balance studies with 200-mEq daily sodium intake, during 12 hr of standing, leg volume was found to increase excessively in orthostatic sodium retainers [by 459 ± 24 ml as compared with an increase of only 129 ± 20 ml ($p < 0.01$) in normal controls]. Theoretically, this abnormal response might have resulted from a primarily cardiac, renal, autonomic, or other cause of inadequate

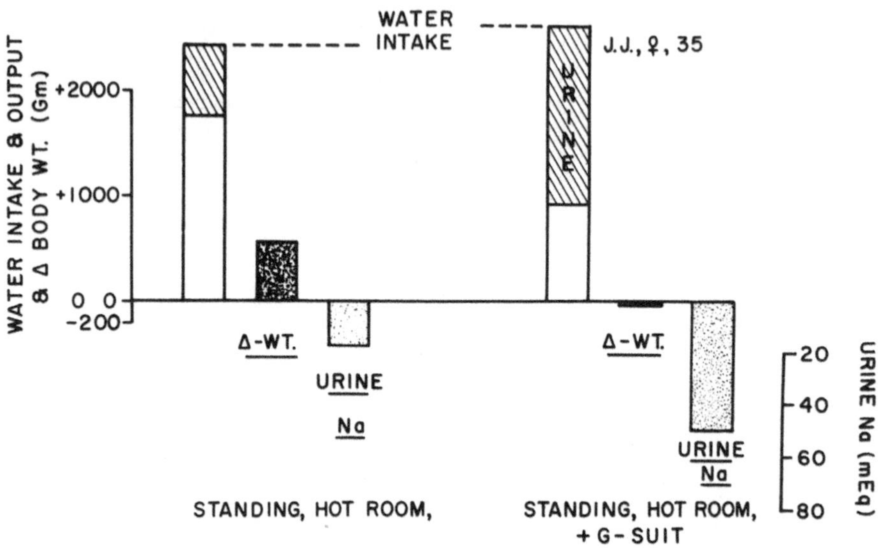

FIGURE 28. Effects of antigravity suit on urine volume, Na output, and weight change in patient with orthostatic sodium retention and heat intolerance (Figs. 24 and 25) during 7-hr days standing in a hot room. The suit increased urine volume and Na output and converted a weight gain of 0.56 kg into a loss of 0.043 kg. (From Streeten *et al.*, 1960.)

sodium excretion, which led to sodium retention, and secondarily, to excessive accumulation of the retained sodium and water in the dependent limbs. In these circumstances, reduction of sodium intake from 200 to 10 mEq/day would have been expected to have reduced the orthostatic leg volume changes into the normal range, since excessive sodium retention could no longer take place. In fact, however, the mean (± SEM) increases in leg volume declined only slightly from 459 ± 24 to 345 ± 24 ml during the 12-hr periods of orthostasis. These findings suggest strongly that a peripheral vascular abnormality causing excessive transudation into the dependent limbs is the primary disorder in orthostatic edema, which leads secondarily to the series of changes described above, ending with renal sodium retention (if there is ingested sodium to be retained), or to a persistent fall in plasma volume (if there are negligible amounts of ingested sodium to be retained).

2.3.4.7. Conclusions

The evidence of orthostatic plasma volume changes, the beneficial effects of external compression of the legs, the harmful effects of external heat, and the lack of improvement in the leg volume changes during restricted sodium intake all support the view that a local vascular defect, leading to excessive intracapillary pooling, is the primary defect in orthostatic edema.

2.3.5. Cause of Excessive Orthostatic Intravascular Pooling

2.3.5.1. Anatomical Site of Lesion

Evidence is still fragmentary and conflicting in this area. Since orthostatic hypotension is very seldom present in untreated patients with orthostatic edema (Streeten *et al.*, 1973), it seems unlikely that excessive arteriolar dilatation could be present in the upright posture in these patients. Disorders of the large veins, such as varicose veins or venous obstruction, can undoubtedly lead to edema (Cooper, 1981). However, varicose veins have been consistently looked for and found in only 10 of 150 (7%) patients with orthostatic edema (see Appendix I, patients #21, 32, 45, 56, 58, 88, 97, 107, 130, and 136). Venograms performed in a consecutive series of patients with orthostatic edema revealed obstruction of the deep veins in none of the 12 patients studied. Similarly, lymphangiograms were normal in all patients examined (Streeten *et al.*, 1973). Kuchel *et al.* (1970) also reported normal lymphangiograms in all six patients with orthostatic edema. It seems most likely, therefore, that increased volume and increased hydrostatic pressure within the capillary bed result in excessive orthostatic pooling caused by subnormal tone in the precapillary sphincters or excessive tone in the muscular venules. There are several postulated abnormalities:

1. Precapillary sphincter dilatation alone with consequent opening up and "flooding" of the capillary bed
2. Precapillary sphincter dilatation associated with venular constriction, such as occurs in animals in response to histamine or serotonin administration (Vanhoutte, 1978)
3. Dilatation of both the precapillary sphincters and the muscular venules.

It is unlikely to result from excessive tone in the venules alone, since one would not expect that such a lesion would be relieved by external compression.

2.3.5.2. Postulated Mechanisms of Disorder

The possible ways in which such a microcirculatory disorder might originate include the following:

a. *α-Adrenergic Innervation or Responsiveness.* The precapillary sphincters might be defective in this respect. If we knew whether the precapillary sphincters of the human peripheral vessels have such adrenergic innervation in the first place—as do the coronary vessels of the dog (Burnstock, 1981)—or receive no adrenergic innervation, like the mesenteric vessels of the rat, the potential role of precapillary sphincter innervation could be more effectively considered.

b. Plasma Concentrations of Norepinephrine and/or Epinephrine. In microvascular control, these concentrations are probably more important than norepinephrine released at sympathetic nerve-endings, and might be subnormal in patients with orthostatic edema. Our own measurements of plasma catecholamines in such patients have disclosed no abnormalities. Similarly, total urinary excretion of norepinephrine and epinephrine has been normal in both the recumbent and the upright posture (Kuchel, 1970, 1977) or has actually been elevated (Gill *et al.*, 1972*b*) in patients with idiopathic edema.

c. Vasodilating Humoral or Tissue Agent. A tissue metabolite or a circulating humoral agent with vasodilatory action on the microvasculature might be present in excessive concentrations, especially in the upright posture, in these patients. This might be histamine, bradykinin, serotonin, one of the prostaglandins, or other agents and might conceivably not always be the same agent in all patients. The possible role of one of these agents is supported by the demonstration that even nonvasodilating doses of these potent dilators are capable of overwhelming the constrictor influence of norepinephrine, angiotensin II, and vasopressin on precapillary sphincters and other microvessels *in vivo* (Altura, 1978*b*). Since H1 and H2 histamine receptor antagonists have had no significant effects on the severity of fluid retention in patients with orthostatic edema, histamine excess seems unlikely to have a pathogenic role. Such drugs as indomethacin and other inhibitors of prostaglandin synthesis have consistently aggravated and never been found to reduce the edema in these patients (Streeten, unpublished observations). Since blood bradykinin concentrations have been found to rise in the upright posture in human subjects (Streeten *et al.*, 1972; Wong *et al.*, 1975), excessive orthostatic release of bradykinin in orthostatic edema seemed possible. Blood levels of bradykinin have been measured in several of our patients. Kinin concentrations were found to be elevated in some patients, especially in those whose orthostatic edema was associated with orthostatic changes in mean arterial pressure or in pulse pressure, causing orthostatic lightheadedness (Auchincloss *et al.*, 1985). Blood kinin concentrations in a series of patients with orthostatic edema are compared with values in normal subjects in Figure 29.

The synergistic action of bradykinin and serotonin in inducing intense venular spasm, capillary stasis, and extravasation of erythrocytes through defects in the capillary walls (Zweifach, 1973) might be relevant to the pathogenesis of orthostatic edema. These responses of the rat mesenteric vessels are attenuated

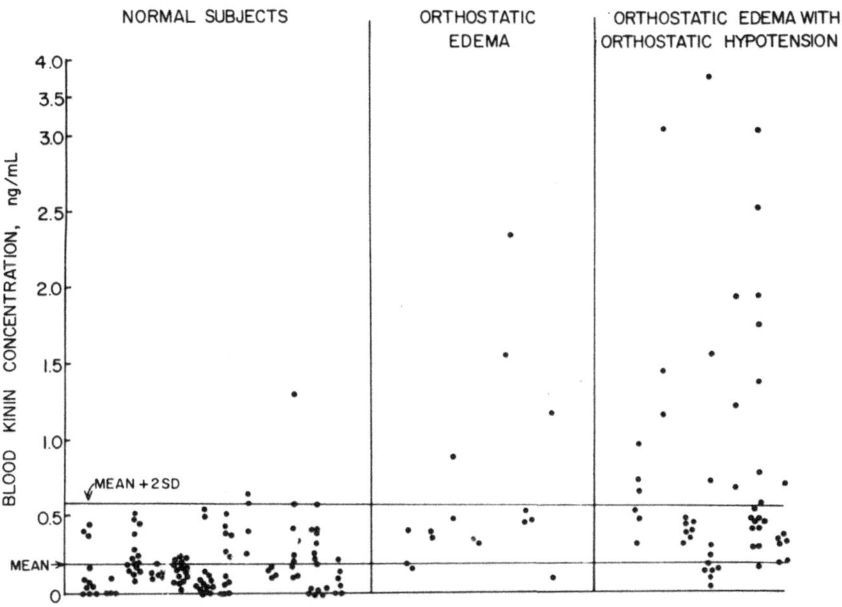

FIGURE 29. Multiple blood kinin levels in patients with orthostatic edema and normal subjects, each studied over a period of several days.

by indomethacin, but this drug has had no favorable effect on the severity of the usual types of orthostatic edema. On the contrary, we have found that administration of most nonsteroidal anti-inflammatory agents has tended to increase the severity of orthostatic edema.

d. Deficient Release of Dopamine. This deficiency has been proposed as an important pathogenetic mechanism in premenstrual edema by Evered *et al.* (1976). It was also proposed as a factor in idiopathic edema by Kuchel *et al.* (1977), who found significantly lower urinary excretion of dopamine in 16 patients with idiopathic edema than in 10 normal subjects, in the recumbent posture. However, these differences were not present in the upright posture, reducing the likelihood that orthostatic edema could be due to dopamine deficiency. Furthermore, urinary free dopamine excretion apparently reflects renal dopamine release more than peripheral vascular turnover of this agent (Alexander *et al.*, 1974; Faucheux *et al.*, 1977). Also, dopamine has insignificant effects on microvascular constriction *in vitro*, except in amounts (>10 μg), which are five or six orders of magnitude greater than minimally constrictive amounts of epinephrine or norepinephrine (Altura, 1978*a*) and probably have little relevance to the effects of physiological dopamine concentrations *in vivo*. Nonetheless, the postulated role of dopamine deficiency in orthostatic edema has stimulated therapeutic trials of the dopamine receptor agonist, bromocriptine. This drug has promoted natriuresis, reduced orthostatic edema, and restored excessive increases in body weight intra diem into the normal range, according to some reports (Sowers *et al.*, 1982*a*). The therapeutic action of bromocriptine has been less impressive in the experience of other investigators (Edwards *et al.*, 1979). The role of dopamine deficiency in the pathogenesis of orthostatic edema rests on rather tenuous evidence. It is unknown whether dopamine might exert an action in orthostatic edema exercised by enhancing cAMP formation through D1 receptors promoting vasodilatation of renal vessels or through D2 receptors (e.g., in the pituitary) that inhibit norepinephrine release (Langer, 1981).

e. Deficient Microvascular Constriction at an Undetermined Site. This appears to be the primary lesion in orthostatic edema, supported by evidence that the disorder can be corrected, often for many months or years, by a variety of vasoconstrictive agents. These have included phenylephrine (Laragh *et al.*, 1960), ephedrine (Streeten, 1978), D-amphetamine (Speller and Streeten, 1964), and, most recently, Midodrine (Streeten, unpublished results). The therapeutic use of these agents is considered in more detail in Chapter 5.

f. Structural Abnormality of Capillaries. This might be responsible for abnormal permeability that would result in excessive fluid loss into the interstitial space during an increase in intracapillary pressure, such as occurs during sitting and standing. Sims *et al.* (1965) reported that the basement membrane of capillaries within the gastrocnemius muscle was thicker in 11 patients with idiopathic edema (mean 4700 ± 1900 Å SD), than in control subjects, seven of whom were not edematous (mean thickness 2600 ± 210 Å), while two had edema that was due to congestive heart failure in one and to systemic lupus erythematosus (SLE) in the other (mean thickness 3730 Å). Although there was slight overlap between the thicknesses of the basement membrane of the capillaries in the idiopathic edema patients and the control subjects, the difference between the two groups was significant ($p < 0.05$). The normal restriction of protein loss from the capillaries probably requires integrity of the basement membrane. The occurrence of similar basement membrane changes in the leaky capillaries of the renal glomeruli of patients with the nephrotic syndrome implies that basement membrane thickening might well cause increased permeability to protein. Sims *et al.* (1965) likened the basement membrane change in patients with idiopathic edema to the lesion seen in many patients with diabetes mellitus. In fact, they found that three of their 11 patients had diabetic glucose tolerance tests, while one patient subsequently developed gestational diabetes, and four had abnormal cortisone glucose tolerance tests (Conn and Fajans, 1961). The prevalence of overt diabetes mellitus in our patients (Appendix I) was only 2.4%, probably no higher than in the general population. Coleman *et al.* (1970) confirmed the finding of thickened capillary basement membranes in a patient with idiopathic edema but pointed out that such abnormalities are nonspecific, having been demonstrated in polymyositis, SLE, scleroderma, arteriosclerosis, and diabetes mellitus. It remains uncertain as to whether the basement membrane thickening in idiopathic edema has any pathogenic significance.

g. Hypoproteinemia. In the older literature, there are occasional reports, such as that of Emerson and Armstrong (1955), of massive edema associated with hypoproteinemia of unknown cause. It is not clear whether the possible role of protein-losing enteropathy was appreciated at that time or was excluded in this patient. However, the observation that the protein concentration in the edema fluid was unusually high (0.8 g/dl) would suggest abnormal capillary permeability to protein. The patient reported by Coleman *et al.* (1970) appears to have had a similar condition in that she had hypoproteinemia of unknown cause, and with evidence against its having resulted from protein-losing enteropathy. In their patient, the protein concentration in the edema fluid was 3.1 g/dl, and microscopic lesions were demonstrable: pericapillary round cell and plasma cell infiltration and thickened capillary basement membranes with laminated split basement membranes in the precapillary arterioles. The low plasma volume and accelerated turnover of labeled serum albumin seem to indicate that the morphologically abnormal capillaries were excessively permeable to protein, causing extravascular protein accumulation and consequent edema formation. More recently, Gill and associates (1972*a,b*) concluded from their studies that mild hypoproteinemia of unknown origin might be the cause of idiopathic edema. The observations that led to these conclusions included the finding of slightly subnormal concentration and pool size of circulating albumin, attributed to accelerated movement of albumin from the intravascular compartment to an enlarged extravascular pool. However, the plasma albumin concentrations in the patients reported were not low enough to constitute a mechanism for edema formation; the findings of hypoproteinemia have not been confirmed in other studies (Sims *et al.*, 1965; Thorn, 1968; Veyrat *et al.*, 1968; Werning *et al.*, 1969; Kuchel *et al.*, 1970; Streeten *et al.*, 1973; Oelkers *et al.*, 1975; Edwards and Bayliss, 1976).

h. Obesity. Most clinicians are probably aware that edema of the legs and feet is commonly seen in extremely obese persons who appear to be otherwise healthy. Edema will frequently disappear in these patients if and when they are able to reduce body fat toward the normal range by caloric restriction. The body weights of two women in whom this was accomplished are shown in Figure 30. There are no data to show whether the pathogenesis of this type of edema of obesity involves mechanical obstructive effects of adipose tissue deposits, un-

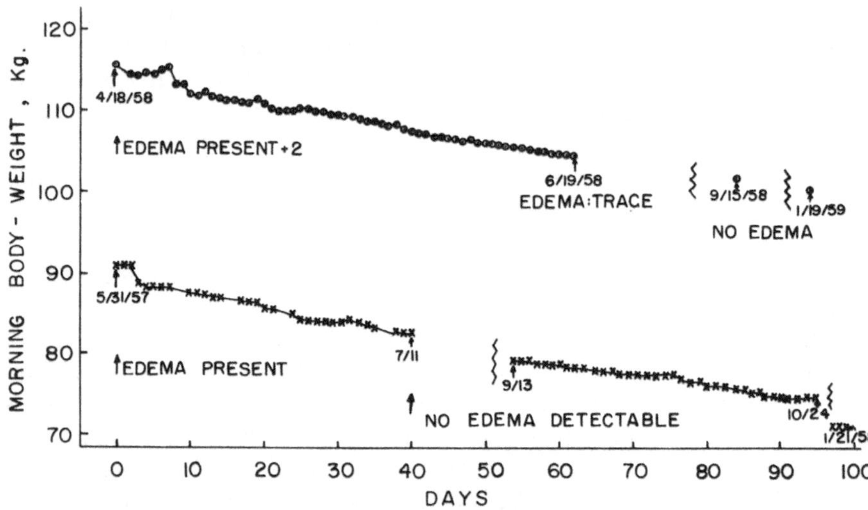

FIGURE 30. Edema of obesity. Curves show disappearance of edema with weight loss in two women with severe obesity. (From Streeten, 1978.)

usual inactivity of the subjects, the mildly subnormal renal plasma flow and GFR (per square meter) associated with obesity (Bansi *et al.*, 1959), or other mechanisms. While only 24% of patients in our studies of the pathogenesis of orthostatic edema (see Appendix I) were severely obese (>15% above the Metropolitan Life Insurance Company range of normal), the frequency of extremely obese individuals in several of the studies in the literature has not been stated. Some of the differences between the findings in reported series of patients with idiopathic edema could be the result of variations in the prevalence of severe obesity among the patients studied.

i. Diuretic-Induced Edema. It has been suggested that idiopathic edema is usually, if not always, an iatrogenic disorder resulting from chronic abuse of diuretic therapy (MacGregor and de Wardener, 1975, 1979*a;* de Wardener, 1981). Their evidence includes the observation that when diuretic treatment was stopped in 10 patients, the edema initially became more severe, reaching a peak at 4–10 days, and then spontaneously receded. The body weight returned to the level present during diuretic treatment in four patients and to within 1.5 kg of this level in another three patients. In the remaining three patients, weight remained elevated by 3–5 kg and edema persisted for at least the 18–19 days of observation in the hospital but gradually subsided after several months of a low sodium diet at home. The diet was then liberalized, without the return of edema, except in one patient.

It is reasonable to believe that diuretic-induced stimulation of the renin-angiotensin-aldosterone system was responsible for aggravating the edema after cessation of treatment with diuretics. It is quite possible that these patients were being overtreated for mild forms of edema or that no edema had been present in the first place, as MacGregor and de Wardener imply. However, these investigators did not determine whether edema was absent after a period of supervised orthostasis lasting several hours. Their claim that the patients were free of edema in the followup visits makes no mention of whether the patients were examined in the morning, or the late afternoon or evening when edema is usually more evident in patients with orthostatic edema, despite being frequently undetectable in the morning. We have often found no pitting edema during morning visits in patients who later developed obvious edema after being on their feet for 8 or 10 hr. There is no indication that the patients of MacGregor and de Wardener were capable of normal activity, such as working on their feet for an 8-hr day, without developing edema. No attempt was made to define the patients' renal responses to posture.

These investigators considered that an inordinate percentage of nurses and paramedical personnel appeared to complain of idiopathic edema, supposedly because diuretics would be easily available to them, although no instances in which this was actually shown to have been the case were described. This evidence and their speculation that idiopathic edema did not exist before oral diuretic therapy first became available do not accord with our experience, since I had seen several patients with this disorder in Dr. Thorn's unit at the Peter Bent Brigham Hospital, as well as several additional patients in the Division of Endocrinology and Metabolism at the University of Michigan, before oral diuretics were first released for clinical use in the United States in about 1957 (Streeten, 1979). Moreover, of the patients we have studied (Appendix I), only 7 of 169 (4.2%) were practising nurses or paramedical personnel who could have had any access to diuretics, except by prescription. If there are more nurses than housewives with orthostatic edema, this might quite possibly result from the fact that nurses in most hospitals spend virtually a complete 8-hr day on their feet, while many housewives might not do so. Furthermore, several physicians, including many in Boston and Ann Arbor with whom I was associated, were very familiar with idiopathic edema for several years before the first effective oral diuretic, chlorothiazide, became available in the United States. When this drug was first marketed, we used it immediately for the treatment of 10 patients whose edema had antedated availability of the drug.

If orthostatic edema were really the consequence of diuretic treatment, it would be difficult to understand why we virtually never see the development of edema in the thousands of hypertensive patients who receive diuretic drugs exclusively, for the treatment of their hypertension, over periods of many years. One would also wonder why edema has seldom if ever been evident, to our knowledge, when diuretic treatment has been stopped in these patients, unless congestive heart failure was present.

j. Deficient Natriuretic Factor. Jones (1973) reported that some patients with idiopathic edema fail to show the normal escape phenomenon in response to the continued administration of the mineralocorticoid, fludrocortisone. Such failure to escape from progressive sodium and water retention during treatment with fludrocortisone is certainly not pathognomonic of orthostatic edema, since it has also occurred in congestive heart failure (Jones, 1973) and in several otherwise normal females whom we have studied. However, the finding does raise the possibility that the release of a natriuretic factor during hypervolemia may be subnormal in these patients. Favre and Mach (1980) measured the effects of a fraction of the 24-hr urines, obtained from 10 patients with idiopathic edema, extracted on Sephadex G-25 columns, on sodium excretion in rats. Without convincing evidence, they concluded that the excretion of "natriuretic factor" was appropriate in the five patients with the smallest amounts and was above normal in the five patients with the largest amounts of this substance in the urine. They wondered whether the patients who excreted excessive amounts of natriuretic factor might be manifesting renal tubular resistance to the action of the factor.

Now that atrial natriuretic peptides have been discovered and shown to cause natriuresis and diuresis (de Bold *et al.*, 1981; Kangawa and Matsuo, 1984), the possibility that deficiency of one or more of these substances or failure of their release or action may be involved in the pathogenesis of orthostatic edema is worthy of study.

2.4. SUMMARY

Orthostatic edema is an excessive accumulation of extracellular fluid that results from abnormal retention of fluid exclusively in the upright posture. The orthostatic disorder has been clearly documented by metabolic studies in the recumbent and standing postures. Some patients with this disorder excrete less than 55% of an administered water load (20 ml/kg) during 4 hr in the upright posture and can excrete the same load normally in recumbency; these individuals are *orthostatic water retainers*. Others excrete water normally but retain sodium excessively as evidenced by an abnormal drop in sodium excretion in the upright posture to less than 33% of the recumbent excretion rate: *orthostatic sodium retainers*. Individuals of a third group have both *orthostatic sodium and water retention*. Leg volume and body weight measurements confirm the presence of excessive leg swelling and fluid retention in the upright posture in these patients. Patients with orthostatic edema can readily be differentiated by these tests from individuals with *nonorthostatic edema*.

The pathogenesis of edema with orthostatic sodium retention appears to be initiated by excessive orthostatic capillary perfusion, since it can be reduced or corrected by leg bandages or pressure suits and is aggravated by warming the legs. Excessive transudation of fluid occurs into the dependent limbs, causing an abnormal orthostatic fall in plasma volume, with consequent orthostatic reduction in RBF and GFR, less filtration of sodium at the renal glomeruli, and excessive tubular reabsorption of sodium often resulting from orthostatic hyperaldosteronism. Thus, the plasma volume is partially replenished by sodium and water retention, only to be reduced once again by transudation if orthostasis continues. In patients with orthostatic water retention, sodium excretion is normal, but a water load is excreted subnormally in the upright posture. The demonstrable failure of normal vasopressin suppression by the water load (judging from urinary excretion of vasopressin) exclusively in the upright posture probably causes the orthostatic water retention in most of these patients, since the defect can be largely or completely corrected by ethanol administration with the water load. Whether posture contributes to the capillary leak syndrome, in which episodic loss of circulating fluid and plasma proteins is severe enough to cause profound hypovolemic shock, is unknown. Since the abnormal orthostatic increase in leg volume in patients with orthostatic edema is aggravated by environmental heat, is often unaffected by reduced sodium intake, and is usually not associated with hypoproteinemia, it probably results from a disorder of microcirculatory function. This may be the result of diminished dopamine release or excessive action of a vasodilator (a humoral or tissue agent such as bradykinin or a prostaglandin), for both of which the evidence is meager, or some other cause of excessive orthostatic capillary pooling and transudation. Administration of diuretics aggravates the response of the renin-angiotensin-aldosterone system to orthostasis, but probably seldom, if ever, plays a primary role in the pathogenesis of orthostatic edema. Some obese women have edema that disappears with weight loss after caloric restriction and is probably not orthostatic in type.

3

ORTHOSTATIC EDEMA

Clinical Features

3.1. GENDER, AGE, AND PREVALENCE

3.1.1. In Women

Orthostatic edema is a disorder seen mainly if not exclusively in females. This fact may or may not be related to ovarian function; although orthostatic edema seldom, if ever, becomes evident before puberty, it frequently persists after the menopause or after bilateral oophorectomy. In fact, the disorder first became evident after the menopause in 13 (7.8%) of our patients (see Appendix I, patients #4, 27, 30, 43, 68, 73, 85, 94, 97, 117, 131, 142, and 155). On the other hand, orthostatic edema is clearly affected by changes in the physiology of the reproductive organs of women, since it commonly appears to start with or to be aggravated by premenstrual fluid retention, and it frequently begins during pregnancy, as it did in 24 of 153 patients (16%) (identified as P in the symptoms column in Appendix I).

3.1.2. In Men

Among the several hundred patients with idiopathic edema we have seen over the past 33 years, only three were males. Data pertaining to the role of posture in the genesis of the edema in two cases are shown in Appendix I (patients #173 and 174).

The first male reported in the literature to have had idiopathic edema (Preston *et al.*, 1962) had recurrent monthly bouts of edema, associated with fever that was suppressible with prednisolone. This patient was apparently entirely free of edema between bouts. Water excretion was normal, even during attacks of edema. Since he was presumably not confined to bed during the edema-free periods, it seems unlikely that this patient's edema was of the orthostatic type, which by definition disappears with recumbency. Among the three males we studied, one had edema that seemed more related to psychic stress than to posture (Streeten, 1978).

The second male (#173, Appendix I) was a teacher who presented with striking signs and laboratory confirmation of the presence of hyperthyroidism, yet he had virtually no symptoms except for weight loss, which did not concern him. He was completely unaware that he had severe (4+) ankle edema until this was pointed out to him at his first office visit. The edema was very slightly, if at all, affected by his becoming *seriatim* euthyroid for several years after radioiodine therapy, then transiently hypothyroid for a few months, and finally euthyroid again on treatment with desiccated thyroid supplements. His mean change in body weight from morning to evening was excessive (1.0 kg), but the limited studies he would allow us to perform at the Clinical Research Center showed no convincing evidence of an important postural component in the causation of his edema. This patient died 18 years after he was first seen; the cause of his edema was never determined.

The third male we studied briefly for unexplained edema is a surgeon whose edema was episodic, lasting 1–4 weeks at a time, with almost complete freedom from edema between attacks. During a typical period of fluid retention, his weight would rise by 4–7 kg in 2–3 days because of a tremendous increase in fluid intake stimulated by sudden, extreme thirst. On at least one occasion, he gained as much as 15 kg within a few days, resulting in fulminating pulmonary edema and coma, requiring intravenous furosemide for relief. When studied over a 2-day period, he excreted 78% of a water load (20 ml/kg) during 4 hr in the upright posture (normal excretion >55%). Urinary osmolality fell only as low as 123 mOsm/kg after the water load (normal <100). When he stood for 2 hr during oral loading with dilute saline solution in one of our posture tests (Streeten, 1978), sodium excretion fell only to 77% of recumbent values (normal 33–100%). Although we did not have an opportunity to study this patient during an attack of severe edema, the episodic nature and the absence of any evidence of postural components in his disorder make it clear that this patient does not have orthostatic edema of the type usually seen in women. We have never seen a convincing example of orthostatic edema in any male patient.

3.1.3. Age of Onset

Orthostatic edema may start at any age after the onset of puberty. From Appendix I it is evident that of the patients with orthostatic edema who were studied, six had first observed abnormal fluid retention before the age of 15; in two the edema first became noticeable after the age of 60; and in 50% of the remaining patients studied, it started between the ages of 18 and 30. The disorder is aggravated by some factors and ameliorated by others (see below). It may not always require treatment, but there is no convincing evidence that it ever disappears spontaneously or that it can be "cured."

3.1.4. Distribution and Prevalence

The pathogenetic role of posture in patients with orthostatic edema has been confirmed (Streeten, 1978) in Syracuse—in individuals from 4 continents—and we know that its occurrence is not limited to Caucasians, as the predominance of reports from America and Europe might lead one to conclude. We have seen typical orthostatic edema in an American-born patient of Chinese descent and in an African student from Ghana. Mild forms of orthostatic edema are probably common, but there have been no attempts to define the prevalence of the disorder. A strong hereditary tendency to orthostatic edema is evident, with rather frequent occurrence of the disorder in mothers and their daughters or among sisters.

3.2. SYMPTOMS AND SIGNS

3.2.1. Evidence of Fluid Accumulation

Characteristically, patients with orthostatic edema notice swelling at the ankles, in the legs, and in the abdomen, either starting in the latter half of each day of normal activity or worsening from morning to evening. Some patients find that if they remove their shoes in the late afternoon, increasing pedal edema may make it difficult for them to get into their shoes again, if they wish to do so later the same evening. Others complain that their skirts become tighter toward the end of the day, sometimes requiring a larger size in the evening. After rest in bed or after a night's sleep, edema in the legs subsides and often disappears. Upon awakening the next morning, there may be visible swelling in the eyelids and the face, as well as edema in the hands and fingers, making it difficult to remove rings from the fingers and causing stiffness, discomfort, and sometimes pain in the hands. Swelling of the breasts may also cause discomfort. These diurnal changes in the site of the edema are clearly gravitational in origin; night workers notice that edema of the legs is most severe when they go off duty in the mornings. The predominant effect of orthostasis compared with purely circadian factors in influencing body weight is shown in the weight changes recorded in a registered nurse during periods of night duty, off-duty days, and periods of day duty (see Fig. 31).

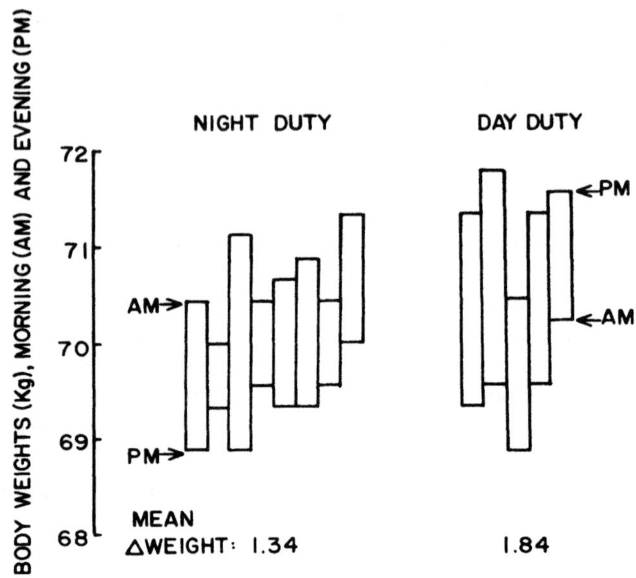

FIGURE 31. Body weight changes during periods of orthostasis and activity in a nurse working on day and night duty. Weight at the end of the work day (upper borders of rectangles) was always abnormally greater than weight before the work day (lower borders of rectangles), indicating that excessive weight gain was work and posture related and not simply a circadian change.

3.2.1.1. Pitting Edema

When the disorder is severe, pitting edema may be detected in the legs during the morning, after recumbency overnight. However, far more commonly no pitting edema is demonstrable at the ankles or over the pretibial areas in the mornings or early afternoons. Patients who consult physicians at these times or who are seen in the hospital, where most patients spend the major part of the day lying down, are often embarrassed and disconcerted when physicians can find no evidence of edema. Pitting edema is usually most easily demonstrable in the pretibial area. In doubtful cases, it is reasonable for the doctor to withhold judgment about the presence or absence of orthostatic edema unless and until the patient has been examined between 5:00 and 8:00 p.m., after being on her feet for 10 or 12 hr. Since it is under such conditions that the edema is usually complained of, it may be essential to examine the patient in the early evening, after prolonged orthostasis at her place of work, in the physician's office, or even in a hospital observation unit, if necessary. By examining patients when the edema of which they complain is likely to be at its worst, we have found that pitting edema is unequivocally demonstrable in the overwhelming majority of patients complaining of swollen legs.

3.2.1.2. Changes in Leg Volume

Verification of the excessive swelling of the legs in the upright posture may be obtained by direct measurement of the changes in the volume of the legs. This can be accomplished inexpensively, easily, and with good reproducibility, using a simple water-displacement technique that we have used for several years (Streeten, 1965, 1973, 1978). The patient stands in a rigid plastic bucket that has been fitted with a wide metal spout 33.5 cm from the bottom. Tepid water is poured into the bucket until it begins to overflow slowly from the spout, at about 1 drop per second. The patient then steps out of the bucket. More water is then added until it overflows again, at the same rate as before; the volume of water added is considered to equal the volume of the patient's legs to a vertical distance of 33.5 cm from the soles. The measurement is routinely performed in duplicate; the agreement between duplicate determinations has been quite satisfactory in thousands of measurements over the past 20 years. Five measurements of leg volume made on the same normal subject by each of six nurses on two successive days (a total of 30 determinations) yielded a mean of 4.05 liters, with a standard deviation of 33 ml (coefficient of variation, 0.82%) (Streeten *et al.*, 1973).

Obviously, the absolute volume of any individual's legs is of little interest, because of the large differences in the mass of the muscle, fat, and bone, apart from the possible presence of edema. However, changes in the volume of the legs from morning to evening, during known periods of orthostasis, are very relevant to orthostatic edema. These changes over 12 hr have been found to average +130 ml, with a range of −60 to +270 ml, in normal females in balance on a 200-mEq Na diet daily (Streeten *et al.*, 1973). Patients with orthostatic edema show larger changes in leg volume over a 12-hr period in the upright posture, varying from 275 to more than 800 ml (see Appendix I). In two of our patients with lymphedema, (not included in Appendix I), leg volume increased by 1200 and 3500 ml during 12 hr of standing. When there has been difficulty in being sure whether there was excessive swelling of the legs after orthostasis, measurements of the changes in leg volume have provided objective diagnostic assistance. Although patients with nonorthostatic edema may sometimes experience an excessive increase in leg volume after standing for 12 hr (Streeten *et al.*, 1973), this apparently paradoxical finding is probably due to gravitational redistribution of edema fluid, the accumulation of which was not the result of orthostasis (as evidenced by the fact that weight gain in the upright posture was normal in these patients). By contrast, when the leg volume shows no more than a normal increase during 12 hr in the upright posture, in the presence of obvious edema before and after standing, there can be little doubt that the edema is of the nonorthostatic type (see patients #136, 146, 149, 151, 152, and 157 in Appendix I).

3.2.1.3. Body Weight Changes

The increases in body weight, which are concomitants of fluid retention, often lead patients to seek the help of a physician. When weight gain is severe and the evidence of edema is minimal, there can be little doubt that adiposity is also present and may actually be contributing to the pathogenesis of the edema, by mechanisms that have not been successfully studied. However, excessive diurnal weight changes are seldom seen in obesity *per se* and are the hallmark of orthostatic edema.

a. Weight Changes Intra Diem in Normal Subjects. A healthy person who is in caloric equilibrium, with no persistent upward or downward trend in body fat content, would be expected to have a similar body weight each morning. In such individuals, weight gain from morning to evening (intra diem) must closely parallel the sum of the weights of voided urine and insensible fluid loss during the night, except if there were unusually bulky fecal excretion during the night. Since the urge to urinate commonly occurs when the bladder contains 400–600 ml of urine, and since most normal persons do not have nocturia, it follows that the average weight loss from bedtime to rising time the next morning must usually be no more than 400–600 g. It would therefore be expected that, except when a large intake of fluid occurs shortly before retiring, the mean weight gain intra diem would be the same: 400–600 g. Clearly, this would vary from day to day. A particularly large intake of salt on one day, stimulating water intake and retention of fluid for several hours, would undoubtedly increase the weight gain from morning to evening that day. But, when natriuresis ensued during the following day(s), there would be a tendency toward weight loss intra diem, so that weight gain from morning to evening, over the course of 2 or 3 weeks should be substantially unaffected and would average about 0.4–0.6 kg. In fact, the mean weight gain intra diem in a series of eight healthy subjects who recorded their weights at home for 13–37 days was found to be 0.455 ± 0.04 kg (SEM), with a total range of 0.31–0.58 kg (Streeten *et al.*, 1960). Furthermore, any unconscious tendency of an individual to over- or underreading of the weights, and any errors in the scale itself, would tend to balance themselves out and should have little effect on the change in weight intra diem, if weight records were continued for 2 weeks or more.

b. Weight Changes Intra Diem in Orthostatic Edema Patients. If a woman were retaining fluid to an abnormal extent because of orthostasis during the day, one would expect her to experience excessive weight gain from morning to evening. Such changes were first described in 1960 in five patients with severe orthostatic edema, in all of whom weight gain from morning to evening averaged between 1.1 and 1.7 kg (Streeten *et al.*, 1960). Subsequent studies by ourselves and others over the succeeding 25 years have confirmed the reliability of this simple indication of pathological fluid retention in the upright posture (Streeten, 1965, 1973, 1978; Thorn, 1968; Kuchel *et al.*, 1970; Rovner, 1972; Edwards and Bayliss, 1976). A comparison of weight changes intra diem in eight normal subjects and five representative patients with moderately severe orthostatic edema is depicted in Figure 10.

Some investigators have espoused the view, without any published evidence to support it, that a weight gain of 1.4 kg from morning to evening should be required for the diagnosis of orthostatic edema (Thorn, 1968; Edwards and Bayliss, 1976). Adherence to this criterion would require that the diagnosis of orthostatic edema be withheld unless patients were retaining more than three times as much fluid as normal subjects, in the upright posture. Such patients would certainly be expected to have the disorder, but most patients whose disorder is fortunately far less severe would be incorrectly considered normal. We have seen a large number of patients whose features correspond in every way with those of others who undoubtedly have orthostatic edema and whose weight gain intra diem consistently exceeds not only the expected normal range but also the observed total normal range and the mean ±2 SD of the normal changes (0.26–0.66 kg), yet averages less than 1.4 kg. Since there seems to be no rational explanation for the choice of the 1.4-kg criterion, we believe it is better to consider that patients whose weight changes from morning to evening average 0.7 kg or more are almost certainly abnormal and might have orthostatic edema. Occasional patients who have edema during orthostasis, which disappears at bed rest, have had mean weight changes of +0.6 kg intra diem, which is still greater than the normal range. Although evidence for orthostatic fluid retention would have to be established firmly on other grounds, we believe that weight gains of 0.6 kg or more are also compatible with the diagnosis of orthostatic edema (see Appendix I).

3.2.2. *Nocturia*

In a patient with excessive fluid retention in the upright posture during the day, there should be an unusually large volume of fluid to be excreted during recumbency overnight. It would therefore be expected that, if she had come into equilibrium, i.e., morning weights were fairly constant over several days or weeks, her overnight urine excretion would be larger than normal. Unless bladder capacity were increased or bladder sensitivity reduced, such a patient would tend to have nocturia. These expectations are satisfied in patients with orthostatic edema who gain excessive amounts of weight from morning to evening and often have nocturia. In fact, many patients even notice and volunteer that they seem to have to void very seldom during the day but almost always have to pass urine once, twice, or more often during the night. Unless cystitis is present, which causes urinary frequency by day as well as by night, the history of daytime oliguria and nocturnal polyuria strongly suggests abnormal fluid accumulation in the upright posture and consequent orthostatic edema.

3.2.3. Symptoms Resulting from the Edema

A large variety of symptoms have been attributed to the local effects of edema. The implied causation (in this instance edema) of patients' complaints cannot always be validated by any objective or scientific procedure. However, there should be little reluctance to accept the possible correctness of the implied causation if symptoms occur consistently when edema is severe, disappear when the edema is reduced or absent, and are complained of repeatedly in the same circumstances by several patients who appear to have the same disorder. The symptoms that our patients have attributed to the presence of edema are listed under each individual in Appendix I. In some instances, these symptoms may have been attributable to potassium depletion or plasma hypovolemia caused by antecedent diuretic treatment. But an attempt has been made to exclude such symptoms from the list, whenever this possibility seemed likely.

3.2.3.1. Discomfort in Legs

An aching tight feeling of discomfort was a frequent complaint of patients with orthostatic edema (D in Appendix I). This was almost invariably worst in the evenings when edema was most noticeable, was frequently complained of after the patients had been standing in our research unit for a full 12-hr day, and was reduced by the relatively rapid decrease in the severity of the edema, which could be accomplished by elevating the legs well above the height of the abdomen for 3 or 4 hr. The edematous legs were frequently somewhat tender to pressure over the tibiae. In about 10 patients, discomfort in the legs was described as severe pain. Patient #89 (Appendix I) was one of these 10 individuals who had required narcotic treatment for the pain, which apparently became excruciating when she was very edematous after sitting for 12 hr (orthostatic hypotension prevented her from standing for long periods of time) at our Clinical Research Center. The pain was strikingly relieved by diuresis, induced rapidly by furosemide, or more gradually by recumbency with elevation of the legs. This phenomenon was observed repeatedly, during three separate admissions, each lasting at least 2 weeks, at intervals of 1 year or more, in this patient.

3.2.3.2. Abdominal Discomfort

A bloated distended feeling in the abdomen is a common complaint in patients with orthostatic edema who have been edematous after having walked about for several hours. Shopping for many hours often aggravates abdominal discomfort as well as leg edema.

Girth measurements, which are notoriously difficult to reproduce, sometimes show enlargement of the abdominal girth, but ascites has never been clinically detectable. There may be slight pitting edema of the abdominal wall, but this too is usually difficult to determine. Excessive extracellular fluid in the abdominal wall is the probable cause of abdominal discomfort.

3.2.3.3. Discomfort in Hands: Carpal Tunnel Syndrome

A sense of fullness and distention in the hands and fingers is often complained of. Interrogation reveals that this is usually most troublesome in the mornings after awakening. It is associated with more severe swelling of the fingers at the same time, manifested by tightness of rings or inability to remove rings, if they have been worn through the night. By contrast, finger swelling is, perhaps somewhat surprisingly, usually less severe immediately after prolonged orthostasis. Numbness and tingling in the hands and fingers are also frequent complaints in severe edema. The combination of pain, paresthesias, and sensory loss in the distribution of the median nerve, together with a positive Tinel's sign (Phalen, 1970), have led to the diagnosis of the *carpal tunnel syndrome* in several patients. Some have been operated on once or repeatedly for the carpal tunnel syndrome before discovering that adequate control of the orthostatic edema that had been causing the syndrome produced satisfactory improvement in these uncomfortable symptoms (see patients #6, 14, 73, 90, 142, 159, 162, and 166 in Appendix I).

3.2.4. Intracranial Symptoms

3.2.4.1. Headache

Headache is a symptom the severity, cause, and significance of which are often difficult to evaluate. Mild headaches are commonly complained of by patients with orthostatic edema, although there is no way of knowing whether the symptom is more or less common than in the general population. In several patients the headaches have had the typical features of migraine. In some instances, however, we have been impressed, particularly during studies of the effects of posture, that headaches would be particularly severe during the mornings after 12 hr of standing and ambulation the previous day. Such headaches sometimes required relief by analgesics and usually tended to disappear spontaneously during the course of the day or when the upright posture was resumed the following day. Whether these headaches might have resulted, in some way, from edema of tissues in the head, we have no way of knowing.

3.2.4.2. Pseudotumor Cerebri

Three patients (#89, 95, and 96 in Appendix I) with subsequently obvious orthostatic edema presented initially with excruciating headaches associated with papilledema. In each case, the possibility of brain tumor led to the admission of these patients to the neurosurgical ward, where the existence of cerebral edema was suggested by elevated cerebrospinal fluid (CSF) pressure and confirmed in two patients by computed tomographic (CT) scans of the head, which were typical of pseudotumor cerebri (Reid *et al.*, 1980). The absence of localizing features and the findings on CT scan of the head led to the diagnosis of pseudotumor cerebri, which was treated with repeated decompression by spinal taps and the administration of dexamethasone. When it became evident, after several weeks of observation, that weight gain from morning to evening was excessive, the possible presence of orthostatic edema was studied. Leg volume was found to increase more than normally during 12 hr in the upright posture, and leg edema became evident after orthostasis, followed by clearly visible edema of the eyelids the next morning. Excretion both of a water load and of administered dilute saline (posture test) was severely subnormal in the upright posture. Because of this evidence of orthostatic fluid retention in a more generalized distribution than only in the brain, administration of diuretics was begun. Dexamethasone therapy was carefully tapered and stopped, with much symptomatic improvement noticeable to the patients as their iatrogenic Cushing's syndrome subsided. Ephedrine or D-amphetamine was later added to the therapy, with further improvement. In the two patients we have followed closely since the onset of their pseudotumor cerebri (patients #95 and 96, Appendix I) weight has fallen over several weeks by 7 and 15 kg, headaches have been few and only once or twice were they severe; these patients have been able to lead normal lives, over the subsequent period of 4 and 8 years, respectively. At least the possibility is worthy of consideration that, in some patients with pseudotumor cerebri, severe intracranial or cerebral edema might result either from excessive capillary transudation into the brain or from gravitational transposition of peripheral edema fluid into the cranium in recumbency.

3.2.4.3. Changes in Cerebration

Some patients complain repeatedly of mental dullness and fogginess in the mornings. These symptoms might well be manifestations of cerebral edema, but we have no proof that this is the case. Others say that they have great difficulty in mental concentration and reduced capacity for intellectual activity, particularly during the early morning after prolonged activity on their feet the previous day. Irritability is complained of by a few. At times, patients will liken their symptoms to those that might result from hypoglycemia, as Sims *et al.* (1965) commented. Food intake is said to improve these symptoms. We have been unable to establish the presence of hypoglycemia even at times when these symptoms were said to be present.

3.2.4.4. Psychological Changes

Psychological abnormalities are present in some, but certainly not all, patients. Lacking obvious physical evidence of serious disease, these patients appear to have complaints that are out of proportion to their relatively mild demonstrable disability. The symptoms described by a few patients are so numerous and so bizarre that they make a profound impression on the patient's family, her physician, and the nursing staff involved in her care at a hospital. Occasionally, the psychic features may be those of depression or even frank psychosis. Some investigators have considered that psychic factors might have a prominent role in the pathogenesis of orthostatic edema (Gordon and Graham, 1959); this might well be the case, although there are no convincing data to show that this is so.

The most striking personality trait in many of these patients is an almost obsessive-compulsive desire for perfection. Some are heavily involved in philanthropic endeavors on which they work long and diligently; others appear to strive compulsively for professional excellence or to meet what they consider to be their social responsibilities. Their physical appearance, or what they perceive it to be, seems to drive some women to attempt to rid themselves of every ounce of seemingly unnecessary fluid by the compulsive and sometimes truly abusive self-administration of diuretics or purgatives.

However, psychic features are neither prominent nor even evident in many patients with orthostatic edema. In those who do manifest them, symptoms often appear to be worsened and progressively amplified as they unsuccessfully seek help and sympathy from a succession of physicians they consult. There is no doubt that effective treatment frequently diminishes complaints in proportion to the therapeutic reduction of the edema. It is still very difficult to be sure to what extent the psychological manifestations might be the results of the edema and its unsuccessful management, rather than the cause of the syndrome.

3.2.5. *Cardiovascular Features*

3.2.5.1. Changes in Blood Pressure and Heart Rate

Some investigators have commented on the occurrence of postural hypotension in patients with orthostatic edema. Reference to Appendix I confirms that a greater than normal drop, particularly in systolic blood pressure, was recorded in several of the patients for whom data are shown. In our relatively prolonged balance studies, during which patients with orthostatic edema consumed a constant weighed diet containing 200 mEq sodium and 65–90 mEq potassium daily (Streeten *et al.*, 1973), blood pressure was measured daily. There was a tendency toward orthostatic hypotension in a few patients upon admission, 4–10 days after cessation of previous diuretic treatment. However, 10–13 days later, after retaining sodium and potassium and coming into balance on the diet, blood pressures and heart rates were normal in recumbency and did not fall abnormally in the erect posture, in any of the patients. Many of the patients whose data are recorded in Appendix I could not be studied after full electrolyte replacement; some of the recorded reductions in blood pressure in the upright posture might well have reflected continuing sodium depletion and hypovolemia.

On the other hand, in a few instances we have good reasons to believe that orthostatic hypotension was a primary phenomenon, unrelated to diuretic-induced hypovolemia. All these patients (Appendix I, patients #18, 26, 31, 47, 77, 89, 90, 112, 116, 132, and 157) were studied when no diuretic treatment had been administered, at least for several weeks. Their previous history of lightheadedness, palpitations, and fainting spells, sometimes dating back to before edema was noted, and the elevated blood bradykinin concentrations measured in most cases, suggest that these patients are different from the others and might have hyperbradykininism (Streeten *et al.*, 1972; Auchincloss *et al.*, 1986). In fact, in these patients edema was a relatively minor part of the symptomatology, whereas orthostatic lightheadedness and syncopal episodes were far more prominent. In the capillary leak syndrome, episodic or sustained loss of plasma volume causes profound and life-threatening reductions in blood pressure.

3.2.5.2. Cyanosis of Legs

Subtle bluish or purplish discoloration of the legs in the standing posture is evident in a large number of patients with orthostatic edema, as it is in patients with orthostatic hypertension and other forms of the pooling syndrome (see Chapter 7). This phenomenon is most readily apparent when, in a good light, the color of the dependent limbs of a patient with any of these disorders is directly compared with that of a normal subject. Occasionally, the legs and even less commonly the fingers, may be deeply cyanotic. Orthostatic cyanosis was most striking in one patient (#72, Appendix I) whose edema was severe (see Fig. 78) and in whom leg discomfort, edema, and fatigue were so severe when she stood for more than a few minutes that our postural studies had to be performed with her sitting rather than standing. The striking orthostatic color changes in another patient, who had autonomic insufficiency associated with hypotension, edema, and cyanosis in the upright posture are shown in Figure 32.

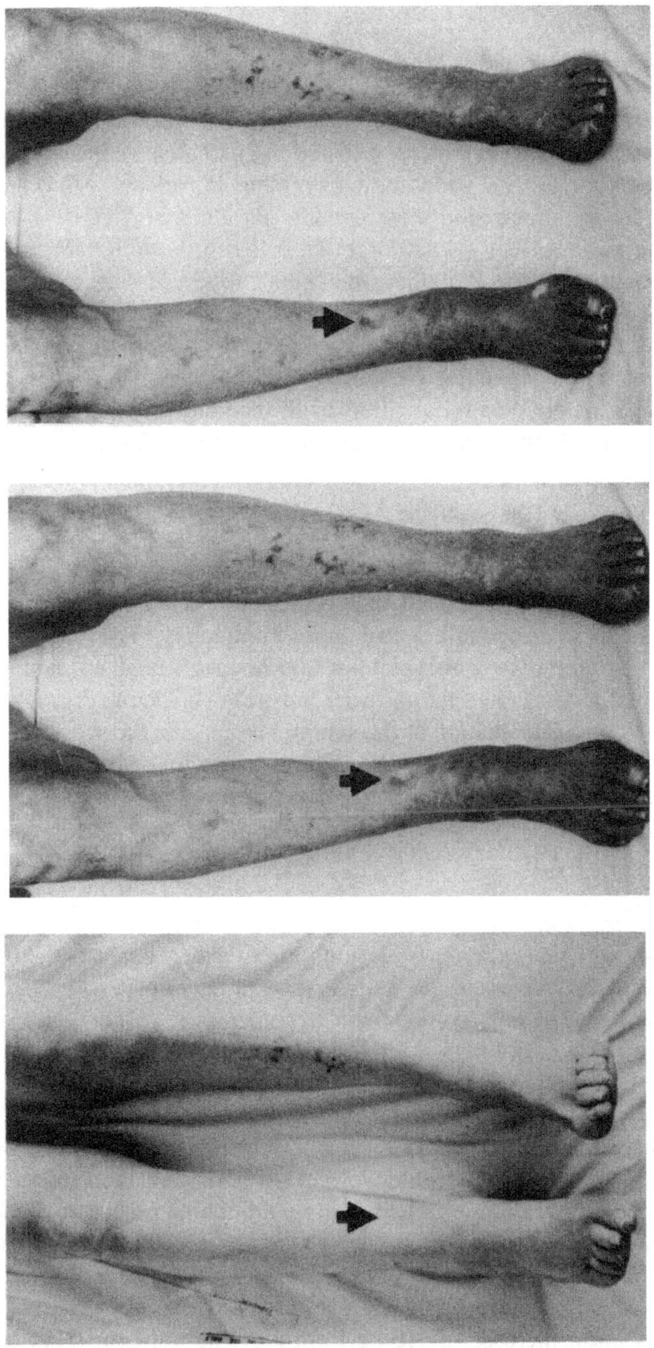

FIGURE 32. Orthostatic cyanosis associated with orthostatic hypotension and edema (arrows point to pitmark over right tibia) in a patient with autonomic insufficiency. Cyanosis is absent after lying down for a few minutes (left), becomes visible after standing for 2 min (center), and intense after standing for 5 min (right).

3.2.6. Other Clinical Features

3.2.6.1. Fatigue, Malaise, Lassitude, and Weakness

Fatigue, malaise, and lassitude are relatively nonspecific symptoms that may result from any of a wide variety of disorders, including orthostatic edema. There is nothing very unusual about these symptoms in patients with orthostatic edema, except for the impression some patients get that their fatigue is entirely related to being on their feet—what might be called orthostatic fatigue. These comments seem to indicate that they feel much relieved, with considerable reduction of their fatigue, if they are able to lie down, whether they sleep or not. We have no evidence of actual muscular weakness, apart from that which often results from potassium depletion caused by diuretic therapy. Tetanic muscle spasms have been reported to follow diuresis in recumbency, and to be associated with losses of calcium and magnesium (Crane *et al.*, 1973).

3.2.6.2. Nonarticular Rheumatism

Musculoskeletal aches, stiffness of the hands and the lower limbs, and backache are present in some patients with orthostatic edema. No fewer than 10 of the 174 patients in Appendix I had these complaints. The nature of the symptoms led to referral to a rheumatologist who had found no evidence of arthritis and usually designated the disorder nonarticular rheumatism (Pinals *et al.*, 1979). The diurnal fluctuation of the symptoms, reaching a crescendo as the day progresses, the aggravation of the symptoms by prolonged orthostasis, and the recognition of pitting edema in the evenings should lead to the diagnosis of orthostatic edema in these patients.

3.2.6.3. Thirst

Occasional patients experience severe thirst, either persistently or episodically. In at least two women, the combination of polydipsia with orthostatic water retention led to severe symptomatic hyponatremia. (Findings in one of these patients are shown in Figure 22.) A third patient (#117, Appendix I) had bizarre eating and drinking habits. For breakfast and while she was at work on her feet for 8–12 hr each day, she would eat egg whites and cucumber salad only and would drink water and two or three cups of coffee. After an evening meal at about 10:00 p.m., however, she would work in her home and attend to the needs of a disabled mother. While so engaged, she would imbibe refrigerated water in large volumes, estimated at 3–4 liters, before retiring at 1:00 or 2:00 a.m. Her weight records revealed a mean change of −0.1 kg from the time of rising until immediately before her late evening meal and the excessive water intake that followed, but a mean increase of 3.6 kg from morning until she went to bed.

Water excretion tests were normal in the upright posture when performed at 8:00 a.m. (60% of the load being excreted in 4 hr) but abnormal when performed while she remained standing from 8:00 p.m., when only 45% of the water load was excreted in 4 hr. This patient probably retained more than one-half the water that she drank each evening; this may have accounted for her edema, which was severe at the time of retiring and still present the next morning. Her nocturnal craving for water appears to have been reduced by treatment with D-amphetamine, with consequent reduction of fluid intake, body weight changes, and edema.

3.2.6.4. Glucose Intolerance

Sims *et al.* (1970) reported a high incidence of abnormal glucose tolerance tests and cortisone-glucose tolerance tests in a small group of patients with idiopathic edema. Frank diabetes mellitus does not seem to be unduly common in the patients with orthostatic edema whom we have studied, however, only three of our 169 patients having had this disorder.

3.2.6.5. Thyroid Disease

It has been reported that thyrotoxicosis may occasionally be associated with edema that disappears when the patient is restored to euthyroidism (Chapman *et al.*, 1956). Eight of the patients listed in Appendix I were found to be hyperthyroid when first seen for edema, but therapeutic correction of the hyperthyroidism seldom made any difference to the severity of the edema. Hypothyroidism was even more common, being present in at least 10% of the patients listed in Appendix I. It is well known that myxedema or even milder degrees of hypothyroidism may be associated with edema that disappears when the hypothyroidism is adequately treated. However, in the patients whose data are summarized in Appendix I, the hypothyroidism was almost always being treated with replacement doses of thyroxine or desiccated thyroid; euthyroidism was confirmed in virtually all instances by the finding of normal serum thyroxine and (often) thyrotropin levels, at the time the patients were seen by us. Thus, although the prevalence of hypothyroidism in patients with orthostatic edema is apparently far higher than in the general population, hypothyroidism is probably not directly involved in the pathogenesis of the edema.

3.3. *FACTORS THAT AGGRAVATE ORTHOSTATIC EDEMA*

3.3.1. *Menstruation*

The severity of edema and of the weight changes is increased premenstrually in less than one-half of patients who are still having menstrual cycles when orthostatic edema is diagnosed. The lack of detectable effect of the menstrual cycle on body weight in most patients suggests that premenstrual and orthostatic edema are generally unrelated pathogenetically. The responses to therapy confirm this conclusion, since premenstrual edema frequently persists unchanged, when orthostatic edema has been measurably improved by treatment with sympathomimetic amines.

3.3.2. Oral Estrogen Therapy

Estrogens given either for menopausal symptoms or as constituents of oral contraceptive preparations sometimes aggravate orthostatic edema.

3.3.3. Pregnancy

Many women have reported that they had been free of edema until its occurrence during one of their pregnancies; also, their subsequently recognized orthostatic edema had been evident ever since that pregnancy. The frequency of this observation, in 27 of 133 women (20%) with known or suspected orthostatic edema, is shown in Appendix I, designated by P. A few patients had experienced severe toxemia in a previous pregnancy, usually relieved by bed rest. One or two others noted that previously diagnosed orthostatic edema became considerably worse during a subsequent pregnancy. These facts seem to indicate that appropriate restriction of orthostasis during pregnancy would be reasonable and probably helpful advice to patients with orthostatic edema who subsequently became pregnant.

3.3.4. Environmental Heat

High environmental temperatures increase the severity of orthostatic edema in a large number of patients. This fact was elicited in the history obtained from no fewer than 37% of patients who were shown or strongly suspected to have excessive orthostatic sodium retention; it was also common in orthostatic water retainers (25%) and in patients with nonorthostatic edema (35%) (see Appendix I, where Ha = edema aggravated by heat). Occasionally, heat was more important than orthostasis. Thus, in patient #162, excretion of sodium and water was entirely normal when she was standing in a walk-in refrigerator (temp. 4°C) for 7 hr but was severely reduced in a hot room (temp. 33–38°C) over the same period of time (Fig. 26). This woman had been well aware of the adverse effects of heat and had attempted for years to counteract this effect by air conditioning her home to temperatures far below what most individuals would find comfortable: 55°F (13°C). In four other patients with orthostatic edema who were exposed to the same changes in posture and temperature, no clear-cut effect of temperature was evident (Streeten *et al.*, 1960).

3.4. LABORATORY FINDINGS

No measurements are available from routine hospital laboratories, which are invariably useful in the diagnosis of orthostatic edema, except by excluding other possible causes of edema. These are discussed under Diagnosis.

3.5. SUMMARY

Orthostatic edema may start at puberty or any time thereafter. It seldom, if ever, occurs in men. The disorder is manifested by abdominal swelling and pitting edema at the ankles and over the tibiae, which may not be clearly detectable in the morning but becomes worse as orthostasis continues during the day. Because the retained fluid is not completely excreted overnight, periorbital puffiness and edema of the hands may be evident upon awakening in the morning. Excessive swelling of the legs (measured by a simple water displacement technique) is associated with excessive weight gain during orthostasis from morning to evening, which is a clinical hallmark of orthostatic edema. Thus, when the mean weight gain from morning to evening (or during the working day) for 2 weeks or more exceeds 0.6 kg (1.3 lb), the normal mean change being 0.455 kg (1 lb), there is a strong possibility that orthostatic fluid retention is excessive and might be causing edema. Fluid retained during orthostasis is partially or completely excreted at rest, often causing nocturia. The edema *per se* may cause discomfort or even pain in the legs, a sensation of fullness or bloating in the abdomen, and paresthesias and pain in the hands resulting from the carpal tunnel syndrome. Headaches are often complained of; we have seen three patients with otherwise typical orthostatic edema who presented with excruciating headaches and papilledema diagnosed as pseudotumor cerebri. Many patients complain of poor cerebration, especially in the mornings; others are correctly or incorrectly considered psychoneurotic by physicians who may not be aware of the need to look for pedal edema after 8–10 hr of orthostasis in these patients. Orthostatic changes in blood pressure are usually within the normal range in untreated patients, but occasionally orthostatic hypotension may be present. When the legs are examined in a good light in the standing position, side by side with those of a normal subject, orthostatic cyanosis is frequently evident. Other clinical features include fatigue, malaise, lassitude, and a subjective complaint of weakness, as well as diffuse aches and pains resembling those of nonarthritic rheumatism. The history will often indicate that menstruation, oral estrogen intake, pregnancy, and hot humid weather conditions tend to aggravate the edema.

4

ORTHOSTATIC EDEMA

Diagnosis

In establishing the diagnosis of orthostatic edema, it is necessary both to exclude the presence of the many other known types of edema and to demonstrate that fluids are retained only in the erect posture. A careful history and physical examination will frequently suffice to indicate the cause and type of edema present in a patient complaining of fluid accumulation. Depending on the information elicited, a number of special inquiries, observations, measurements, and laboratory tests may be needed to exclude specific types of edema and to make a positive diagnosis of orthostatic edema.

4.1. EXCLUSION OF KNOWN TYPES OF EDEMA

4.1.1. Congestive Heart Failure

This condition is usually obvious at the bedside. The history of exertional dyspnea, orthopnea, and paroxysmal nocturnal dyspnea, reinforced by the finding of tachycardia, jugular venous distention, cardiomegaly, gallop rhythm, basal pulmonary rales, and hepatomegaly, indicates the presence of classic CHF. Many of these features may be absent in exclusively right-heart failure, in failure associated with constrictive pericarditis, and in a number of other special types of heart failure, but the use of ancillary procedures, e.g., chest radiographs, electrocardiography (ECG), and isotopic ventriculography, will generally enable the clinician to recognize that heart failure is present and is presumably causing the edema.

4.1.1.1. Occult Heart Failure

There is a particularly subtle form of heart failure, however, that may be associated with few, if any, of the classic manifestations. This was described by

Gill *et al.* (1965) in a 26-year-old woman thought to have idiopathic edema. She was found by cardiac catheterization to have raised left ventricular end-diastolic pressure and a subnormal increase in cardiac output in response both to exercise and to elevation of the afterload by infusion of angiotensin II. These findings, indicating subnormal left ventricular function, were supported by evidence of excessive sodium retention and weight gain in response to the mineralocorticoid, deoxycorticosterone acetate (DOCA). Treatment with digoxin resulted not only in restoration of a normal response to DOCA but in disappearance of the edema as well. Gill and co-workers concluded that an occult form of heart disease was responsible for this type of idiopathic edema.

Stimulated by these findings of Gill *et al.* (1965), we performed a hemodynamic study in 11 patients with orthostatic edema (Obeid *et al.*, 1974). This revealed moderate elevation of the mean pulmonary arterial and capillary wedge blood pressures and elevated stroke volume while the patients were on a controlled 200-mEq sodium diet, with further elevations in the same measurements after exercise in 10 of the 11 patients studied. The findings showed no evidence of intrinsic cardiac dysfunction in these 10 patients. In the eleventh woman, however, whose stroke volume failed to rise normally during exercise on the high-sodium diet, the findings were interpreted to indicate occult heart failure. In striking contrast with the other 10 patients, this one patient with idiopathic edema experienced dramatic improvement when given a trial of treatment with digitoxin. Her edema disappeared completely and has remained absent without the need for diuretic therapy as long as she has continued to take digitoxin regularly, during the subsequent 19 years. Unfortunately, we did not discover any simple means (short of cardiac catheterization) of diagnosing the occult form of heart failure seen in this patient, most of whose findings (patient #136, Appendix I) were similar to those of other patients with orthostatic water retention.

4.1.2. Renal Edema

This condition may occur in at least three ways. In acute glomerulonephritis, the typical clinical picture is associated with characteristic abnormalities in the urinary sediment. The mechanism of edema formation is probably related to increased capillary permeability and, to some extent, renal insufficiency. In the nephrotic syndrome, glomerular damage causes proteinuria, resulting in hypoproteinemia, which is the primary mechanism of the severe edema usually seen in this disease. Chronic renal insufficiency may also be associated with edema that appears to be the consequence of nonspecifically impaired renal excretion of sodium, water, urea, creatinine, and many other substances. Appropriate blood and urinary determinations leave little doubt as to the presence or absence of these renal causes of edema.

4.1.3. Hepatic Disease

Seldom if ever does hepatic disease cause peripheral edema before there is obvious ascites and/or clear evidence of abnormal blood tests of liver function.

4.1.4. Other Generalized Disorders

Peripheral edema may also result less frequently from a number of causes that can be diagnosed without much difficulty by the use of appropriate studies.

Anemia is evident from the blood count.

Hypothyroidism (Al-Khader and Aber, 1979) and hyperthyroidism (Chapman *et al.*, 1956) are diagnosed by measuring serum thyroxine, thyrotropin (TSH), and, when necessary, triiodothyronine (T3) concentrations.

Cushing's syndrome, which often causes edema, requires steroid measurements (Streeten *et al.*, 1969) but is frequently recognizable clinically.

Thiamine deficiency (beri-beri) in the Western world occurs mainly in alcoholics, food faddists, and other malnourished individuals.

Hypoproteinemia may result from inadequate protein intake (in malnutrition and debilitating chronic diseases), inadequacy of plasma protein synthesis (in liver diseases), or excessive protein losses in the urine (evidenced by urinary protein determinations) or stool (as in chronic diarrheas and protein-losing enteropathy). Protein-losing enteropathy is an occult cause of hypoproteinemic edema, the recognition of which requires specialized studies such as the measurement of radioactivity recovered in the stool after an intravenous injection of ^{51}Cr-labeled human serum albumin (Waldmann, 1961). These complex procedures are occasionally of great value when the cause of mildly hypoproteinemic edema is not apparent after measurements of urinary protein loss and hepatic function.

Drug-induced fluid retention must be ruled out. The possibility that, without the physician's knowledge, the patient might be taking sodium-retaining drugs, such as indomethacin, nonsteroidal anti-inflammatory agents, fludrocortisone, and (occasionally) phenothiazines, or water-retaining drugs such as chlorpropamide, should be determined.

Allergies may certainly cause edema but should seldom present diagnostic difficulties because of the usual presence of urticaria, the episodic occurrence, and the absence of any suggestion that orthostasis aggravates the edema.

Lymphedema is easily recognized in severe cases by the brawny consistency of the swelling, the frequently asymmetrical distribution (Figs. 33 and 34), the familial incidence (in many patients with lymphedema praecox), and the frequent history of recurrent attacks of lymphangitis. There is a widespread misconception that lymphedema is always brawny and never associated

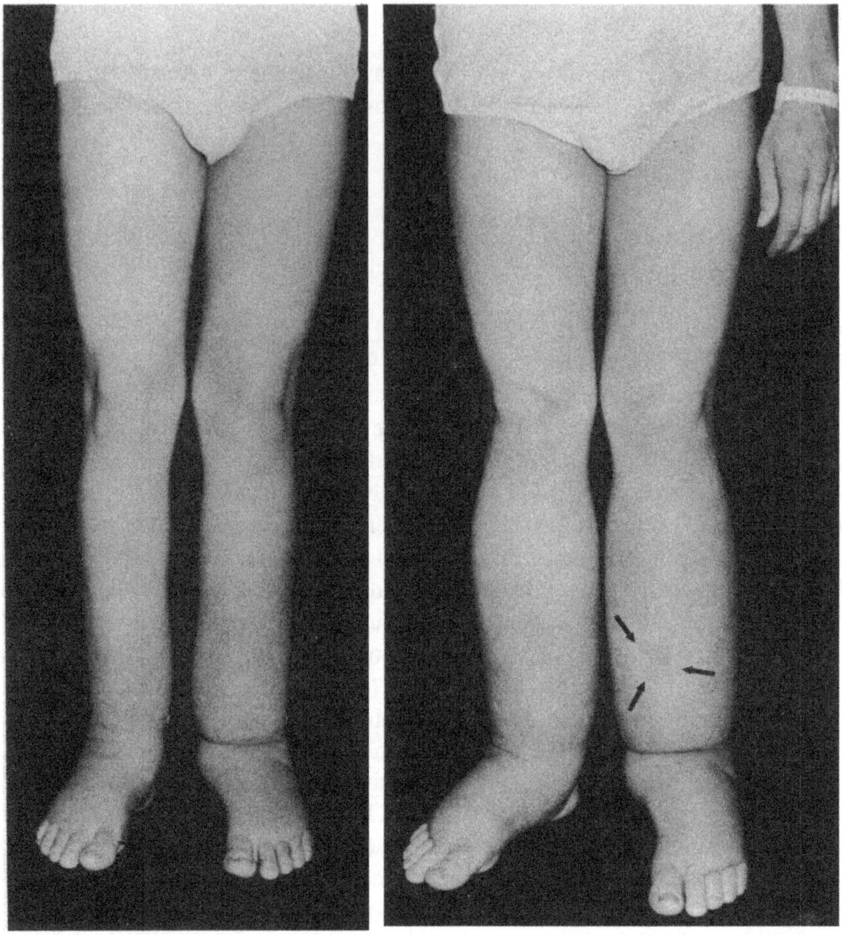

FIGURE 33. Lymphedema in a young male, showing the presence of an acutely variable, pitting component of the edema (illustrated between the arrows) which resulted in a change in measured leg volume from 7105 ml after 3 days of recumbency (left) to 10,255 ml after standing for 12 hr the following day (right). The irregular contour of the legs and the asymmetry of the swelling are evident.

with pitting edema. On the contrary, many patients with lymphedema have demonstrable pitting, usually superimposed on more persistent elephantiasiform swelling. These patients may show large increases in the degree of leg edema during orthostasis. Two of our patients with severe congenital bilateral lymphedema have had obvious pitting edema which was severely

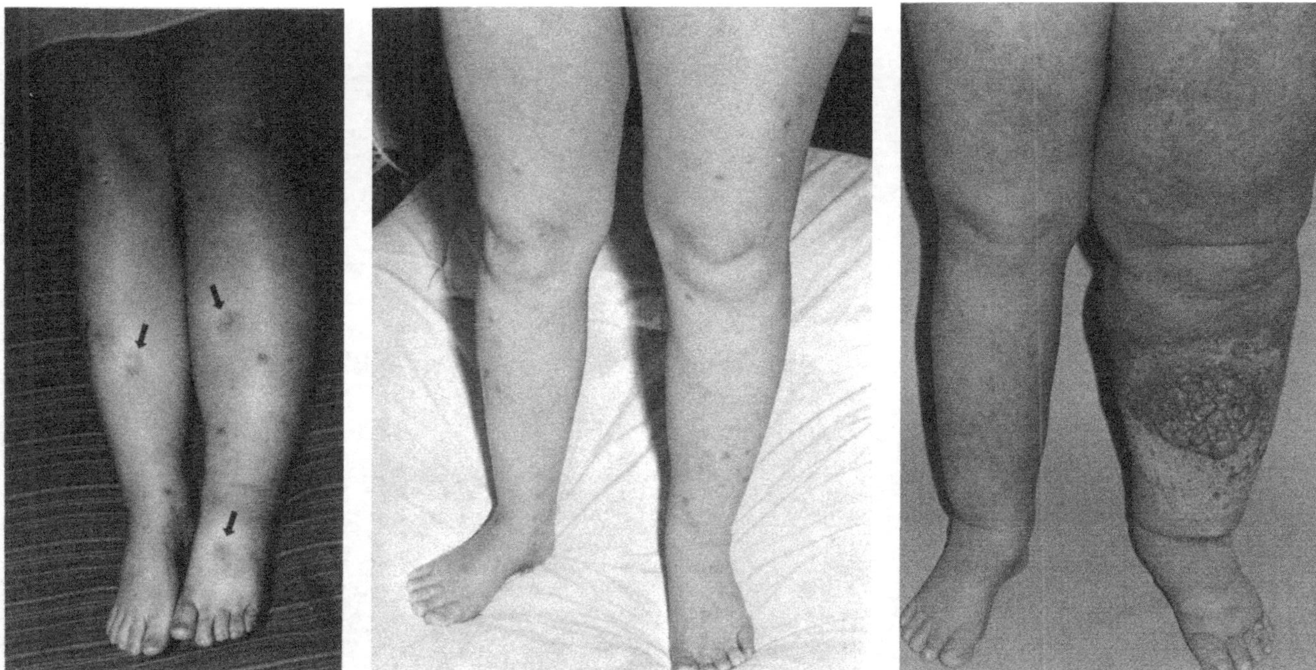

FIGURE 34. Lymphedema of the legs associated with pitting (arrows) when the patient was first seen at age 16 (left). The pitting component disappeared after treatment with a rigorous low-fat diet and a supplement of medium-chain triglycerides for 2 months (middle), but the edema progressed inexorably, with the development of fungating papillomatous lesions (right) over the next 15 years.

aggravated by orthostasis. The increase in their leg volume after 12 hr of standing was greater, by far, than in any of our patients with simple orthostatic edema: approximately 1000 ml in one patient and 3150 ml in the other (see Figs. 33 and 34). When there are doubts about the possible presence of lymphedema, lymphangiography will usually provide definitive information. It is important to appreciate, however, that this procedure often causes discomfort and may sometimes aggravate the lymphedema which it is being used to diagnose.

Scleroderma may present with pitting edema (Fig. 35) before the characteristic shiny tense induration of the skin is obvious.

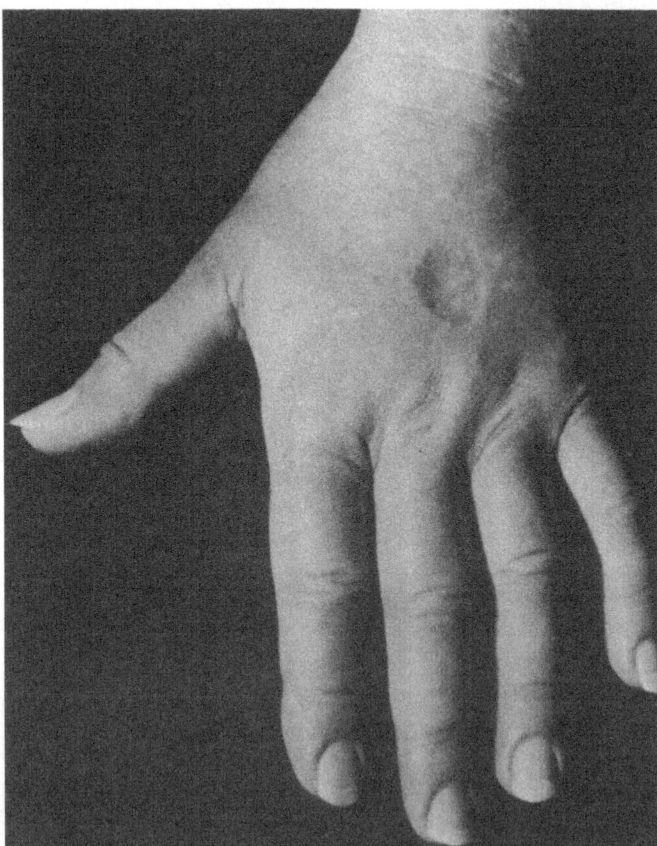

FIGURE 35. Edema as an early sign of scleroderma, shown on the dorsum of the hand, but also involving the legs.

4.1.5. Local Causes of Edema

Local etiologies of edema should not be overlooked. These include traumatic and inflammatory lesions (such as acute arthritis, cellulitis, and abscesses), venous obstruction (resulting from venous thrombosis, thrombophlebitis, massive thrombosis of the type of phlegmasia coerulea dolens, external pressure on or constriction of veins), lymphatic obstruction (by neoplastic metastases, from surgical section of lymphatics, e.g., after venous bypass surgery), and a few metabolic causes (e.g., gout). Most of these conditions are easily recognized by classic clinical methods. Venous obstruction resulting from relatively gradual, slowly developing venous thrombosis may cause diagnostic difficulties, requiring phlebography for their solution. Whether varicose veins are always the cause of associated edema is often impossible to determine. While there is little doubt of the frequent association of varicose veins with edema, there are also innumerable patients who manifest no edema in spite of the presence of prominent venous varicosities. When varicose veins or local venous obstructive lesions in the legs are the cause of edema, there is never, as far as is known, any edema in other parts of the body, similar to the early morning periorbital edema and finger swelling seen in patients with orthostatic edema.

4.1.6. Capillary Leak Syndrome

This episodic, acutely developing form of edema is associated with profound falls in blood pressure. It seldom causes diagnostic difficulties.

4.2. POSITIVE DIAGNOSIS OF ORTHOSTATIC EDEMA

4.2.1. History

A strong clinical suspicion of the presence of orthostatic edema is frequently derived from the history; this is usually valid as long as the pons asinorum of leading questions is avoided. Answers to the questions, "At what time of day is the swelling in your legs most severe?" and "Do you notice any swelling in parts of your body other than the legs?," with an affirmative answer to the latter followed by, "Where and when do you notice swelling elsewhere than in your legs?," are often helpful. They should give a strong indication of the presence or absence of gravitationally dependent leg edema in the evenings and periorbital together with finger edema in the early morning. Inquiry about the effects of prolonged orthostasis, such as during long shopping sprees, and unusual recumbency, such as during a day spent in bed because of an intercurrent infection or other ailment, should also provide helpful indications of the potential role of posture in the genesis of the edema.

4.2.2. Screening Test

If the history suggests a role of posture in the causation of the edema, strong support for the possibility may be obtained by having the patient measure body weights every morning, on arising, and every evening immediately before retiring, on both occasions after voiding, and either in the nude or in identical underclothing each day. Three or four measurements should be obtained by the patient at each weighing, and the average recorded in writing immediately. It is best not to inform the patient that the weights will be used to determine mean weight change intra diem, so that bias is avoided, as far as possible. The almost ubiquitous availability of bathroom scales in this country facilitates obtaining this information. Body weights should be recorded initially while the patient is receiving no diuretic treatment, over a period of at least 2 weeks. If the mean weight change from morning to evening exceeds 0.6 kg (1.3 lb), and certainly if it is above 0.9 kg (2 lb), the strong suspicion of orthostatic edema is supported. Changes smaller than 0.6 kg make the likelihood of orthostatic edema remote.

4.2.3. Definitive Tests

Clinically, the undoubted presence of pitting edema, evident on firm pressure with the examining finger over the medial surface of the tibia and/or below the malleoli, should be sought after several hours (up to 10 or 12 hr, if necessary) of ambulation and standing, sitting being allowed only for meals. The finding of minimal or no pitting edema at a subsequent appointment before 9:00 a.m. provides the best purely clinical evidence that edema is, in fact, slight after recumbency, and more marked after orthostasis.

4.2.3.1. Water Excretion Tests

These tests can easily be performed as outpatient or office procedures. The patients should always have been off diuretic treatment for at least 4 or 5 days, preferably 10 days or more. On an empty stomach, at between 8:00 a.m. and 10:00 a.m., the patient is asked to drink a water load of 20 ml/kg ideal body weight (and certainly never more than 1500 ml) during the space of about 15 min. Such water loads should preferably be of tap water, without ice. The patient should empty the bladder both before drinking the water, and every hour after the beginning of the water intake, for 4 hr, while she walks about or stands at her leisure in a quiet, undisturbed atmosphere. Micturition is permitted before the end of any hour but should then be repeated at the end of the hour. The total volume of urine passed in the 4 hr and the osmolality of the hourly urine samples are measured. The volume excreted in 4 hr is expressed as a percentage of the water load administered. The occurrence of severe headache, nausea, or vomiting during the tests should be considered to invalidate the results, since any of these symptoms will increase vasopressin release and reduce water excretion, even in an otherwise normal subject.

Normal limits. In normal persons, total excretion during 4 hr in the upright posture exceeds 55% of the load administered (Fig. 36), and lowest urinary osmolality (usually in the second hour) should be below 100 mOsm/kg. Vasopressin measurements, if performed on urine samples (after acidification to pH 4 with acetic acid), should fall below 1.0 μU/ml in one of the hourly urines (usually the second or third).

Patients whose results are abnormal in the test performed while standing should have the test repeated under identical conditions, 1 or more days later, but during recumbency, with only one pillow. Most normal subjects will excrete more than 100% of the administered water load in the supine posture, but occasional normal individuals have excreted no more than 65% of the load, within 4 hr. Patients whose water excretion is abnormal even in recumbency may have renal insufficiency, adrenal insufficiency, SIADH, or other disorders, and do not have simple, orthostatic edema. Subnormal water excretion in the upright posture, with normal excretion in recumbency, indicates edema with orthostatic water retention (Fig. 36). By definition, patients with nonorthostatic edema and those with orthostatic sodium retention excrete the water load normally (Fig. 36).

If vasopressin measurements are unavailable, patients who excrete less than 55% of the load when upright and more than 65% when reclining should be given a third water load test, again in the upright posture, in which the patient drinks 25 ml 95% ethanol, flavored with fruit juice, together with the water load. Mild symptoms of alcoholic intoxication may result from this amount of ethanol. An increase in the water excreted after the ethanol and water administration, to above 55% of the load (i.e., into the normal range), confirms the diagnosis of orthostatic edema with orthostatic water retention and strongly implies that the previously subnormal water excretion resulted from excessive vasopressin release in the upright posture.

4.2.3.2. Orthostatic Sodium Excretion: The Posture Test

In this procedure, the patient is again tested in the morning, after an overnight fast, and at least 1 week after the cessation of diuretic therapy. She empties the bladder immediately before and every 30 min during the intake, by mouth, of 150 ml of a 0.14 % NaCl solution, every 30 min, for 6 hr. The first 4 hr are spent in recumbency, and the last 2 hr in the upright posture. The urine passed during the last 2 hr in recumbency and during the 2 hr of standing is collected in two separate pools for measurements of volume, sodium, and creatinine content. The precise periods in recumbency and in the upright posture may have to be varied somewhat, if the patient passes no urine at all during the last half-hour in

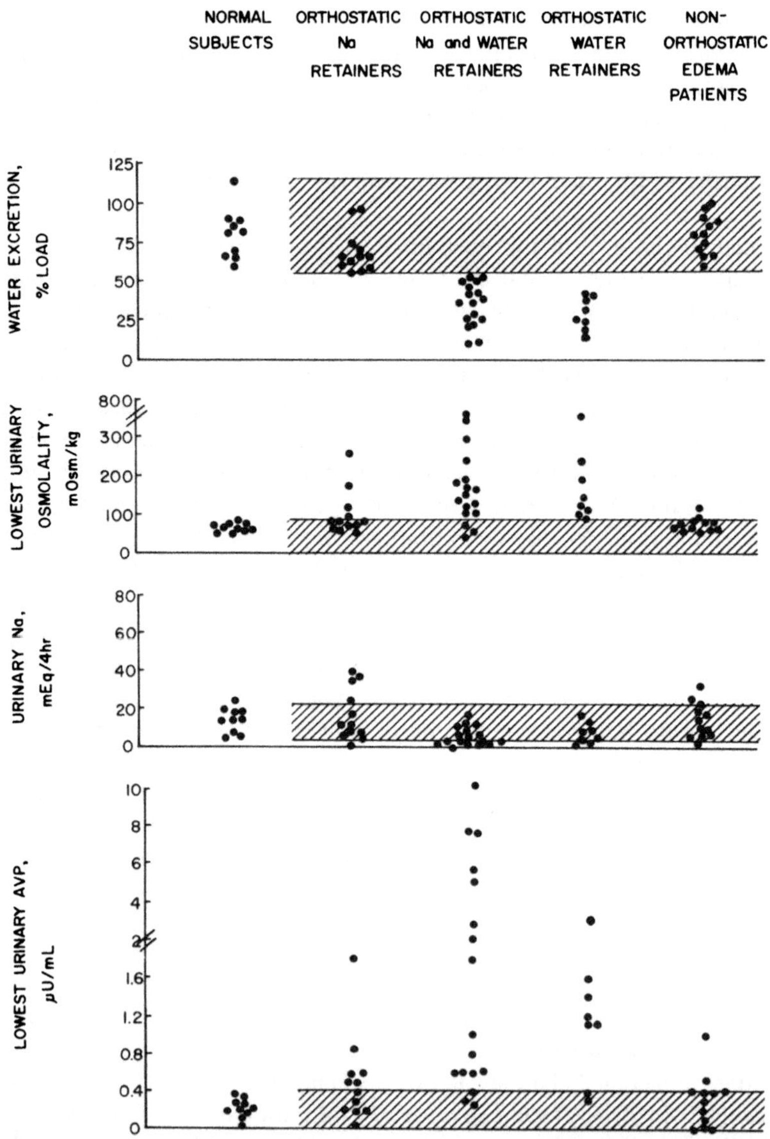

FIGURE 36. Results of water excretion tests in the standing posture in normal subjects and patients with edema. Patients with orthostatic water retention excrete less than 55% of the administered water load in 4 hr and usually fail to dilute any one of the four hourly urines below 100 mOsm/kg, or to decrease urinary vasopressin below 1 μU/ml.

recumbency or the last half-hour in the upright posture, with appropriate arithmetic corrections applied to the results.

Normal Limits. Urinary Na upright/urinary Na recumbent × 100 should fall between 33 and 100% (see Figs. 8 and 37). Urinary creatinine upright/urinary creatinine recumbent × 100 should exceed 80%.

Patients are considered to have edema with orthostatic sodium retention if upright Na excretion is less than 33% of recumbent Na excretion (Fig. 37). An associated excessive orthostatic fall in creatinine excretion strengthens the evidence that orthostatic sodium retention results from an excessive fall in GFR in the upright posture, which is the usual finding in these patients. This test should not be performed in patients who have been on a low-sodium diet or diuretic therapy during the week before the test.

Some patients have excessive retention both of sodium and of water in the upright posture. They appear to have the most severe forms of orthostatic edema, in terms of clinical symptoms. Orthostatic water retainers and patients with nonorthostatic edema excrete sodium normally in the posture test (Fig. 38).

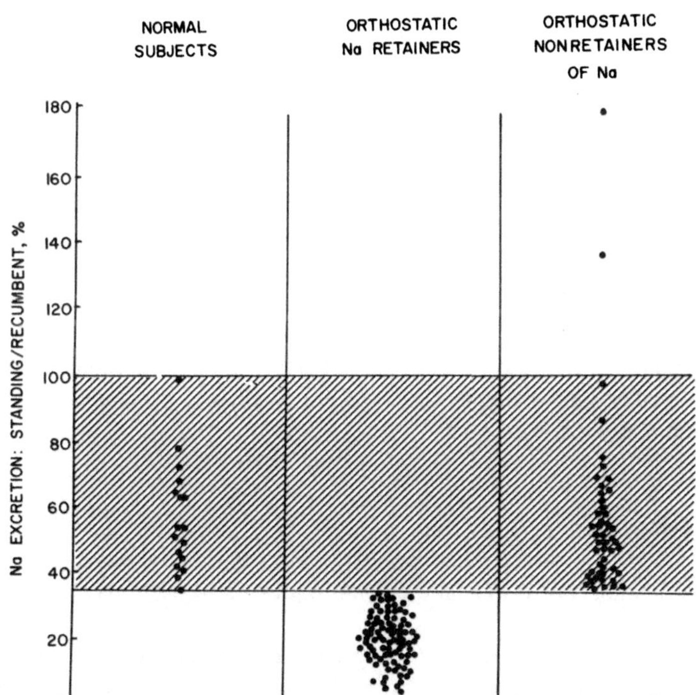

FIGURE 37. Sodium excretion results in the posture test. Upright/recumbent sodium excretion is less than 33% in orthostatic sodium retainers.

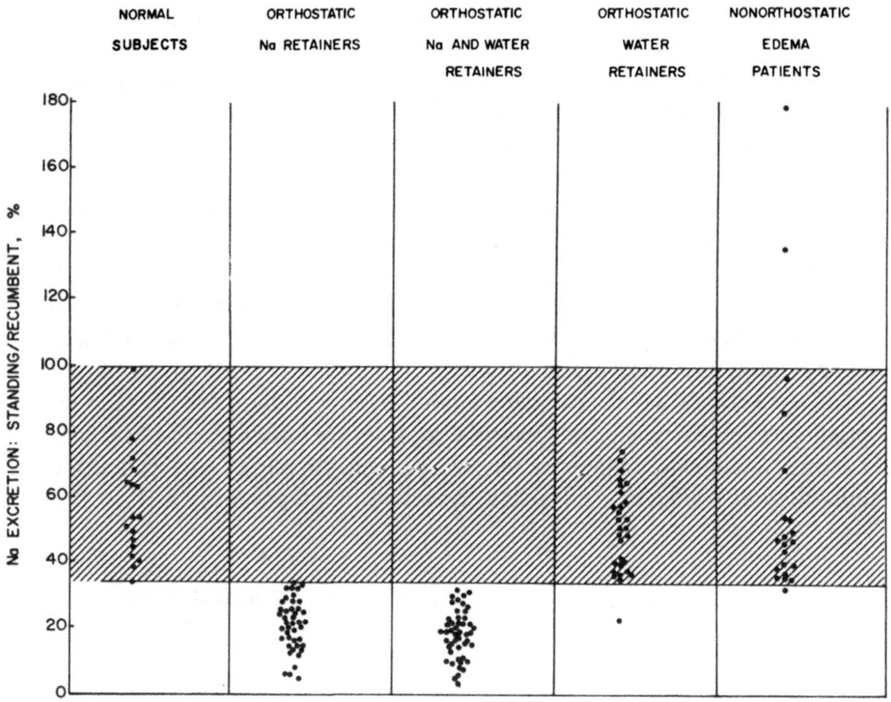

FIGURE 38. Sodium excretion results in the posture test together with water excretion test results in these 158 subjects differentiate normal subjects and patients with nonorthostatic edema from those with orthostatic sodium and/or water retention.

If further confirmation of the role of posture in the fluid retention is desired, and the facilities of a metabolic ward are available, a balance study can be performed (Streeten *et al.*, 1973).

4.3. SUMMARY

The diagnosis of orthostatic edema requires several steps:

1. *Exclusion of known causes of generalized edema*, such as congestive heart failure, renal diseases, cirrhosis and ascites, anemia, hypothyroidism and hyperthyroidism, Cushing's syndrome, thiamine deficiency, kwashiorkor, hypoproteinemia, allergic edema, lymphedema, scleroderma, and edema resulting from the intake of sodium-retaining drugs

2. *Exclusion of known local causes of edema,* including trauma, inflammation, venous obstruction, lymphatic obstruction, and gout
3. *Positive diagnostic measures,* including body weight measurements each morning and evening for 2–4 weeks, water excretion tests (20 ml/kg by mouth) over 4 hr in the upright and recumbent postures, and a posture test comprising measurement of sodium excretion during 4 hr of recumbency followed by 2 hr in the upright posture while imbibing 150 ml 0.14% sodium chloride solution every half-hour

When patients complain of swelling of the legs, which is not apparent at an early afternoon office visit, the diagnosis of orthostatic edema cannot be excluded until the patient has been seen again after having been on her feet for several (preferably 8–12) hr.

5

ORTHOSTATIC EDEMA

Treatment and Prognosis

5.1. GENERAL ASPECTS

It is important, both for the physician and for the patient, to be aware that, although orthostatic edema is an uncomfortable and sometimes distressing disorder, it seldom, if ever, shortens life or incapacitates the patient. Unfortunately, no cure is available, and remissions, both spontaneous and therapeutically induced, are rare. It is therefore obviously essential to prescribe treatment that will reduce discomfort but will not have serious side effects when used daily for several years. Fortunately, there are several ways in which gratifying reduction in discomfort can be accomplished, with negligible long-term hazards to the patient. Many patients are relieved when they are reassured that the disorder seldom worsens with the passage of time and has no grave implications with regard to their longevity.

Several general principles may be of help in guiding the physician in treatment of this condition:

1. Use the mildest therapy and the lowest doses of medications that will produce an acceptable improvement in the patient's comfort.
2. Encourage continuation of a normal life-style, except for need to reduce the daily duration of orthostasis as much as practicable.
3. Be aware of and try to discourage or prevent the tendency of a few patients to escalate their dosages of medications to the point where drug side effects become more serious than the disorder that is being treated.
4. Ask the patient to keep records of body weight twice daily (immediately after rising and before retiring, after emptying the bladder) and of potentially pertinent events such as dates of menstruation, days of unusually prolonged or reduced orthostasis, extreme changes in environmental

temperature, and vacation periods. These records are used to monitor the efficacy of each therapeutic modality used. They may indicate the presence or absence of a downward trend in morning weights, any change in body weight intra diem, and the effects of menstruation, temperature changes, and other factors that might aggravate fluid retention.

5.2. CONTROL OF POSTURE

An understanding of the pivotal role of posture in causing orthostatic edema is helpful to the doctor and should be communicated to the patient. She should be urged to reduce the amount of time spent sitting or standing each day to the maximum extent compatible with maintenance of a reasonable style of living. An afternoon rest on a couch or in a comfortable chair with the feet elevated on a footstool for 1–3 hr should be recommended whenever possible. Avoidance or reduction of social or business requirements for prolonged sitting or standing may be necessary. A conscious effort should be made by the patient to lie down on a couch or to sit with the legs elevated, for as many hours as possible during the afternoon or after the evening meal, before retiring at night. The understanding and cooperation of her family should be enlisted.

5.3. DIETARY AND FLUID RESTRICTIONS

Despite some undoubted exceptions to the general rule, orthostatic edema usually accounts for less than 7 kg (15–16 lb) of excess body weight. Obese women require disciplined caloric restriction and should be encouraged to expect that reduction of adiposity will often decrease fluid retention and usually increase comfort. Moderate reduction of sodium intake, at least to the extent of avoiding obviously salty foods, may be useful in reducing the need for the administration of diuretics and minimizing consequent potassium depletion. When edema is severe, more rigorous adherence to an intake of 10–35 mEq sodium (0.5 or 2 g salt) daily is worthwhile, particularly in patients with pronounced orthostatic sodium retention.

Some patients complain of intense thirst (e.g., patients #117, 127, 138, 143, and 145, all designated by T in Appendix I); they may be conscious of drinking large volumes of fluid during the day. In occasional patients with orthostatic water retention, the concomitant presence of severe polydipsia greatly increases the magnitude of their orthostatic fluid retention. In the three or four patients in whom we have recognized this combination (e.g., patient # 117 in Appendix I; see Fig. 22), voluntary restriction of fluid intake to 1000–1200 ml/day has been more successful than in most patients with psychogenic polydipsia, and appears to have been assisted by the administration of sympathomimetic drugs or small doses of Captopril.

5.4. CONVENTIONAL DIURETICS

Except in the mildest cases, diuretics are usually needed for the treatment of orthostatic edema. Patients often find, however, and their weight records confirm, that thiazides or even loop diuretics such as furosemide, lose their effectiveness when taken each day in the upright posture. This is understandable, as no drugs can be expected to induce diuresis in the presence of profound orthostatic reductions of renal blood flow and GFR. The usual response of patients and of many doctors to such an experience is to look for the most potent diuretic available and to increase the dosage progressively, without benefit in many instances. We have seen some patients who have taken furosemide in doses as high as 560 mg/day without controlling their edema but usually at the cost of hypokalemia. In all these instances, an excellent diuretic response was subsequently demonstrated when administration of 40 mg of the drug was followed by recumbency for 4 hr.

For these reasons, the best diuretic program comprises the administration of the drug concomitantly with the start of a 4-hr period of recumbency, usually after supper, either every evening, or as often as is practicable. We have found the long-acting drug chlorthalidone particularly useful, but there is no objective evidence of its superiority over other diuretics in the treatment of patients with orthostatic edema. Rapidly acting drugs, such as furosemide, may be useful in inducing an acute, profuse diuresis in recumbency, between 7:00 or 8:00 p.m. and bedtime, 3–5 hr later. In this way, nocturia, a frequent complaint in untreated orthostatic edema, is decreased, rather than increased by the diuretic therapy.

5.5. TREATMENT OF POTASSIUM DEPLETION

Since potassium depletion is a frequent, potentially serious complication of diuretic therapy, often causing coupled ventricular ectopic beats (Holland *et al.*, 1981; Nordrehaug *et al.*, 1983; Kaplan, 1984), it should be sought by periodic measurements of serum potassium concentration. When the serum potassium is found to have fallen below 3.5–3.7 mEq/l, it may be treated by administering either (1) a potassium-sparing diuretic, or (2) potassium supplements, but not both together, since hyperkalemia might result.

5.5.1. Potassium-Sparing Diuretics

Since secondary hyperaldosteronism is an important component of the pathogenesis of orthostatic sodium retention in many patients, it is appropriate to administer the aldosterone receptor antagonist, spironolactone (Aldactone R). This drug has been used with good effect ever since it first became available (Streeten, 1960*a*). When given in small doses, spironolactone is a slow-acting diuretic with prolonged activity (Streeten, 1961), which may be given once daily at any time of day. It produces a gradual decline in morning body weight, without reducing the weight gain from morning to evening, as is evident from the

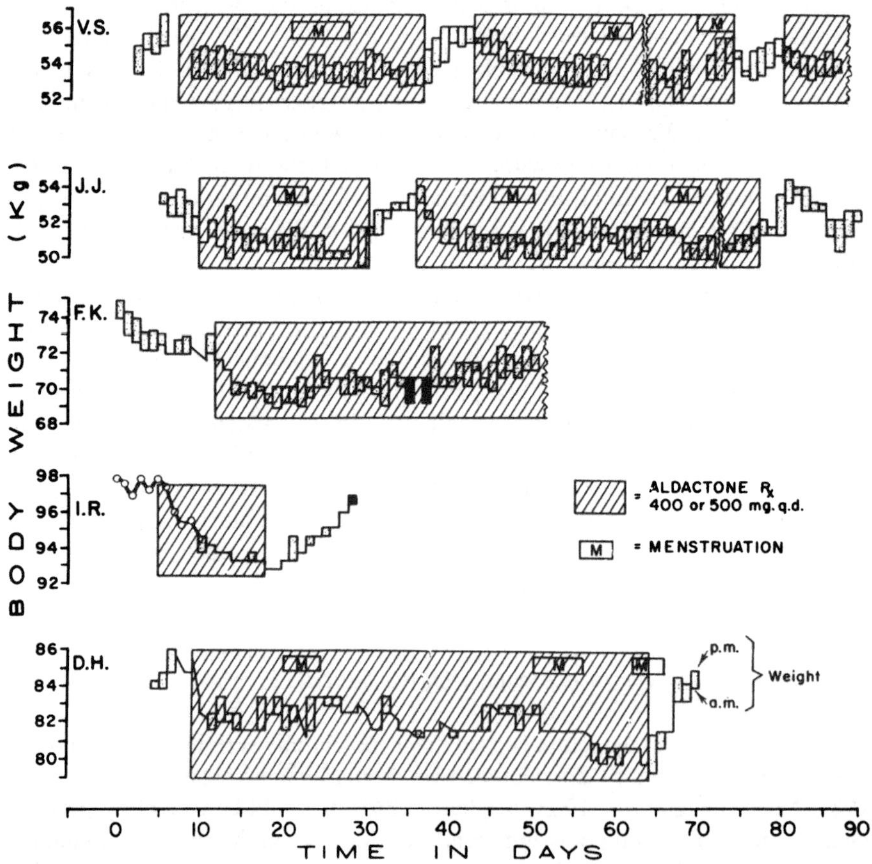

FIGURE 39. Effects of spironolactone therapy on body weight changes from morning to evening in five patients with orthostatic edema. During therapy the morning body weight (lower borders of rectangles) declined, but weight gain from morning to evening (height of the rectangles) was substantially unchanged. (From Streeten *et al.*, 1960*b*.)

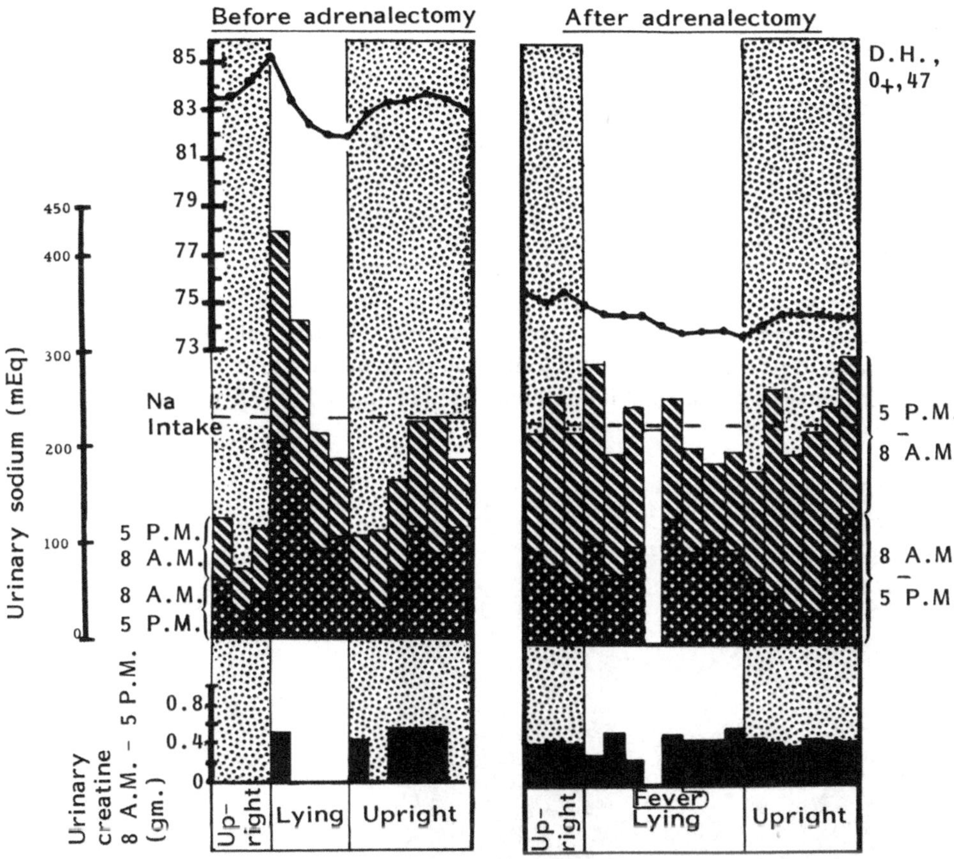

FIGURE 40. Effects of bilateral adrenalectomy in a patient with severe orthostatic edema studied while in balance on a 200-mEq Na intake. During 3-day periods of standing from 8:00 a.m. to 5:00 p.m. before surgery, sodium excretion was less than one-half the sodium intake and body weight rose progressively. After the subtotal adrenalectomy, sodium excretion approximately equaled daily intake, even on the days when the patient stood for 7 hr. This was mainly due to increased Na excretion between 5:00 p.m. and 8:00 a.m. the next morning, while the patient was recumbent.

weight records of patients treated with spironolactone alone, in Figure 39. In these respects, as might be expected, its action is identical with the effects of subtotal adrenalectomy, observed in two patients treated before spironolactone became available (Streeten *et al.*, 1960*b*), as shown for one of these patients in Figure 40. Because of its tendency to cause menstrual irregularity and breast discomfort when used in larger doses, spironolactone should be used, we believe, in doses of 75–150 mg/day. In these doses, it is still a valuable agent for the treatment of orthostatic edema, especially of the orthostatic sodium-retaining type. Triamterene may also be used, and amiloride has been effective in several patients. Combinations of these drugs with hydrochlorothiazide, marketed as Aldactazide, Dyazide, and Moduretic, provide increased diuretic potency but sometimes at the cost of inducing hypokalemia because of the predominance of the potassium-losing effect of the thiazide over the potassium-sparing action of the other drug.

5.5.2. Potassium Supplements

These are available in a large variety of preparations. In general, potassium chloride is preferred, and can be given as a 10% solution or elixir. The unpleasant taste of potassium chloride solution and its frequently irritative effect on the gastric mucosa require that it be administered during or immediately after meals,

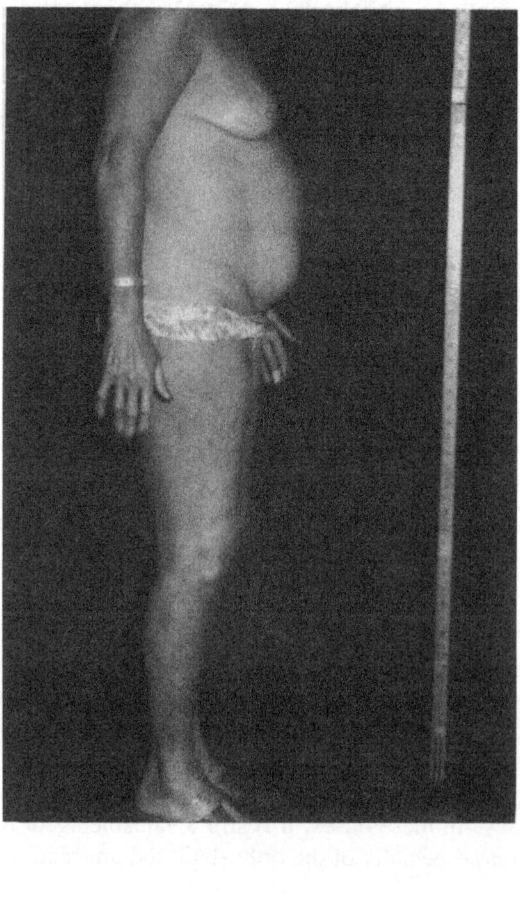

FIGURE 41. Abdominal distension resulting from megacolon due to potassium depletion in a patient with orthostatic sodium retention who greatly exceeded her prescribed dosage of diuretic.

in doses of about 20 ml of the 10% solution (i.e., 2 g or 27 mEq), two or three times per day. Slow-release tablets containing potassium chloride in wax matrix (Slow-K) are a convenient, palatable, and often effective form of potassium supplementation. Unfortunately, gastric and upper intestinal ulceration is not uncommon in patients treated with Slow-K and may lead to hemorrhage, or to abdominal pain and vomiting, sometimes resulting from intestinal obstruction that has had fatal consequences very occasionally. The most recent addition to the forms of potassium supplements available contains small particles of crystalline KCl, microencapsulated in a polymer coating, and all contained within a hard gelatin capsule, marketed as Micro-K Extencaps. Potassium chloride is slowly released from this preparation, which appears to be well tolerated by most patients, with less gastrointestinal side effects than are seen with Slow-K. One of our patients in whom potassium depletion had been a troublesome effect of her diuretic program for many years actually developed such severe obstipation and abdominal distention (Fig. 41) that she was considered at another medical center to have megacolon, for which treatment by colectomy was under consideration. Fortunately, this operation was not performed. The patient experienced dramatic abdominal deflation when given potassium chloride in large amounts. Since then, she has been treated with Micro-K Extencaps, to which she has responded extremely well. Whereas hypokalemia was almost always demonstrable when she was being supplemented with KCl solution, or Slow-K, it has been consistently absent since she has been taking Micro-K.

5.6. ELASTIC GARMENTS AND STOCKINGS

Inflated antigravity suits or elastic bandages wrapped around the legs and thighs greatly reduce the edema formation and weight gain, while increasing the excretion of administered sodium and water in the upright posture, in patients with orthostatic edema. These findings support the other evidence that a microvascular disorder (? inadequate precapillary sphincter constriction) is the primary defect causing excessive transudation of fluid into the limbs of patients with orthostatic edema, while they are in the upright posture. These facts strongly suggested that chronic use of elastic garments or stockings would constitute the most direct and effective therapy of orthostatic edema, obviating the need for drugs. Such customized elastic garments, as manufactured by the Jobst Company and more recently by others, have been used by several of our patients. In cool weather, the results have been generally good. In warm weather, however, when the edema often becomes more severe spontaneously, the garments are uncomfortable and poorly tolerated, perhaps because they tend to increase the temperature of the limbs further.

5.7. DOPAMINE AGONISTS

Kuchel *et al.* (1977) reported that patients with idiopathic edema excreted less dopamine in the urine than did normal subjects, in the reclining but not in the upright posture. Since dopamine is known to have natriuretic properties (Cuche *et al.*, 1972), and since urinary dopamine excretion increases during sodium loading (Alexander *et al.*, 1974; Faucheux *et al.*, 1977), the possibility was suggested that deficient dopamine release might be the cause of idiopathic edema. Although the evidence for this view was never strong, several physicians have used the dopamine D2 agonist, bromocriptine, for the treatment of patients with orthostatic edema. Some researchers have reported that bromocriptine, administered in doses of 5–7.5 mg/day, results in reduction of edema and body weight, and even in a decrease of the weight gain from morning to evening into the normal range (Sowers *et al.*, 1982*a*). Bromocriptine may have some acute natriuretic action that is useful for a short while in the treatment of orthostatic edema. Dent and O. M. Edwards (1979*a*) initially found in seven patients with idiopathic edema that two patients could not tolerate the side effects of bromocriptine (because of nausea and postural hypotension) and that five showed some improvement in sodium and water excretion upright but no improvement in the excessive fall in plasma volume on standing. In a subsequent letter the same year, Dent and Edwards (1979*b*) expressed doubt that bromocriptine would provide major benefit to most patients with idiopathic edema. At about the same time, C. R. W. Edwards *et al.* (1979) reported that continued treatment with bromocriptine had been of little value to 10 of 12 patients but that two had experienced a reduction in weight gain from morning to evening, without reduction in morning body weight. Therapeutic trials of bromocriptine in six of our patients with orthostatic edema have been disappointing. None of the patients has enjoyed continued improvement in morning body weight, weight gain intra diem, or symptoms.

5.8. CONVERTING ENZYME INHIBITORS: CAPTOPRIL

Whether PRA levels are elevated in association with the orthostatic hyperaldosteronism that some patients with orthostatic sodium retention manifest is still unclear, since such an increase has not been found by most investigators. Because of the reasonable possibility that PRA might be too high in the presence of fluid overload in these patients, in spite of being technically within the normal limits, the use of captopril has been investigated in patients with orthostatic edema, in the hope that it might reduce the excessive aldosterone production. Mimran and Targhetta (1979) reported that captopril (50 mg three times daily) reduced the weight gain intra diem from 1.13 and 1.7 kg to 0.5 and 0.4 kg, in a single patient with idiopathic edema. Docci *et al.* (1983) treated four patients with captopril (50 mg bid) and observed a reduction in weight gain from morning to evening, an increase in sodium excretion (although the patients were on a free diet, treated as outpatients) and disappearance of edema in all four individuals. Our own studies have revealed no evidence that captopril significantly reduced orthostatic sodium retention, weight gain, or increased leg volume in the upright posture in 11 patients studied on a constant high-sodium (200 mEq/day) diet in our Clinical Research Center. As anticipated, we found that the drug frequently caused severely symptomatic orthostatic hypotension in spite of our using far smaller doses: 12.5 mg two or three times during the 12-hr period of orthostasis. When used for the treatment of outpatients, the drug has decreased neither weight gain intra diem nor morning body weight. However, three patients have felt clinically improved, less thirsty, and almost euphoric on captopril used in small doses (12.5 mg tid) over a period of several months. We also have some evidence from acute balance studies that captopril may enhance the natriuretic action of D-amphetamine and might constitute a useful adjuvant to therapy, if its potentially serious toxic effects can be avoided. As of this writing, its use in orthostatic edema should be considered experimental.

5.9. VASOCONSTRICTORS

Greenough *et al.* (1962) administered large doses of ephedrine, phenylephrine, and hydroxyamphetamine in an attempt to correct the hypotension in a patient with severe idiopathic edema. Unexpectedly, they found that the drugs induced natriuresis and controlled the edema more effectively than the hypotension. In an attempt to improve the apparently defective orthostatic constriction of the responsible segment of the microvasculature (? the precapillary sphincters), we used a variety of vasoconstricting drugs for the treatment of orthostatic edema. The results have been excellent in many instances.

5.9.1. Ephedrine

This agent is sometimes very effective in reducing the weight gain from morning to evening and lowering morning body weight in patients with orthostatic edema. If it is shown in the individual patient to be effective in these ways and is well tolerated, it can be safely prescribed and will usually retain its efficacy for many years. Unfortunately, the large doses used with great effectiveness by Greenough *et al.* (1962) often cause severe palpitations and are not tolerated by most patients. An exception to this general rule appears to be the patient with edema associated with autonomic insufficiency. Edmonds *et al.* (1983) reported that ephedrine in doses of 60 mg three times daily was well tolerated and brought about a dramatic reduction in edema that had been present in four diabetic patients with autonomic neuropathy. The mean body weight of the patients fell from 85.6 ± 16.1 to 78.1 ± 14.6 kg ($p < 0.05$), with persistent improvement for at least 12–15 months. In one of their patients (#1), weight gain from morning to evening averaged about 1.2 kg during acute retention of

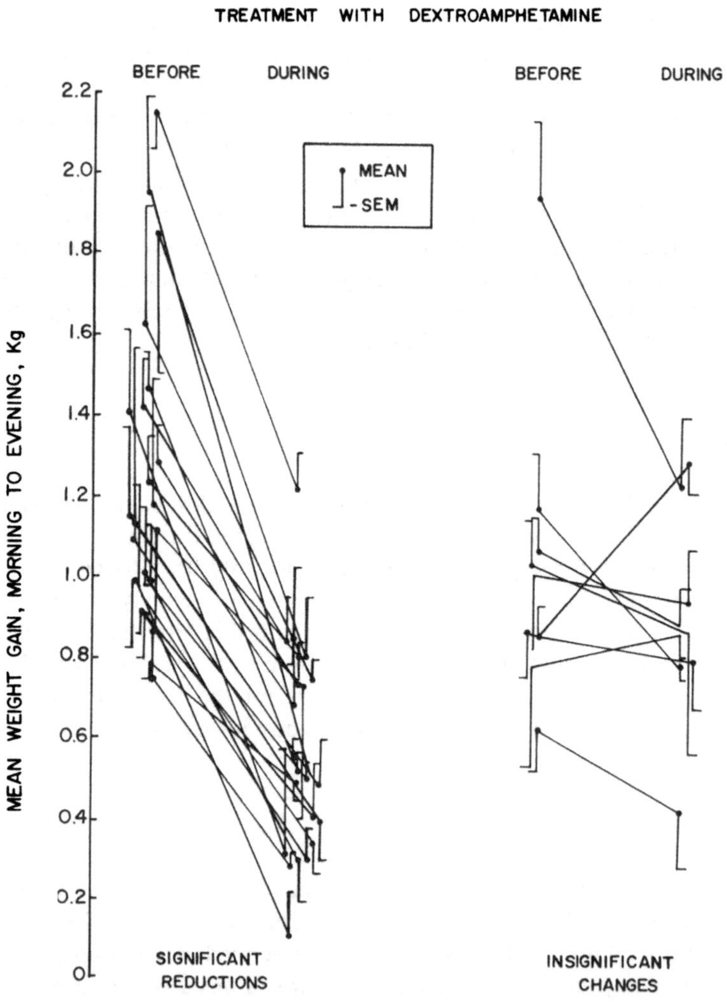

FIGURE 42. Effects of dextroamphetamine on body weight changes from morning to evening in patients with orthostatic edema. Mean ±SEM of body weight changes intra diem over 10–50 days are shown both before and during administration of D-amphetamine (10–25 mg/day) in 21 patients whose weight changes were significantly reduced (p at least <0.05) by D-amphetamine and in nine patients in whom these changes did not reach statistical significance.

fluid for 6 days after ephedrine withdrawal, while an average of about 1.2 kg was lost from morning to evening when ephedrine therapy was resumed for 5 days (see Fig. 1 in their paper). These patients had severe peripheral vasodilatation and arteriovenous (A-V) shunting resulting from their sympathetic denervation. Edmonds *et al.* (1983) point out that such phenomena could lead to excessive venous pooling, a mechanism of edema formation similar to that probably responsible for the development of orthostatic edema. In some of our patients (#76, 77, 91, and 100 in Appendix I) ephedrine, in doses of 25 mg, three times daily, has reduced weight gain intra diem from 1.35 to 0.73 kg (mean) and decreased morning weight by an average of 1.8 kg. Ephedrine has also been a useful adjuvant to other therapeutic agents in several additional patients (see Appendix I).

5.9.2. Amphetamines

In patients who failed to respond to or experienced adverse effects of ephedrine therapy, D-amphetamine frequently, although not invariably, induced gratifying natriuresis. Changes in mean (±SEM) weight gain from morning to evening, in a large number of women treated with D-amphetamine contained in sustained-release capsules (Spansules), in doses of 10–25 mg/day, are shown in Figure 42. In 21 of the 30 patients whose weight changes are depicted, there was a statistically significant reduction in the weight gain from morning to evening (Fig. 42, left). In the remaining nine patients (Fig. 42, right) weight gain either rose (in two) or fell insignificantly. Among the responders, the weight gain intra diem fell into the normal range (<0.6 kg) in 13 patients, or 43% of the entire group treated.

These effects of D-amphetamine have been compared, in a group of 11 patients with orthostatic edema, with the effects of other drugs known to be devoid of vasoconstrictor actions. In Table I, it is evident that 10 of the 11 patients experienced a significant reduction in weight gain from morning to evening when treated with D-amphetamine, whereas none showed a significant response in weight gain to spironolactone, phenergan, propranolol, L-amphetamine, digitoxin, chlorthalidone, or chlorpromazine. Responses to the D-amphetamine and to the other drugs used in the same patients were highly significantly different ($p < 0.001$).

5.9.3. Midodrine

We have compared the acute effects of a new vasoconstrictor, Midodrine, with those of D-amphetamine on changes in body weight, leg volume, and electrolyte balance in groups of patients with orthostatic edema. The studies commenced when the patients had come into sodium balance after 4–8 days on a constant, weighed diet, containing 200 mEq Na, 60–80 mEq K, and 3 liters

TABLE I. Comparison of Weight Changes Intra Diem in 11 Patients Being Treated for Orthostatic Edema[a]

Patient no.	D-Amphetamine[b] Mean ± SEM	p	No drug therapy Mean ± SEM	p	Other agents[c] Mean ± SEM	Drug
162	0.59 ± 0.11	<0.02	1.18 ± 0.22	NS	1.10 ± 0.05	Spironolactone
65	0.73 ± 0.11	<0.001	1.28 ± 0.09	NS	1.23 ± 0.03	Spironolactone
19	0.84 ± 0.11	0.05	1.23 ± 0.12	NS	1.40 ± 0.29	Phenergan
2	0.88 ± 0.10	NS	1.06 ± 0.09	NS	0.98 ± 0.10	Propranolol
61	0.83 ± 0.05	<0.001	1.42 ± 0.12	NS	1.28 ± 0.11	L-Amphetamine
112	0.30 ± 0.07	<0.001	0.91 ± 0.12	NS	0.93 ± 0.17	L-Amphetamine
162	0.59 ± 0.11	<0.02	1.18 ± 0.22	NS	1.32 ± 0.12	Digitoxin
107	0.39 ± 0.09	<0.05	0.85 ± 0.09	NS	0.94 ± 0.13	Phenformin
15	1.22 ± 0.07	<0.001	2.16 ± 0.10	NS	1.90 ± 0.09	Spironolactone
98	0.70 ± 0.08	<0.05	1.01 ± 0.10	NS	1.0 ± 0.11	Chlorthalidone
—	0.85 ± 0.36	<0.01	1.63 ± 0.32	NS	1.59 ± 0.12	Chlorpromazine
Mean	0.72 ± 0.08	<0.001	1.27 ± 0.11	NS	1.24 ± 0.09	

[a]Weight gain from morning to evening during 2–3-week periods of measurements.
[b]10 mg/day.
[c]No vasoconstrictive action.

water, given at consistent times of the day in our Clinical Research Center at the SUNY Health Science Center in Syracuse. On alternate days, the patients were either recumbent in bed for the 24 hr or were on their feet, standing and walking at their leisure, but sitting for three meals, from 8:00 a.m. until 8:00 p.m. In random order, various therapeutic agents, including placebos, were administered on the days spent in the upright posture. Urinary electrolytes and catecholamines, body weights, and leg volumes were measured at 8:00 a.m. and 8:00 p.m. each day.

The results of these studies (Fig. 43) showed that D-amphetamine, in a dose of 10–25 mg/day, significantly reduced the weight gain between 8:00 a.m. and 8:00 p.m. from control values of 1.45 ± 0.11 to 1.18 ± 0.11 kg (mean ±SEM) in the 18 patients studied. The mean change in leg volume during the 12 hr of orthostasis was reduced from 506 ± 44 to 456 ± 75 ml ($p < 0.01$). Urinary excretion of sodium during the period in the upright posture was not significantly increased, changing from 59.9 ± 13.6 to 78.5 ± 17.4 mEq/12 hr. In the same studies performed on eight patients with orthostatic edema (Fig. 43), midodrine (5 mg given at 8:00 a.m., noon, and 4:00 p.m.) reduced the orthostatic increase in leg volume (from 519 ± 67 to 336 ± 77 ml, $p < 0.05$), but its effect on the changes in body weight (from 1.81 ± 0.25 to 1.27 ± 0.45 kg, $p < 0.1$) did not reach statistical significance. Again, the changes in sodium excretion (from 33 to 38 mEq in 12 hr) were not significant.

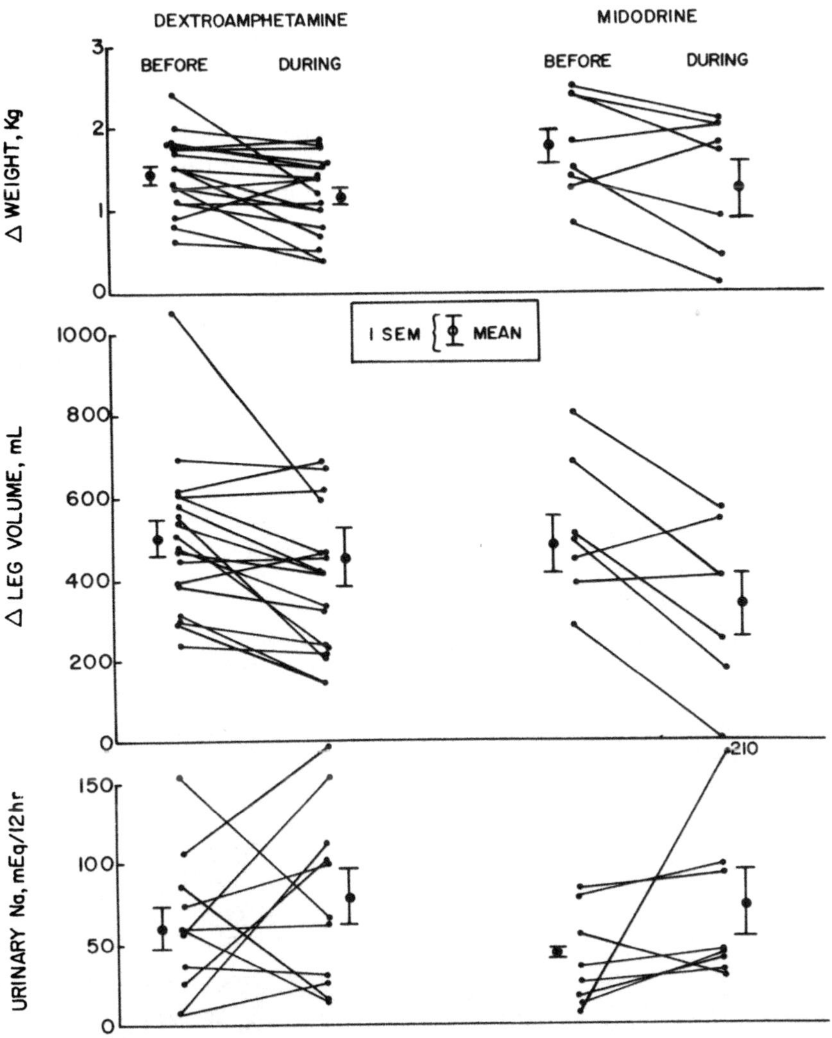

FIGURE 43. Comparison of acute effects of dextroamphetamine and midodrine on weight and leg volume changes and urinary sodium excretion during 12 hr of standing, while in balance on a 200-mEq Na diet. The changes in leg volume induced by both drugs were significant, while the effects of dextroamphetamine on body weight were also significant.

These results indicate that the severity of the swelling measurable in the legs after orthostasis for 12 hr—presumably resulting from excessive transudation into the subcutaneous tissue—was significantly reduced by both D-amphetamine and midodrine, while the excessive orthostatic weight gain was reduced significantly by D-amphetamine but not by midodrine. These effects of the two agents appeared to result from a direct action on the abnormal fluid transudation into the extracellular space and not from a primary action on renal sodium excretion, since this did not increase significantly during the 12-hr period.

In many patients, although certainly not in all, the administration of long-acting D-amphetamine capsules in doses of 10–25 mg/day will result not only in reduction in the weight gain from morning to evening but also in a rapid drop in morning weight (Fig. 44). These amphetamine-induced reductions in body weight sometimes occur more rapidly than can be accomplished by zero caloric intake, clearly indicating that the weight loss results largely from sodium excretion and not from an extreme decrease in food intake.

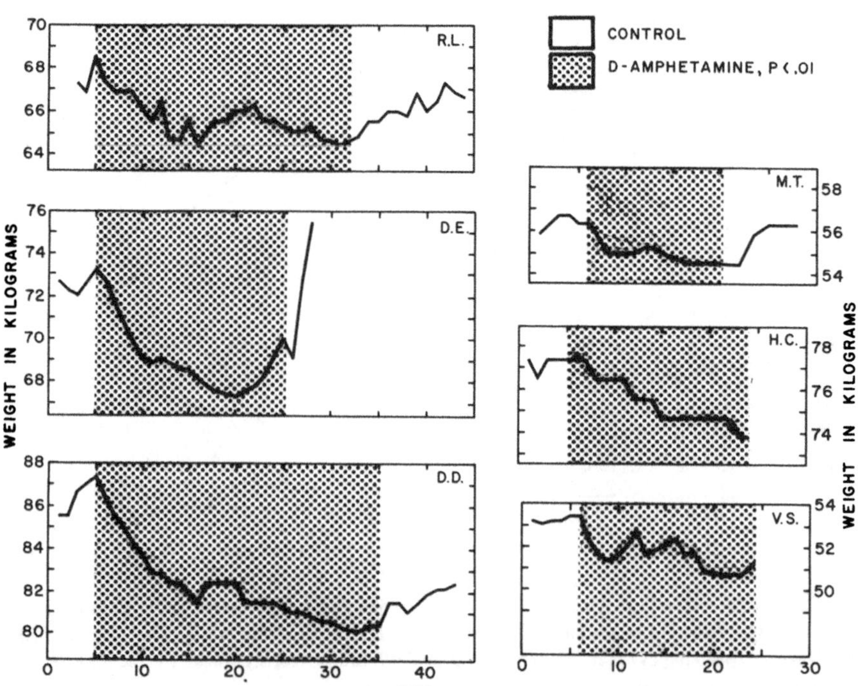

FIGURE 44. Acute effects of D-amphetamine on morning weight in six patients with orthostatic edema. Note the rapidity of weight loss, which in most instances exceeded changes that might have resulted from decreased food intake. (From Speller and Streeten, 1964.)

It is important to appreciate that while D-amphetamine and other drugs that increase dopamine release are often useful in reducing fluid retention, neuroleptic drugs such as phenothiazines, and haloperidol, which block dopamine release, frequently promote the retention of fluid and aggravate orthostatic edema. The use of such neuroleptic agents as tranquilizers is usually counterproductive in patients with orthostatic edema and blocks the beneficial action of sympathomimetic drugs.

5.9.4. Mechanism of Action of Vasoconstrictors in Orthostatic Edema

In a patient with orthostatic hypotension associated with severe edema, Greenough *et al.* (1962) found that the sympathomimetic amines, phenylephrine and ephedrine, had potent natriuretic effects. These effects were not attributable to the improvement in blood pressure that resulted from the use of the two drugs, since natriuresis could not be reproduced by intravenous infusion of norepinephrine at 20 μg/min for about an hour, which raised blood pressure to levels at least as high as those that followed the use of the two oral vasoconstrictors used. Failure of norepinephrine to induce natriuresis was surprising in view of the demonstration by the same group (Laragh *et al.*, 1960) that both norepinephrine and epinephrine infusions often reduce the aldosterone secretion rate profoundly, when it has been raised previously by physiological or pathological stimuli.

Our own observations have shown that L-norepinephrine and L-epinephrine infusions at rates as low as 1 μg/min blunt the increase in aldosterone excretion stimulated by sodium deprivation or by venesection in normal subjects (Streeten, 1966). D-Amphetamine, which acts by releasing catecholamines from sympathetic nerve endings, was also found to reduce aldosterone excretion and to promote natriuresis, with negligible effects on potassium excretion, both in normal subjects and in patients with orthostatic edema (Speller and Streeten, 1964). There was a significant negative correlation between the effects of D-amphetamine on aldosterone and on sodium excretion ($r = -0.66, p < 0.001$). It seemed likely, therefore, that the natriuretic effects of D-amphetamine resulted, at least in part, from the reduction of aldosterone secretion caused by this drug. This conclusion was strongly supported by the later finding (Streeten and Speller, 1966) that D-amphetamine enhanced the excretion of sodium, in the recumbent and in the upright posture, during posture tests, both in normal subjects and in patients with orthostatic edema, but not in adrenalectomized patients treated with hydrocortisone alone.

Since a drop in aldosterone excretion and secretion rates accompanies the natriuresis that results from the administration of norepinephrine and epinephrine (Laragh *et al.*, 1960; Streeten, 1966), ephedrine (Greenough *et al.*, 1962), phenylephrine (Greenough *et al.*, 1962), and D-amphetamine (Speller and

Streeten, 1964), and since the last three drugs are known to release norepinephrine and epinephrine from adrenergic neurons, it is likely that all these compounds have a similar mechanism of action on sodium excretion. The fact that some of them (e.g., norepinephrine and epinephrine) do not pass the blood–brain barrier suggests that the inhibitory action on aldosterone secretion is exerted peripherally and not through the central nervous system (CNS).

Although the effect of D-amphetamine and of other sympathomimetic amines on daily sodium excretion in orthostatic edema is similar to that of the aldosterone antagonist, spironolactone, and resembles the consequences of subtotal adrenalectomy in these patients (Streeten *et al.*, 1960*b*), the effects on weight gain intra diem are quite different. The excessive rise in body weight from morning to evening in patients with orthostatic edema is not affected by spironolactone or by subtotal adrenalectomy (Streeten *et al.*, 1960*b*) (see Figs. 39 and 40) but is significantly reduced, frequently into the normal range, by vasoconstrictors (see Table I). This action of D-amphetamine and other sympathomimetic agents is clearly not mediated through changes in aldosterone secretion and does not result from the administration of other classes of drugs, including conventional diuretics, in patients with orthostatic edema. Since excessive weight gain intra diem is the hallmark of orthostatic edema, it seems likely that the reduction of weight gain intra diem results from correction of the primary defect in orthostatic edema, i.e., from constriction of the segment of the microvasculature that appears to fail to contract normally in the upright posture, in these patients.

5.9.5. Side Effects of Sympathomimetic Amines

Complications associated with sympathomimetic amines have been mild. Nervousness, excitement, and insomnia may require the concomitant administration of a barbiturate, such as amobarbital, or may make it undesirable to persist in the use of these drugs. The generally improved attentional performance, manifested by faster reaction times, superior memory, improved vigilance, both in normal and hyperactive individuals (Rapoport *et al.*, 1978), are side effects that are usually more advantageous than harmful. Palpitations, resulting from tachycardia, are sometimes troublesome, more frequently with ephedrine than with D-amphetamine therapy. Allergic reactions have not been encountered. Since these drugs do not increase potassium excretion, they have never been found to cause potassium depletion, a distinct advantage over the conventional diuretics. Neither D-amphetamine (10–25 mg/day) nor ephedrine (25–50 mg tid) has raised blood pressure noticeably, or into the hypertensive range, but we have avoided the use of these drugs in those very few patients (4 of 135 patients with orthostatic edema in Appendix I) in whom orthostatic edema has been associated with a recumbent diastolic blood pressure of $\geqslant$98 mm Hg. Although I have prescribed the use of D-amphetamine for periods of from several months to 30 years at a time, in well over 200 patients with orthostatic edema, I have encountered no patient who became dependent on the drug or who developed any of the psychiatric complications seen in drug abusers. The only adverse consequences observed when the drug has been withdrawn for a few days or a week have been fluid retention and sleepiness for 1 or 2 days. The complications of thiazide diuretics—dysrhythmias, weakness, orthostatic syncope, and paralytic ileus—have been more frequent and more serious than the complications of sympathomimetic drugs in the doses we have used. It is important to know that amphetamine dependency, psychoses, and depression upon withdrawal of the drug are common among those who abuse amphetamines for their euphoric or other effects on the brain. Since such central effects, like the anorectic action, decline after 3 or 4 weeks, individuals who abuse amphetamines almost invariably escalate the dosage of the drugs to levels at which the well-known psychiatric complications are likely to occur. These complications are never seen, as far as we know, in patients who continue to take D-amphetamine in doses of 10–25 mg/day for orthostatic edema, narcolepsy, or pediatric hyperkinesis (Cantwell, 1975), even after 20–30 years of continued use for these disorders (Food and Drug Administration, 1979). Moreover, unlike the central and the anorexigenic actions of amphetamines, the effects on orthostatic edema, narcolepsy, and hyperkinesis do not diminish even after many years (see Fig. 45) and therefore

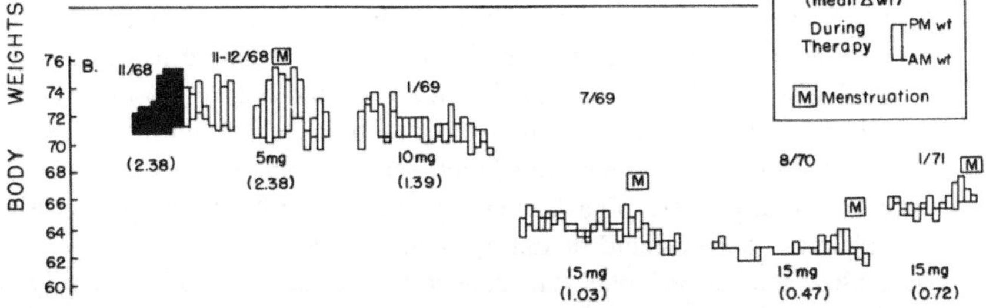

FIGURE 45. Chronic effects of D-amphetamine on morning and evening body weights (bottoms and tops of each rectangle) in two patients with orthostatic edema. The drug consistently and persistently reduced the mean weight changes intra diem (shown in parentheses) for several years in both patients. M, menstruation. (From Streeten, 1978.)

should not lead to dangerous progressive increases in dosage. It is most unfortunate that the abusers of these drugs are making it increasingly difficult for physicians to prescribe these valuable therapeutic agents for the many patients with orthostatic edema in whom they still constitute the most effective and safest form of treatment.

5.9.6. Long-Term Administration of Sympathomimetic Agents

D-Amphetamine has been effective in maintaining reduced or even normal morning-to-evening body weight changes in patients with orthostatic edema for many years. Unlike the effects of conventional diuretics given during the daytime, the beneficial action of D-amphetamine on weight gain intra diem has been sustained for 20 years or more in at least five or six patients we have treated. Changes in morning and evening body weights in two of these patients are shown in Figure 45.

5.10. SUMMARY OF THERAPEUTIC PROGRAM

1. If the orthostatic origins of the edema have been documented by history, twice-daily weight measurements, or posture tests, explain to the patient the need to reduce the amount of time spent sitting and standing each day.
2. Have the patient keep daily written records of body weights on arising and at bedtime, after voiding.
3. Institute moderate sodium restriction, with avoidance of foods with extremely high salt content. If the patient is a water retainer, inquire about daily fluid intake; if excessive, recommend reduction.
4. If the degree of edema and symptoms is mild, the patient might try wearing elastic stockings, such as the Jobst waist-high garment.
5. If complaints and excessive diurnal weight gain persist, add a diuretic, such as chlorthalidone, 50 mg. If the diuretic response to this agent is inadequate, insist that the medication be taken before a 4-hr period of recumbency on a bed, a couch, or a reclining chair, with the feet elevated. This can be done after lunch each afternoon or after supper and before going to sleep each evening. Recommend that the patient elicit help from her husband or family with the evening chores.
6. Follow the serum potassium concentration approximately monthly for the first few months. If it falls below 3.5 mEq/liter and diuresis is adequate, prescribe potassium supplements (see pages 96–97). If edema is still poorly controlled, add a potassium-sparing diuretic, preferably spironolactone (50–100 mg/day).

7. If edema persists and morning-to-evening weight gain continues to be excessive, add ephedrine, 25 mg tid. If this is poorly tolerated or fails to lower morning weights and weight gains from morning to evening, change from ephedrine to D-amphetamine sustained-release capsules, increasing from 10 to 25 mg each morning, if necessary, until weight gain intra diem falls towards 0.5 kg and morning weight is adequately reduced.
8. If all these measures prove ineffective, the following oral vasoconstrictors may be tried: phenylephrine (Neosynephrine), midodrine (Gutron), methamphetamine (Desoxyn), or diethylpropion (Tenuate). Alternatively, a trial of bromocriptine may be instituted, starting with 2.5 mg at bedtime and increasing, as required, to tolerance.
9. Recommend an exercise program, preferably including swimming as often as possible each week.

5.11. SUMMARY

The treatment of orthostatic edema should include use of the lowest doses of drugs that will produce acceptable improvement, as reflected in the patient's complaints and in the continuing record of twice-daily weight measurements. Prolonged orthostasis should be avoided as far as possible. Mild to moderate sodium restriction is helpful. Thiazides, chlorthalidone, or other "conventional" diuretics often lose effectiveness if taken during orthostasis but almost invariably retain potency if taken before a 2–6-hr period of recumbency during the day or before bedtime in the evening. Potassium-sparing diuretics or potassium supplements are often needed. Elastic stockings or garments (e.g., Jobst waist-high garments) may be used but often prove uncomfortable, especially in hot weather. Bromocriptine may be helpful initially but seldom for more than a few weeks. Vasoconstrictors are the most effective agents in reducing weight gain from morning to evening. Ephedrine (25 mg tid) is sometimes useful and should be tried first. Midodrine (5 mg tid) may be helpful but has not yet been approved for this indication by the FDA. D-Amphetamine is still generally the most effective and best tolerated drug.

These vasoconstrictors have few side effects, do not deplete potassium reserves, and retain their efficacy for many years, because they come closest to correcting the probable underlying pathogenetic disorder: excessive dilatation of the precapillary sphincter, causing overdistention of the capillary bed in the dependent limbs.

6

ORTHOSTATIC DISORDERS OF BLOOD PRESSURE CONTROL

Definitions and Classification

The detection and investigation of orthostatic blood pressure disorders are completely dependent on accurate and reliable blood pressure measurements in the upright posture. This chapter discusses technical details of these simple measurements, the range of changes in healthy subjects, and definable orthostatic disorders of blood pressure control.

6.1. TECHNIQUE OF BLOOD PRESSURE MEASUREMENT IN THE UPRIGHT POSTURE

To ensure uniformity in the technique of measuring blood pressure, it is important to adhere to standard recommendations, such as those of the American Heart Association (Kirkendall *et al.*, 1980). These recommendations include (1) use of a narrow cuff for children and a wide cuff (20 cm) for persons with exceptionally large (obese or muscular) upper arms, (2) a periodic check for the accuracy of aneroid gauges against a mercury manometer, and (3) use of the fifth phase of the Korotkoff sounds (disappearance of the sounds) to indicate the diastolic blood pressure. In addition, the patient's elbow should be slightly flexed (at least to about 175°) while auscultating over the antecubital fossa; this technique avoids spuriously low diastolic pressures that can result from compression of the brachial artery if the elbow is hyperextended (especially in women). The subject's antecubital fossa should be as close as possible to the horizontal level of the sternal angle (angle of Louis), both in the reclining and in the upright postures (Grill, 1937; Berry, 1941; Currens, 1948; Green *et al.*, 1948), in order to minimize the slight error that can result from the difference in hydrostatic pressure when the site of the cuff is a considerable distance below the heart. This

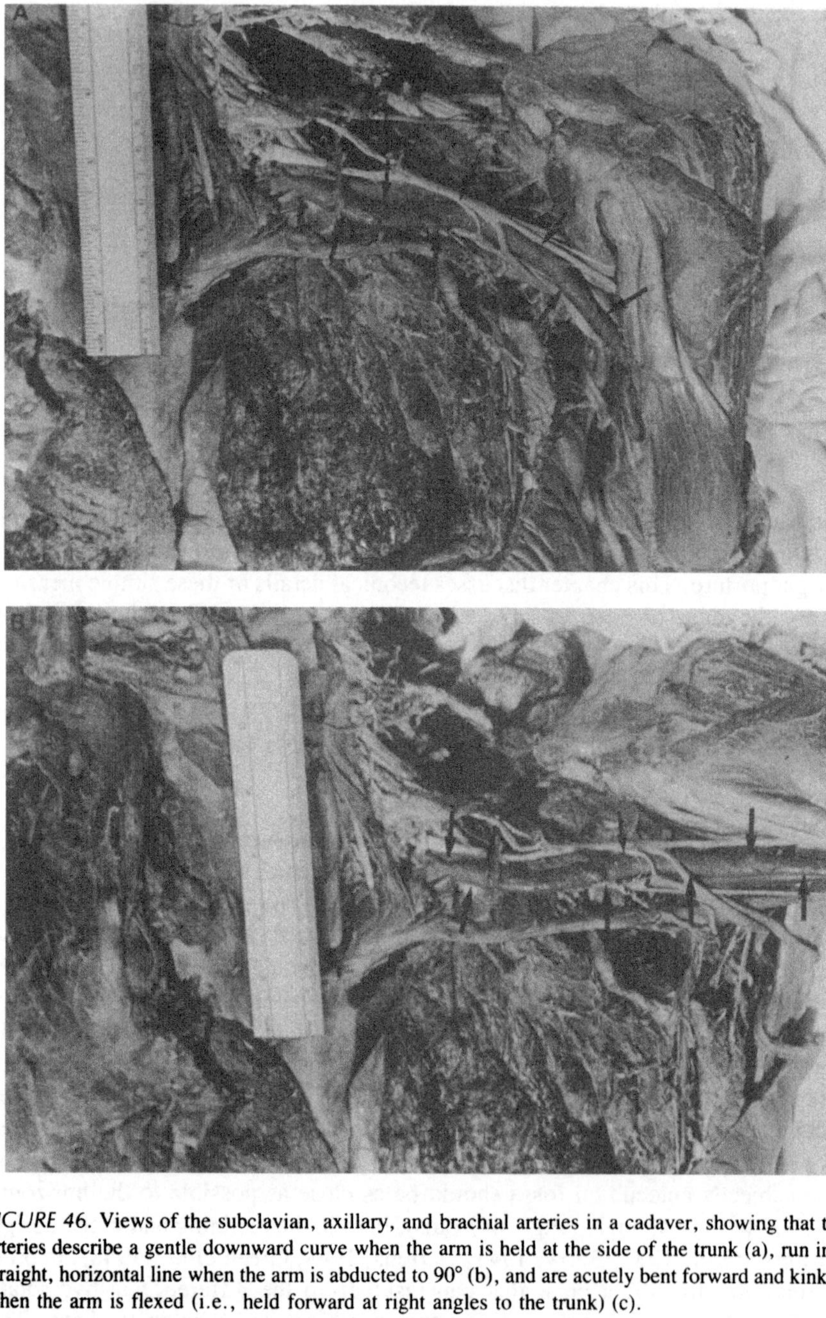

FIGURE 46. Views of the subclavian, axillary, and brachial arteries in a cadaver, showing that the arteries describe a gentle downward curve when the arm is held at the side of the trunk (a), run in a straight, horizontal line when the arm is abducted to 90° (b), and are acutely bent forward and kinked when the arm is flexed (i.e., held forward at right angles to the trunk) (c).

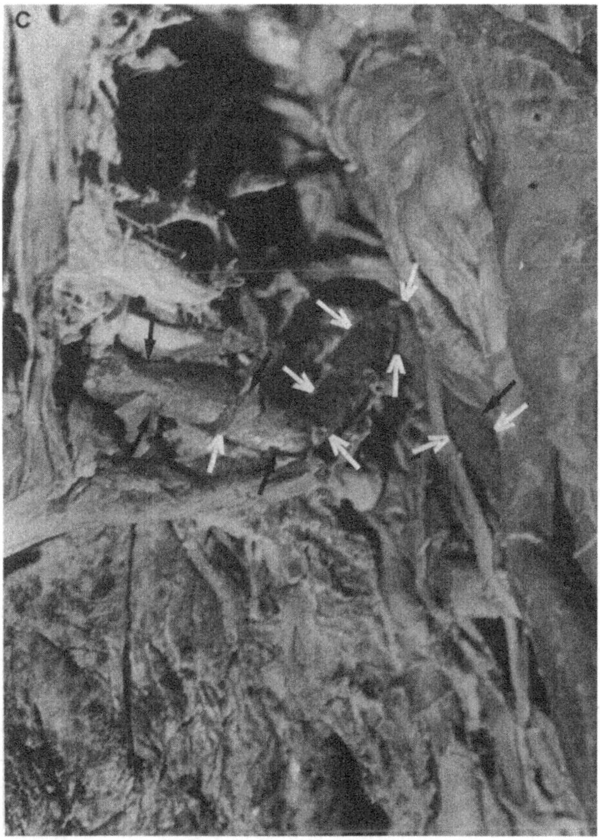

FIGURE 46. (Continued)

potential error may amount to 10–20 cm H_2O or 7–15 mg Hg, the larger errors occurring in persons with unusually long arms. If this precaution is not observed, orthostatic hypotension may be minimized or overlooked and the frequency of orthostatic hypertension greatly exaggerated.

We investigated possible errors that might result from kinking of the subclavian artery when the arm is held forward (i.e., flexed at the shoulder) or laterally (i.e., abducted at the shoulder) in a cadaver. When the arm is held at the side, the course of the subclavian and brachial arteries describes a gentle curve as the vessel passes from the chest to the arm (Fig. 46a). When the arm is abducted to 90 degrees (Fig. 46b), the subclavian and brachial arteries run almost exactly horizontally, just above the level of the atria. However, when the arm of the cadaver is flexed to 90° degrees at the shoulder (i.e., pointing forward) (Fig.

46c), the artery shows an obvious kinking at the lateral border of the chest, before the artery enters the arm.

There is no reason to believe that these appearances are artifactual and that a similar condition would not be found in living patients. We have not yet encountered a patient in whom the standing blood pressure was spuriously low because of kinking of an atherosclerotic subclavian artery when the blood pressure was measured with the arm flexed at the shoulder (i.e., pointing forward, parallel to the floor). However, one would not recognize such an error unless one were to measure the blood pressure routinely both with the arm flexed at the shoulder and with the arm abducted at the shoulder, in a large group of patients—which we have not done. In view of this theoretical possibility, however, we have routinely measured the standing blood pressure with the patient's arm abducted at the shoulder, supported on furniture or on the examiner's shoulder or tucked under the examiner's arm (for short patients and tall examiners), and flexed at the elbow so that the cuff was approximately at the level of the patient's sternal angle, as shown in Figure 47.

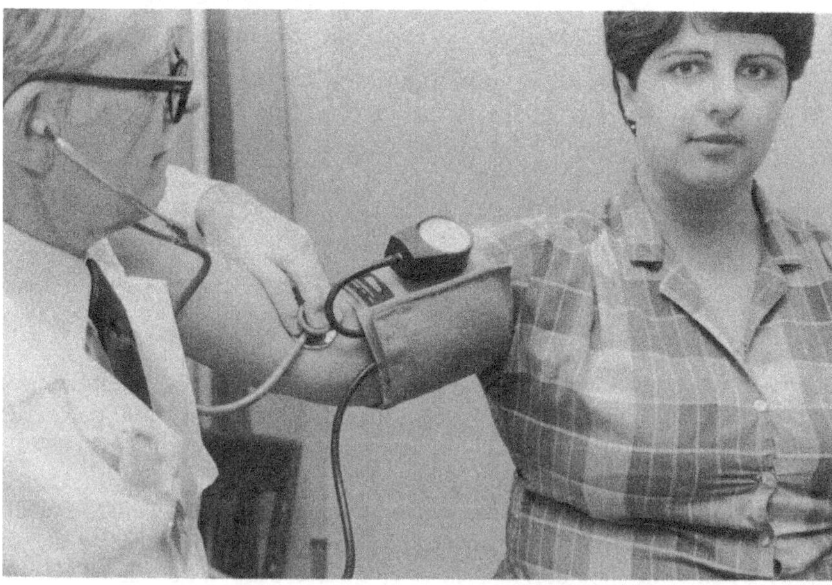

FIGURE 47. Blood pressure measurement in the standing subject, showing one appropriate technique, with the arm abducted approximately at right angles, resting on the shoulder of the examiner and slightly flexed at the elbow. The antecubital fossa is close to the horizontal level (estimated) of the right atrium.

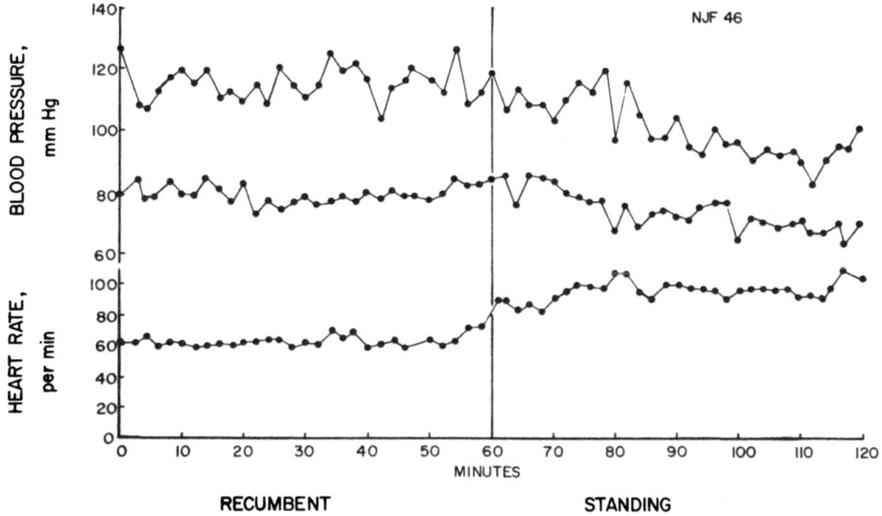

FIGURE 48. Record showing an unusual, delayed, and gradual fall of systolic and diastolic blood pressure (measured automatically by Dinamap every minute), starting 20 min after the change from recumbency to standing. In recumbency mean BP was 115/81 and heart rate was 64 beats/min. During the first 20 min of standing, mean BP was 109/84, and heart rate was 87 beats/min, but in the last 20 min of standing mean BP fell to 93/69; while heart rate rose to 96 beats/min. Prior to these measurements, this patient's (patient #157, Appendix II) complaints of profound fatigue, sleepiness, irritability and impaired cerebration while working as a charge nurse in a busy hospital had been labeled neurotic or "unexplained." Improvement resulted from the use of a Jobst Leotard.

Most orthostatic disorders of blood pressure and heart rate persist or increase in severity as long as the upright posture is maintained. For this reason, documentation of the presence of these orthostatic derangements requires the following steps:

1. Measurement of blood pressure and heart rate in recumbency two or three times or until it is clear that recumbent levels are stable.
2. Measurement of blood pressure and heart rate repeatedly for at least 3 min or for longer periods of time if the levels appear to fluctuate or to drift upward or downward, in the standing posture. [In occasional instances, blood pressure may be normally maintained after 1–3 min of standing but will gradually drift downward to levels that produce orthostatic symptoms, e.g., lightheadedness, blurred vision, fatigue, after 10–30 min or more (see Fig. 48).]

6.2. ORTHOSTATIC BLOOD PRESSURE AND HEART RATE CHANGES: NORMAL LIMITS

An orthostatic acceleration of the heart rate in normal persons was known to such early workers as Knox (1815, 1837) and Guy (1838). Dietlen (1909) recognized that the erect posture was associated with a fall in systolic blood pressure and a rise in diastolic pressure.

Modern studies have shown that, during the first 0.5–3 sec after a change from the reclining to the upright posture, the contraction of postural muscles compresses the arteries and veins in the abdomen and legs, causing a rise in systolic pressure (+29 ± 26 mm Hg) (Borst *et al.*, 1984). These changes are followed, at 6–7 sec after standing, by a transient fall in systolic and diastolic blood pressures to the extent of about 28/15 mm Hg, after which there is a rise to or toward the control levels within 30 sec. Many of these transient orthostatic changes were first described by Wald *et al.* (1937) and have been precisely defined with direct, intra-arterial measurements by others (Green *et al.*, 1948; Borst *et al.*, 1982, 1984). After the immediate transient fall in blood pressure in

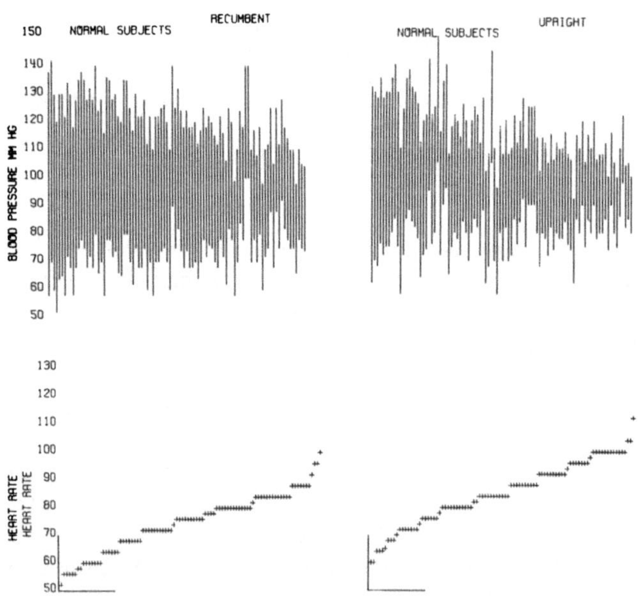

FIGURE 49. Blood pressure and heart rate measurements in 92 normal subjects in the recumbent and standing postures. Results are arranged in descending order of magnitude of the pulse pressure and ascending order of heart rate.

TABLE II. Orthostatic Changes in Blood Pressure and Heart Rate in 92 Normal Subjects (Mean ± SEM)[a]

	Systolic bp (mm Hg)	Diastolic bp (mm Hg)	Heart rate (beats/min)	Pulse pressure (mm Hg)	Mean bp (mm Hg)
Recumbent	129.7 ± 1.0	78.6 ± 0.5	80.2 ± 0.6	51.0 ± 0.7	95.7 ± 0.6
Standing	123.2 ± 0.9	84.2 ± 0.5	92.5 ± 0.7	39.0 ± 0.7	97.2 ± 0.6
Change	−6.5 ± 0.5	+5.6 ± 0.4	+12.3 ± 0.5	−12.0 ± 0.5	+1.5 ± 0.4
P	<0.001	<0.001	<0.001	<0.001	NS
Recumbent range	90–142	52–100	56–100	20–80	
95% limits	100–142	55–90	54–96	25–72	
Standing range	92–150	58–106	60–112	18–70	
95% limits	94–141	61–97	62–108	19–59	

[a]bp, blood pressure; NS, not significant.

the standing position, both the blood pressure and the heart rate stabilize, in healthy subjects, remaining substantially unchanged for several hours.

In 92 healthy male and female subjects, mainly physicians, nurses, secretaries, and laboratory technicians, aged 17–61 years, we have measured blood pressure and heart rate, both after recumbency for 3–4 min and after standing for 3 min. The results are shown in Figure 49, blood pressures being arranged in descending order of magnitude of the pulse pressures and heart rates in ascending order. Table II shows that there was a slight but significant fall in systolic blood pressure, a rise in diastolic blood pressure (by 5.6 ± 0.4 mm Hg), a fall in pulse pressure, and a rise in heart rate in the upright posture; in addition, the change in mean arterial blood pressure was not significant.

The mean orthostatic changes in systolic and diastolic blood pressure and in heart rate, shown in Table II, are very similar to the results reported in healthy subjects by Erlanger and Hooker (1905), Åkesson (1936, 1946), Nordenfelt (1941), Hammerström (1947), Sundin (1956), and Frohlich *et al.*, (1967). Our results confirm the conclusions of Erlanger and Hooker (1905) (and most of the other investigators) that the change from the recumbent to the standing posture is associated with "(1) a rise of the minimum (i.e., diastolic) pressure as a rule; (2) no change of the maximum (i.e., systolic) pressure as a rule; (3) an invariable diminution of the pulse pressure; and (4) an invariable increase of the pulse rate."

Although there is considerable variation between individual responses, it is evident from Table II that the range of blood pressure in 95% of normal subjects studied was 100–142/55–90, in recumbency, and 94–141/61–97 in the upright posture. Although the 95% confidence limits for pulse pressures were as shown in Table II, pulse pressure fell below 20 (to 18) mm Hg in the erect posture, in

TABLE III. Orthostatic Parameters in Normal Subjects

Standing systolic blood pressure	94 to 141 mm Hg
Standing diastolic blood pressure	61 to 97 mm Hg
Standing pulse pressure	19 to 59 mm Hg
Standing heart rate	62 to 108 beats/min
Orthostatic changes:	
Systolic BP	−19 to +11 mm Hg
Diastolic BP	−9 to +22 mm Hg
Pulse pressure	−27 to +6 mm Hg
Heart rate	−6 to +27 beats/min

only one of the 92 normal subjects. In eight subjects the diastolic pressure fell in the upright posture; this drop was more than 8 mm Hg in only two cases. Heart rate showed an orthostatic rise in 86 of the 92 subjects; this rise exceeded 20 beats/min in eight patients and exceeded 24 beats/min in only two patients. We have used these results to define the 95% confidence limits of the ranges of the orthostatic parameters in normal subjects shown in Table III.

6.3. DEFINABLE DISORDERS OF BLOOD PRESSURE AND HEART RATE CONTROL

Using the normal ranges shown in Table III and recognizing that there are wide fluctuations in blood pressure and heart rate measurements made at different times in the same normal subject, five types of orthostatic disorders of blood pressure control can be recognized. These are based on finding the following abnormalities on at least three separate determinations, preferably on different days:

Orthostatic diastolic hypotension: orthostatic fall in diastolic blood pressure of ≥10 mm Hg, with or without an excessive fall in systolic pressure

Orthostatic systolic hypotension: excessive orthostatic fall in systolic pressure only, by ≥20 mm Hg, or to <94 mm Hg

Orthostatic hypertension (diastolic): diastolic BP of ≤90 mm Hg in recumbency and ≥98 mm Hg in the standing position

Orthostatic narrowing of pulse pressure: pulse pressure of ≤18 mm Hg in the standing position

Orthostatic tachycardia: heart rate increased by ≥28 beats/min, or to ≥110 beats/min, after standing for 3 min

These definitions are based directly on the observed orthostatic variations in blood pressure and heart rate in the 92 normal subjects. They differ from the more variable, and sometimes admittedly arbitrary, definitions of orthostatic hypotension, previously proposed by various investigators, without documentation of the normal ranges on which they were presumably based. Various workers have used (1) a fall in systolic pressure alone of 30 mm Hg (Campbell *et al.*, 1976; Ewing *et al.*, 1980) or 20 mm Hg (Overstall *et al.*, 1977); or (2) a fall in systolic and diastolic pressures of at least 30 and 20 mm Hg (Schatz *et al.*, 1963) or 25 and 10 mm Hg (Schatz, 1984) or 30 and 10 mm Hg (Thomas *et al.*, 1981), respectively; or (3) a fall in mean blood pressure of ≥20 mm Hg (Cryer, 1979).

6.3.1. Orthostatic Arterial Anemia

The phenomenon of an abnormally reduced pulse pressure associated with severe tachycardia in the upright posture was first described by Sewall (1919). This phenomenon appears to have received scant subsequent attention in the American and British literature, having been reported only in papers by Meyer *et al.* (1956) and Hickler *et al.* (1959*b*, 1960). Figure 50 shows the dramatic fall in systolic and rise in diastolic blood pressure that resulted in progressive shrinkage

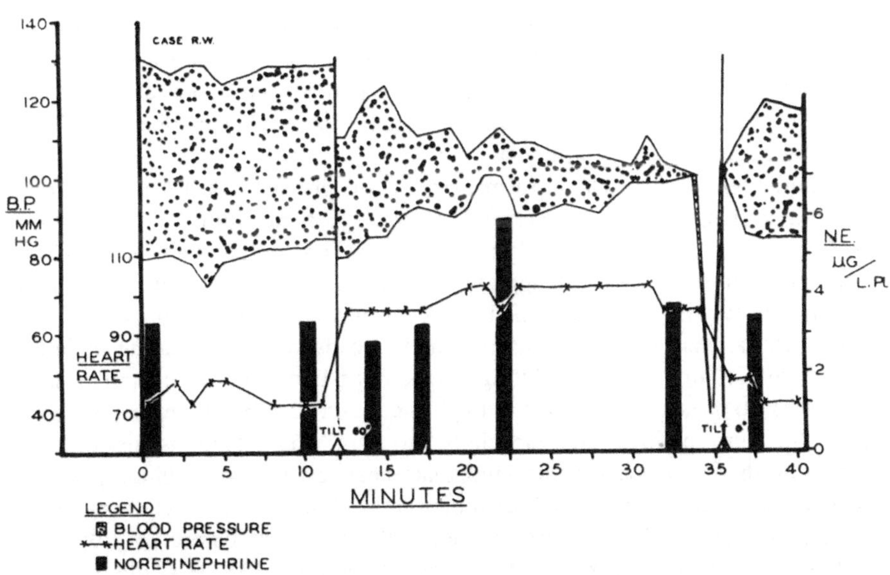

FIGURE 50. Orthostatic shrinkage of pulse pressure of the type described as orthostatic arterial anemia, in one of Hickler's subjects during 60° head-up tilt. Syncope occurred when the pulse pressure was almost immeasurable. (From Hickler *et al.*, 1959*b*.)

of the pulse pressure to the vanishing point—when the individual fainted—during a 60° head-up tilt in one of Hickler's subjects with blood pressure changes typical of orthostatic arterial anemia. Scandinavian and German investigators have long recognized this as a manifestation of a clinical abnormality, described as orthostatic arterial anemia by Bjure and Laurell (1927) and others (Laurell, 1936; Hammerström, 1947; Sundin, 1956). Unfortunately, this disorder has been ignored in our best modern textbooks of medicine and cardiology, and its description in the older literature is not accessible to most computer printouts. Similarly, although orthostatic hypertension was observed in 4.2% of 2000 healthy young American airmen, shortly after World War I (Schneider and Truesdell, 1922), we still know virtually nothing about its significance, whether it has any adverse effects, and whether we should be treating it. This has not deterred physicians from treating such patients in large numbers, relying on authoritative advice to measure the blood pressure in the sitting position (Kirkendall *et al.*, 1980) but forgetting that the pressure must be measured in the reclining position as well.

6.3.2. Neurocirculatory Asthenia

In the disorder variously designated as da Costa's irritable heart syndrome (1871), effort syndrome, or soldier's heart (Lewis, 1918, 1919), and neurocirculatory asthenia (Oppenheimer *et al.*, 1981*a,b*), it seems possible that the symptoms in many of these patients might have resulted from the orthostatic disorders of blood pressure mentioned earlier. However, the roles of posture and of orthostatic changes in blood pressure were never clearly described in publications on neurocirculatory asthenia.

Although he was unable to measure blood pressure, da Costa (1871) did observe striking orthostatic tachycardia in his patients (most of whom were soldiers) who complained of lightheadedness, precordial pain, palpitations, headache, and indigestion, all aggravated by physical effort and fatigue. Similarly, Thomas Lewis (1919) described the occurrence of dyspnea and fatigue, chest pain, palpitations, giddiness, fainting spells, headache, and sweating in British troops with effort syndrome during World War I, but he did not relate these symptoms to orthostasis as much as to physical exertion. He did report, however, that "in some patients and especially those in whom there is giddiness on assuming the erect posture, the immediate change (in systolic blood pressure) may be much more pronounced (than in normal subjects), in one case amounting to 30 or 40 mm Hg." Lewis also reported that in the effort syndrome, "the pulse shows an exaggerated response to posture." In spite of these findings, Lewis appears to have made no attempt to determine the magnitude or the prevalence of the orthostatic changes in blood pressure and heart rate in the large numbers of patients with this syndrome whom he studied during World War I. His findings emphasized the exaggerated cardiovascular responses to exertion in these individuals and their freedom from intrinsic heart disease—more pressing considerations, perhaps, at that time.

6.4. CLASSIFICATION OF ORTHOSTATIC DISORDERS OF BLOOD PRESSURE CONTROL

6.4.1. Role of the Autonomic Nervous System

There are sound reasons to believe that a functionally intact baroreceptor reflex and sympathetic nervous system are essential for maintenance of the diastolic blood pressure in the upright posture:

1. The almost instantaneous rise in heart rate and the extremely rapid appearance of norepinephrine in the circulating blood result from rapid loss of vagal tone (Ewing *et al.*, 1980) and immediate stimulation of a sympathetic nervous discharge.
2. The diastolic blood pressure falls within a few seconds of assumption of the upright posture; it virtually always remains below reclining levels in patients (a) who show other evidence of severely impaired sympathetic nervous system function in the Shy–Drager syndrome (multiple system atrophy), (b) with peripheral autonomic insufficiency, (c) who have had lumbodorsal sympathectomy (Hammerström, 1947), and (d) receiving large doses of ganglion-blocking, catecholamine-depleting, or α_1-adrenergic-blocking drugs.

Repeated measurements of the blood pressure in both the recumbent and the upright posture have always, literally without exception, shown an orthostatic fall in diastolic blood pressure, in every one of our patients with severe central or peripheral autonomic insufficiency, as shown for eight patients in Figure 51. In contrast, patients with several other types of orthostatic hypotension have been found on different occasions to have an orthostatic fall or an orthostatic rise in diastolic blood pressure, associated with consistent or variable orthostatic falls in systolic blood pressure and excessive increases in heart rate (Fig. 51).

On the basis of this evidence, it is concluded that (1) when diastolic blood pressure falls consistently, by $\geq$10 mm Hg, during 3 min of standing, on at least three separate occasions over a period of several days, autonomic insufficiency might be present, whereas (2) when diastolic blood pressure does not fall *consistently* by $\geq$10 mm Hg, during 3 min of standing, on each of three or more occasions, autonomic insufficiency due to structural neuronal lesions cannot be incriminated. These generalizations do not exclude the theoretical possibility that

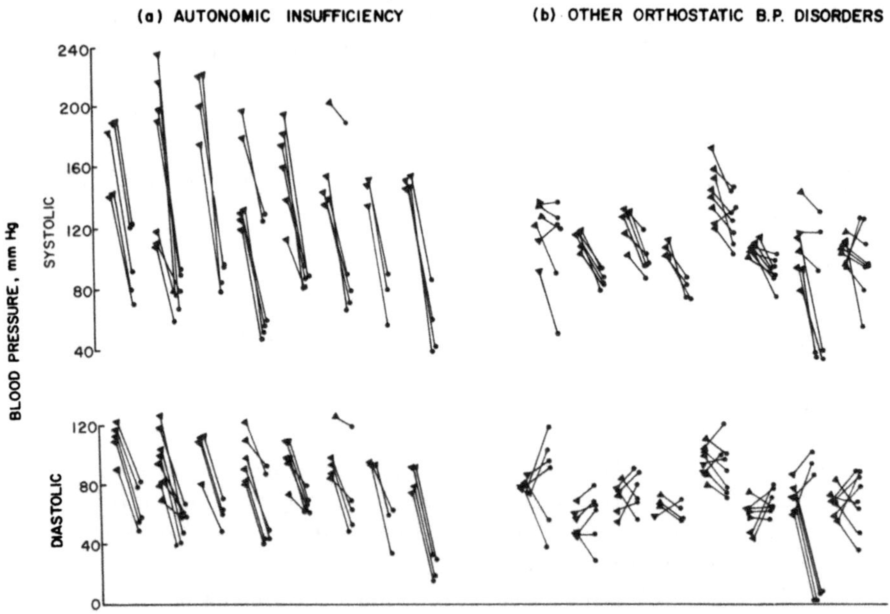

FIGURE 51. Systolic and diastolic blood pressures recumbent (▲) and standing (●) recorded on several occasions (a) in patients with autonomic insufficiency ($N = 9$) and (b) in patients with other orthostatic disorders of the blood pressure ($N = 8$). Systolic and diastolic blood pressure both fell on every occasion of their measurement in the patients with autonomic insufficiency, but orthostatic blood pressure changes (especially in diastolic pressure) were variable and did not always fall in the patients whose orthostatic blood pressure abnormalities were subsequently shown to be associated with intact autonomic nervous system function, which was frequently hyperactive in the upright posture.

"transient autonomic insufficiency" might cause intermittent or inconsistent orthostatic decreases in diastolic blood pressure in patients who have taken sympatholytic drugs or in those suffering from some type of functional or early structural disorder of the sympathetic nervous system. However, if the prior intake of sympatholytic drugs can be excluded, there is no good evidence that an inconsistent orthostatic decrease in diastolic pressure has been the result of transient impairment of sympathetic nervous function.

6.4.2. Heart Rate Changes

When insufficiency of the sympathetic nervous system involves innervation of both the peripheral arterioles and the heart, the orthostatic fall in blood pressure is accompanied by lack of the normal rise in heart rate in the upright posture. In contrast, when a consistent orthostatic fall in diastolic pressure is accompanied by orthostatic tachycardia, the implication is that (1) autonomic insufficiency might involve the peripheral microvasculature but not the heart, or (2) (more commonly) that autonomic insufficiency is not the cause of the persistent orthostatic hypotension.

6.4.3. Effects of Adrenocortical Insufficiency

Adrenocortical insufficiency may involve deficiency of either cortisol (hydrocortisone) or of aldosterone production, or both. Glucocorticoid deficiency (i.e., hypocortisolism in man) has long been known to cause orthostatic hypotension, which is, in fact, one of the most useful signs of adrenocortical insufficiency. In animals, the normal vasoconstrictive action of norepinephrine applied directly to the mesoappendicular vessels is lost after bilateral adrenalectomy (Fritz and Levine, 1951; Zweifach *et al.*, 1952–54). "Permissive amounts" (Ingle, 1942–43, 1954*a,b*) of adrenal glucocorticoid are therefore necessary for the normal contractile response of the vasculature to norepinephrine. It may be concluded that the orthostatic hypotension of hypocortisolism—which is always associated with orthostatic tachycardia—results from failure of the arterioles (and perhaps other parts of the microvascular tree) to contract in response to norepinephrine released in the upright posture.

A direct effect of aldosterone on the muscular function of the arterioles is certainly possible, since aldosterone has a direct positive inotropic action on the myocardium *in vitro* (Tanz, 1962) and stimulates peristaltic contractions of the intestinal smooth muscle, both *in vitro* and *in vivo* (Streeten *et al.*, 1954). However, hypoaldosteronism might be more likely to affect orthostatic changes in blood pressure by its classic effect through impaired renal sodium conservation on total body sodium and plasma volume (Liddle, 1957). As is well known, volume depletion *per se* invariably causes orthostatic tachycardia and, when mild or moderate, increases the normal orthostatic rise in diastolic blood pressure, with consequent narrowing of the pulse pressure. Thus, deficiency of either adrenocortical secretion of cortisol or aldosterone, or both, can usually be differentiated from primary impairment of the autonomic nervous system, as the cause of orthostatic hypotension, by the presence of orthostatic tachycardia.

6.4.4. Excessive Orthostatic Rise in Diastolic Blood Pressure

This problem may present to the clinician as follows:

1. *Orthostatic diastolic hypertension* (≥98 mm Hg):
   a. *Orthostatic hypertension:* hypertension may be evident only in the upright posture (Sapru *et al.*, 1979; Streeten *et al.*, 1985),
   b. *Orthostatic aggravation of persistent hypertension:* may represent

persistent hypertension (i.e., recumbent and orthostatic hypertension) with increased severity when the subject is sitting or standing (Frohlich *et al.*, 1967)

2. *Orthostatic narrowing of the pulse pressure (≤18 mm Hg): without an orthostatic rise in diastolic blood pressure above 97 mm Hg*

It is likely that (1) and (2) might often depend on the same pathogenetic mechanisms, being differentiated merely by the level of diastolic blood pressure arbitrarily chosen as the diagnostic indicator of the presence of hypertension. Both presentations may result from orthostatic reduction of the return of venous blood to the heart consequent upon hypovolemia (e.g., due to hemorrhage or dehydration) or excessive orthostatic pooling of blood in the capacitance vessels. High blood bradykinin levels can lead to excessive orthostatic pooling in the syndrome of hyperbradykininism (Streeten *et al.*, 1972).

6.4.5. Types of Orthostatic Blood Pressure Disorders

Orthostatic disorders of blood pressure have been classified into five groups:

1. *Orthostatic diastolic hypotension:* when diastolic blood pressure falls consistently, in the upright posture, by ≥10 mm Hg, with or without abnormal changes in systolic pressure; causes are as follows:
   a. *Autonomic insufficiency:* when accompanied by absence of the normal orthostatic rise in plasma norepinephrine concentration
   b. *Hypocortisolism:* when associated with laboratory evidence of subnormal plasma levels or production of cortisol
   c. *Idiopathic:* when catecholamine measurements and adrenocortical function are normal
2. *Orthostatic systolic hypotension:* when systolic pressure alone falls by ≥20 mm Hg or to <94 mm Hg in the upright posture; causes are as follows:
   a. *Hypoaldosteronism:* demonstrated by appropriate laboratory tests
   b. *Idiopathic:* no cause has yet been demonstrated
3. *Orthostatic diastolic hypertension:* when diastolic blood pressure rises from <90 mm Hg in the reclining posture to ≥98 mm Hg after standing for 3 min
4. *Orthostatic narrowing of pulse pressure:* to ≤18 mm Hg; causes are as follows:
   a. *Hyperbradykininism*
   b. *Plasma hypovolemia*
   c. *Idiopathic:* no demonstrable cause

5. *Orthostatic tachycardia:* when heart rate rises by ≥28 beats/min and to >108 beats/min without abnormal changes in blood pressure, after 3 min of standing; causes are as follows:
   a. *Hypocortisolism:* established by appropriate laboratory tests
   b. *Hyperbradykininism:* established by finding elevated blood kinin concentrations and/or subnormal plasma bradykininase concentrations
   c. *Idiopathic:* no demonstrable cause

The pathogenesis, clinical features, diagnosis, treatment, and prognosis of each of these disorders are discussed in Chapters 7–10 based on findings in 159 patients (see Appendix II) and on the relevant literature.

6.5. SUMMARY

Because differences in the position of the arm on which the blood pressure is being measured may affect the pressure recorded, the arm should be resting at the approximate vertical height of the atria when the blood pressure is measured. The elbow should be slightly flexed; to avoid possible kinking of the subclavian–axillary artery transition, the arm is best abducted to 90° sideways and not flexed (anteriorly) at the shoulder. Blood pressure and heart rate should be measured at least two or three times in recumbency and three to four times over a 3–5-min period in the standing posture. The normal ranges of systolic and diastolic blood pressures and heart rates in the recumbent and upright postures, measured in this way, have been defined in 92 healthy hospital workers, aged 17–61 years. Using these normal data, we have defined the several types of orthostatic disorders of blood pressure and heart rate control:

1. *Orthostatic diastolic hypotension:* orthostatic fall in diastolic pressure of ≥10 mm Hg
2. *Orthostatic systolic hypotension:* orthostatic fall in systolic blood pressure by ≥20 mm Hg or to ≤94 mm Hg
3. *Orthostatic hypertension:* diastolic blood pressure of ≤90 mm Hg in recumbency and ≥98 mm Hg in the standing position
4. *Orthostatic narrowing of the pulse pressure:* pulse pressure of ≤18 mm Hg in the standing posture
5. *Orthostatic tachycardia:* heart rate increased by >28 beats/min or to 110 beats/min or more while standing for at least 3 min

Multiple measurements of blood pressure lying and standing in 18 patients with well-documented autonomic insufficiency showed the presence of orthostatic diastolic hypotension on every single occasion, confirming the expectation that sympathetically mediated arteriolar contraction in the upright posture requires a normally functioning sympathetic nervous system. In many patients with other types of orthostatic blood pressure abnormalities, however, orthostatic diastolic hypotension might be present consistently, sometimes, or never.

The role of cortisol and aldosterone deficiencies, plasma hypovolemia, hyperbradykininism, and idiopathic lesions in the pathogenesis of the different types of orthostatic blood pressure abnormalities is discussed as the basis for classifying the pathogenesis of the disorders observed in 159 patients, whose findings are reported in Appendix II.

7

ORTHOSTATIC DISORDERS OF BLOOD PRESSURE CONTROL

Pathogenesis

During a change from the lying to the standing position, gravitational forces would cause rapid accumulation of blood in the dependent parts of the body were it not for the constriction of arterioles and capacitance vessels that normally takes place almost instantaneously. Arteriolar constriction is essential for orthostatic maintenance of the diastolic blood pressure, whereas venous and venular constriction is required for the uninterrupted return of blood from the lower parts of the body to the heart, so that stroke volume continues to be adequate to maintain the systolic blood pressure at normal levels. Since increased activity of the sympathetic nervous system is the prime stimulus for constriction of the peripheral vessels, it follows that deficient catecholamine action at these vascular sites is the most important potential mechanism of orthostatic diastolic hypotension.

7.1. ORTHOSTATIC HYPOTENSION

Orthostatic hypotension due to autonomic failure was first reported by Bradbury and Eggleston (1925). Ellis and Haynes (1936) pointed out that orthostatic hypotension was not accompanied by orthostatic tachycardia in these patients; these workers drew attention to the association of neurological diseases with orthostatic hypotension. Sympathetic functions of various types were found to be abnormal by Stead and Ebert (1941). Luft and von Euler (1953) described decreased urinary excretion of norepinephrine in two patients with severe postural hypotension, both in the unstimulated state and after stimulation by subcutaneous histamine injections and insulin-induced hypoglycemia. Absence of the normal rise of plasma norepinephrine concentration in patients with orthostatic hypotension in a standing position was first reported by Hickler *et al.* (1959*b*).

The return of blood to the heart during orthostasis may be inadequate for many reasons other than sympathetic insufficiency. In fact, orthostatic disorders of blood pressure result far more frequently from reduced cardiac preload—caused by anemia, dehydration, excessive pooling of blood in the venous system—and even from inadequate myocardial contractility than from autonomic insufficiency.

7.1.1. Autonomic Insufficiency

The normal response of the sympathetic nervous system to assumption of the upright posture requires integrity of the baroreceptor reflexes. The body "senses" a change from the supine to the vertical position through reduced volume of the vascular lumen at the sites of the low-pressure receptors in the right and left atria and the pulmonary vessels and through reduced pressure at the sites of the high-pressure baroreceptors in the aorta and the carotid sinuses. Diminished stretch at the receptor sites greatly reduces the firing rate of the receptors and the number and strength of the afferent impulses traveling *via* the glossopharyngeal and the vagus nerves to reach the medulla oblongata, particularly the integrating center in the nucleus tracti solitarii. Reduction of the impulses reaching this center increases the activity of the sympathetic neurons supplying the heart, the peripheral arterioles, the veins, and the adrenal medullae. It follows that failure of the arterioles or the capacitance vessels to contract in the erect posture may result from malfunction at any site in this baroreflex, from the receptors, *via* the connecting nervous pathways, to the brainstem, and thence *via* the efferent sympathetic nerves to the peripheral blood vessels (Thomas *et al.*, 1981). Thus, orthostatic hypotension due to autonomic dysfunction may result from any of the causes listed in Table IV.

Many of the disorders listed in Table IV are associated with morphological lesions at the respective sites in the baroreflex pathway. Thus, for example, acute demyelination of sympathetic nerves may be seen in Guillain-Barré syndrome; there is usually severe degeneration in the extrapyramidal tracts, the basal ganglia, and the dorsal nucleus of the vagus in Shy–Drager syndrome. The causes and cellular mechanisms of these and many other forms of damage to the sympathetic nervous system are still unknown. Similarly, although it is well known that diabetes mellitus and alcoholism often cause profound neuropathy involving the sympathetic nervous system, the precise mechanism of these and other types of metabolic nerve damage remains to be discovered. In the case of diabetic neuropathy, the pathogenic role of sorbitol and other polyol accumulations, causing edema of the nerves, has been suggested (Gabbay *et al.*, 1966). Dysautonomia (Riley and Moore, 1966) is inherited as an autosomal recessive disorder. It is

TABLE IV. Causes of Autonomic Insufficiency

I. Baroreceptor failure
II. Disorders of the afferent nerves (glossopharyngeal and vagal neuralgia)
III. Central disorders (preganglionic), resulting from infection, trauma, neoplasms, vascular accidents, demyelinating diseases, or toxic encephalopathy sometimes associated with:
  A. Parkinsonism (Graham and Oppenheimer, 1969)
  B. The Shy–Drager syndrome or multiple system atrophy (Shy and Drager, 1960; Bannister *et al.* 1977)
  C. Strionigral or cerebellar degenerations
  D. The Riley–Day syndrome or familial dysautonomia (Riley *et al.* 1949; Riley and Moore, 1966); not always accompanied by orthostatic hypotension
IV. Peripheral (postganglionic) dysfunction of the sympathetic nerves, caused by:
  A. General disorders, e.g., diabetic, alcoholic, amyloid (Wagner, H. N., 1959), other polyneuropathies, Guillain-Barré syndrome, porphyria, and beriberi
  B. Spinal cord disorders, e.g., syringomyelia (Ellis and Haynes, 1936), subacute combined sclerosis, tabes dorsalis (Ellis and Haynes, 1936), pernicious anemia (Eisenhofer *et al.* 1982), spinal cord trauma, and others
  C. Surgical sympathectomy, especially lumbodorsal (Hammarström, 1947)
  D. Pharmacological causes
    1. Ganglionic blocking drugs, e.g., pentolinium
    2. Drugs which block norepinephrine release from noradrenergic neurons, e.g., guanethidine, bethanidine (Bannister *et al.* 1977), and debrisoquine
    3. α_1-Adrenergic receptor antagonists, e.g., prazosin
    4. α_1- and α_2-Adrenergic antagonists, e.g., phentolamine and phenoxybenzamine
    5. α_2-Adrenergic agonists, e.g., clonidine, methyldopa, and guanabenz
    6. Dopamine antagonists, e.g., phenothiazines and haloperidol
    7. Tricyclic psychotropic drugs, e.g., imipramine and others
    8. L-Dopa
    9. Vincristine (Carmichael *et al.* 1970)
    10. Angiotensin converting enzyme inhibitors, e.g., captopril (Cody *et al.* 1982)
V. Old age
  A. Orthostatic hypotension is common in elderly subjects, occurring in 17% of one population of geriatric inpatients (Johnson, R. H., *et al.* 1965). Impaired elasticity of the peripheral vessel walls probably plays a role (Gross, 1970; Thulesius, 1976).
  B. Johnson; R. H., *et al.* (1965) have presented evidence that the common autonomic defect in the elderly is neither in the afferent nor the efferent pathways, and, therefore, is probably central.

characterized by sensory and autonomic disorders, including orthostatic hypotension without orthostatic tachycardia, low or normal vanillylmandelic acid (VMA) excretion, and normal plasma norepinephrine concentrations in recumbency, which fail to rise in the standing posture (Ziegler *et al.*, 1976), although plasma epinephrine concentration usually increases in response to insulin-induced hypoglycemia (Smith and Dancis, 1967).

Drug effects on the sympathetic nervous system are usually transient, disappearing after the metabolic action of the drug has been dissipated. A few currently used drugs block both α- and β-adrenergic receptors (e.g., labetolol) or block sympathetic ganglia (pentolinium); thus, administration of these agents results in orthostatic diastolic (and systolic) hypotension together with loss of the normal rise in heart rate in the upright posture. Some of the newer, more selective drugs, such as prazosin, however, will block α_1-adrenergic receptors only; thus, the heart rate rises appropriately when orthostatic hypotension results from use of these drugs. Phenothiazines block the actions of epinephrine and norepinephrine (Ibrahim *et al.*, 1975). Autonomic insufficiency of the peripheral type is associated with denervation supersensitivity of the vasculature to the constrictive action of administered norepinephrine and other α-adrenergic agonists (Bannister *et al.*, 1979), which results from an increase in the α-adrenergic receptor number (Davies *et al.*, 1982).

Although it is extremely difficult to prove, it seems likely that some patients may have a disturbance in the autonomic nerve supply to the arterioles of the lower limbs without loss of cardiac innervation. In these circumstances, one would expect orthostatic hypotension to be associated with pronounced orthostatic tachycardia, since the sympathetic fibers to the S-A node of the heart would be intact, as in patients who have undergone lumbodorsal sympathectomy (Hammarström, 1947). Whether this abnormality would be associated with a normal rise in plasma norepinephrine concentration in the standing posture has not been determined. Increased norepinephrine activity in the peripheral vasculature, whether induced by (1) reflex sympathetic nervous stimulation (Page *et al.*, 1955; Shadle *et al.*, 1958; Sharpey-Schafer, 1961, 1963; and Gauer and Thron, 1962), or (2) intravenous infusions of norepinephrine (R. S. Alexander, 1954; Eckstein and Hamilton, 1957; Wood and Eckstein, 1958; Shadle *et al.*, 1958; Glover *et al.*, 1958; Sharpey-Schafer, 1961; Rose *et al.*, 1962), or (3) orthostasis (Wood and Eckstein, 1958; Sharpey-Schafer, 1961) has consistently been shown to induce venous constriction. Since ganglionic blocking agents dilate forearm veins (Sharpey-Schafer, 1961) and autonomic failure results in loss of reflex constriction of veins (Page *et al.*, 1955; Bannister, 1971), the consequent venous pooling and diminution of venous return almost certainly contribute to the orthostatic hypotension in patients with autonomic insufficiency.

7.1.2. Hyperadrenergic Postural Hypotension

Some patients with diabetic neuropathy manifest orthostatic hypotension associated with an excessive orthostatic rise in plasma norepinephrine concentration, called hyperadrenergic postural hypotension by Tohmeh *et al.* (1979). Whether they might fall into the category of patients with microvascular but not cardiac denervation is unknown. With deficient norepinephrine release at the sympathetic nerve endings on the arterioles, or perhaps with some receptor or postreceptor defect in arteriolar response to locally released norepinephrine at these sites, such patients would experience a profound fall in diastolic blood pressure in the upright posture that might be expected to result in the excessive release of norepinephrine from intact neurons and a consequently supranormal rise in plasma norepinephrine concentration in the upright posture.

Tohmeh *et al.* (1979) found a severe reduction in red blood cell (RBC) mass in the four patients they studied. This severe anemia was considered likely to be the cause of the hyperadrenergic postural hypotension, since it was shown that excessive orthostatic increase in plasma norepinephrine concentration could be induced experimentally by decreasing the RBC mass in a normal subject.

7.2. ORTHOSTATIC HYPERTENSION AND OTHER TYPES OF ORTHOSTATIC BLOOD PRESSURE DISORDERS

In the absence of independent evidence to suggest the presence of autonomic insufficiency, some patients will be found consistently, at least for several days or weeks, to manifest an excessive orthostatic fall in diastolic blood pressure (by ≥10 mm Hg). This may result from a variety of different causes. More commonly, however, in patients whose sympathetic nervous system is intact, orthostatic diastolic hypotension is not consistently present. Instead, it may be found to be present on some examinations, while on other occasions there may be either orthostatic hypertension, excessive orthostatic narrowing of the pulse pressure, orthostatic systolic hypotension, or only orthostatic tachycardia (see definitions in Chapter 6), or occasionally no orthostatic changes outside the normal limits. This variability in the findings is not merely related to the time of day at which the measurements are made, although no doubt most of the abnormalities described (certainly orthostatic diastolic hypotension) are worst in the mornings and become less severe as the day progresses (Cranston and Brown, 1963; Mann *et al.*, 1983) (see Clinical Features, Chapter 8). The different abnormalities from day to day and even from minute to minute seem, at least in part, to be related to variations in hydration and can certainly be dramatically altered by acute sodium depletion and repletion (see pages 137–143).

Varying degrees of severity of the underlying pathogenic mechanism may influence the nature of the observed changes as well, as we have found in adrenal insufficiency. Since there is strong evidence that these various blood pressure derangements may coexist in the same patients at different times and that the pathogenetic mechanisms of these varieties of orthostatic disorders share common pathways, their pathogenesis is discussed together.

7.3. CAUSES OF ORTHOSTATIC BLOOD PRESSURE DISORDERS

The potential causes of orthostatic derangements in blood pressure control may be classified as follows:

1. Autonomic insufficiency affecting arteriolar innervation:
   a. With cardiac involvement
   b. Without cardiac involvement
2. Pheochromocytoma: Orthostatic hypotension occurs in 44% and orthostatic tachycardia in 50% of patients with pheochromocytoma (Smithwick *et al.*, 1950), through an unknown mechanism.
3. Hypocortisolism: Characteristically causes orthostatic hypotension, partly by preventing the normal contractile responses of the microvasculature to norepinephrine and epinephrine (Fritz and Levine, 1951; Zweifach *et al.*, 1952–1954)—the "permissive action" of cortisol (Ingle, 1942–1943, 1954*a,b*)—and probably partly through other mechanisms. This form of orthostatic hypotension is often profound when cortisol production is severely reduced; it persists as long as the cortisol deficiency remains uncorrected. It is important to appreciate that orthostatic hypotension may result from both primary adrenocortical disease and adrenal insufficiency secondary to hypopituitarism. Moreover, whereas severe and (probably) primary adrenal insufficiency usually appears to cause orthostatic diastolic hypotension (see patients #19–24 in Appendix II), milder and secondary hypocortisolism (due to hypopituitarism) more commonly seems to present with orthostatic systolic hypotension or with orthostatic narrowing of pulse pressure or orthostatic tachycardia (as in patients #135–140, in Appendix II).
4. Reduction of blood volume: By decreasing cardiac output to the point at which seemingly no amount of arteriolar contraction could possibly maintain the blood pressure, this effect will cause orthostatic diastolic hypotension. Milder decreases in blood volume tend to cause the other disorders in orthostatic blood pressure control described below. Low blood volume may result from:
   a. Blood loss: Such as in bleeding hemorrhoids, peptic ulcers, esophageal varices, neoplasms, or other internal or external lesions, repeated venesections, hemorrhage resulting from spontaneous or iatrogenic defects in blood coagulation, postoperative hemorrhages, or anemias of other types, such as that found in some diabetic patients with hyperadrenergic postural hypotension (Tohmeh *et al.*, 1979).
   b. Severe dehydration and plasma hypovolemia: Caused by anorexia nervosa and other types of starvation, profuse diarrhea and/or vomit-

ing, hypoaldosteronism, renal sodium losses (due to diuretic therapy or intrinsic renal disease), chronic hemodialysis (Schatz, 1984), or excessive sweating, especially when associated with inadequate sodium intake (Streeten *et al.*, 1960*a*).

5. Cardiac dysfunction: May cause mild or severe reductions in blood pressure even in recumbency. The changes are often aggravated or may become evident exclusively during orthostasis in the following conditions:
   a. Severe myocardial disease: Especially massive myocardial infarction, and pump failure.
   b. Heart block and dysrhythmias of many types: We have encountered a few patients in whom a large number of premature ventricular beats have occurred exclusively in the upright posture (see patients #33, 118, 123, and 147, in Appendix II). Although sick sinus syndrome is not generally associated with any orthostatic abnormality of blood pressure control, it often causes syncope because of sinus bradycardia (Ferrer, 1980); presumably, numerous ectopic beats in the upright posture could have the same effect.
   c. Mitral valve prolapse: May be associated with orthostatic blood pressure disorders (Depace *et al.*, 1981), although there is no evidence to establish a cause-and-effect relationship. It may also cause syncope by the dysrhythmias which are often present (Winkle *et al.*, 1976).
   d. Pericarditis and cardiac tamponade.
   e. Aortic or pulmonic stenosis: Especially after exercise (Richards *et al.*, 1984) and other obstructive causes of reduced cardiac output.
6. Debility and inactivity: Especially in bedridden patients (Hickler, 1977), and chronic alcoholics.
7. Transient increases in intrathoracic pressure: Resulting from prolonged vigorous coughing, straining to pass urine, and other forms of prolonged maintenance of the Valsalva maneuver, all are potential causes of orthostatic hypotension and syncope.
8. Excessive orthostatic pooling of blood in the venous system: This may result from any of several factors:
   a. Severe venous obstruction: Such as from massive venous thrombosis (usually involving the inferior vena cava).
   b. Extremely large varicose veins.
   c. Functional inadequacy of venous contractility.
   d. Hyperbradykininism (Streeten *et al.*, 1972).
   e. Pregnancy: Perhaps because of venous obstruction by the gravid uterus.
9. Idiopathic.

The variability in orthostatic blood pressure abnormalities is shown (Fig. 52) in a record of blood pressure (obtained automatically with an Arteriosonde) and heart rate in a 46-year-old man, while he changed from the supine to the standing, the sitting, and again the supine posture. It is evident that most of this patient's blood pressure readings and heart rates in recumbency were normal (mean blood pressure 146/88, heart rate 76–80). In the standing posture, there was an immediate fall in the systolic and a rise in the diastolic blood pressure, with a mean blood pressure of 134/108 for the first 22 min, while the heart rate was 116–128. Since these changes exceed the normal ranges, the findings might be described as indicating the presence of orthostatic diastolic hypertension and tachycardia. During the last 23 min of standing, the blood pressure averaged

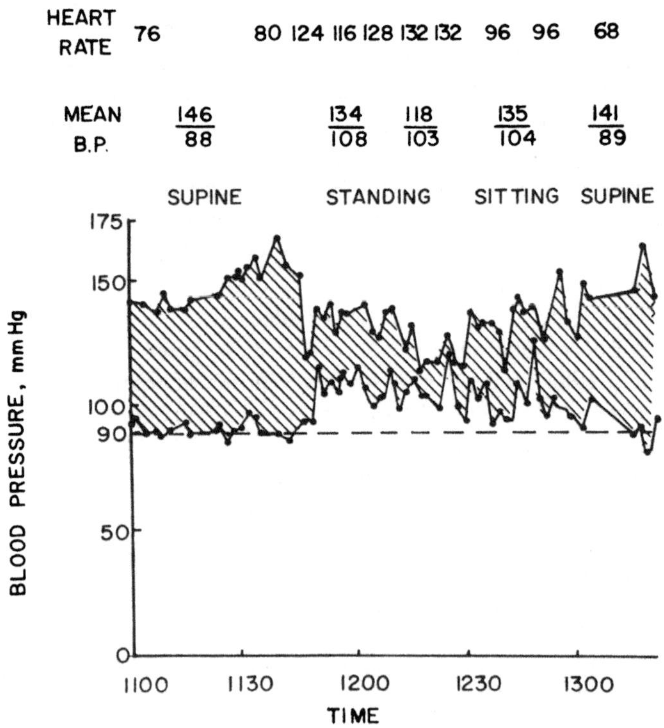

FIGURE 52. Record showing variability of orthostatic blood pressure abnormalities evident in the same subject within a short period of time. This patient's normal recumbent blood pressure changed shortly after standing to values (mean 134/108) that would be described as those of orthostatic hypertension. However, systolic pressure fell gradually thereafter, until the mean of several blood pressure determinations (118/103) satisfied the criteria both for orthostatic systolic hypotension and for excessive orthostatic narrowing of the pulse pressure, while orthostatic tachycardia was present throughout.

118/103, and heart rate 132 beats/min, findings indicating orthostatic systolic hypotension, diastolic hypertension, excessive narrowing of pulse pressure, and tachycardia. Yet, some of the individual blood pressure recordings showed only orthostatic narrowing of the pulse pressure, whereas others showed only orthostatic hypertension; the last reading in the standing position (116/94) would have been described as showing only orthostatic systolic hypotension. All the abnormal changes were attenuated in the sitting position, and normal values returned rapidly once the patient was in a recumbent position.

Incidentally, this patient complained of a worrisome headache for much of the time spent in the standing position (actually his presenting complaint), with remission of the headache shortly after he lay down. In spite of the variety of his changes during a single morning, he was classified as having orthostatic hypertension, since this was the most consistent finding at repeated outpatient visits, but it is clear that he might have been said to have had orthostatic narrowing of the pulse pressure, orthostatic tachycardia, or orthostatic systolic hypotension.

7.4. PATHOGENESIS OF ORTHOSTATIC BLOOD PRESSURE DISORDERS ASSOCIATED WITH INTACT AUTONOMIC FUNCTION

This section presents the evidence that has led to the conclusion that most orthostatic blood pressure disorders (with the exception of those due to autonomic insufficiency) are the result of various pathogenetic mechanisms, all of which produce an abnormally decreased cardiac preload (i.e., excessive reduction of venous return and cardiac filling) in the upright posture. If this view is correct, the orthostatic blood pressure derangements (1) should be seen during acute blood loss, and (2) if not due to low blood volume, should be associated with excessive gravitational pooling of blood in the dependent parts, the prevention of which should correct the orthostatic disorders. These postulates will now be examined.

7.4.1. Effects of Changes in Blood Volume Induced by Venesection

7.4.1.1. Venesection in Animals

Neil (1958) showed in cats that slowly continuing hemorrhage resulted initially in a fall in cardiac stroke volume. This was associated with tachycardia and peripheral vasoconstriction—both *via* reflex stimulation of sympathetic activity mediated by the carotid baroreceptors and chemoreceptors (Landgren and Neil, 1951), which sufficed to maintain the mean blood pressure virtually unchanged. Because of the fall in stroke volume, however, there was a reduction in systolic blood pressure, hence a drop in pulse pressure. Since the mean blood pressure did not fall at any point during these experiments, it was clearly the reduction in stroke volume or the fall in systolic pressure or the narrowing of pulse pressure that activated the baroreflex in these animals. In another study, Ead *et al.* (1952) showed that it is mainly pulsatile pressure changes that activate the baroreceptors. On the basis of these findings, Heymans and Neil (1958) concluded that the diminution in pulse pressure resulting from the hemorrhage-induced fall in stroke volume must have increased sympathetic activity, thereby aggravating the tachycardia, in turn reducing stroke volume and pulse pressure still further—a sort of vicious circle. Guyton *et al.* (1958) described similar responses to more acute venesection in dogs: decreased venous return leading to reduced cardiac filling, producing a fall in stroke volume.

7.4.1.2. Venesection in Humans

Green and Metheny (1947) showed in patients subjected to venesection that the extent of rise of the heart rate in the upright posture is directly related to the volume of blood withdrawn. The blood pressure response to orthostasis after the removal of increasing volumes of blood in their experiments is shown in Table V. As blood volume was progressively reduced by venesection, orthostasis induced a progressive increase in heart rate and a decrease in systolic blood pressure. Simultaneously, diastolic blood pressure gradually increased until the volume of blood removed exceeded 14 ml/kg, when systolic and diastolic blood pressures dropped precipitously in the upright posture. Before the occurrence of orthostatic diastolic hypotension, the progressive reduction of blood volume was associated with *pari passu* narrowing of the pulse pressure in the standing posi-

TABLE V. Effects of Increasing Volumes of Blood Removed by Venesection on Orthostatic Changes (Mean ± SD) in Heart Rate and Blood Pressure

	Vol. blood removed (ml/kg)			
	0	5–9	9–14	14–21
Number of subjects	56	17	9	5
Change in heart rate (per min)	+6 ± 7.8	+20 ± 10	+42 ± 8.3	+36 ± 8.9
Change in systolic BP (mm Hg)	−6 ± 11	−9 ± 10	−10 ± 13	−82 ± 32
Change in diastolic BP (mm Hg)	+4 ± 11	+6 ± 8	+10 ± 7.1	−66 ± 27
Change in pulse pressure (mm Hg)	−10	−15	−20	−16

[a]Data from Green *et al.* (1947).

tion. Gullbring *et al.* (1960) confirmed the occurrence of a rise in heart rate immediately after venesection.

Our own studies in normal subjects donating 500 ml of blood to the transfusion service have shown that venesection aggravates the normal orthostatic rise in diastolic blood pressure, shrinkage in pulse pressure, and increase in heart rate in most persons. In some instances, the orthostatic changes in blood pressure and heart rate approached the abnormal findings described as orthostatic hypertension, orthostatic systolic hypotension, orthostatic narrowing of pulse pressure, and orthostatic tachycardia. These physiological responses to mild reductions in blood volume in healthy subjects indicate that spontaneous orthostatic disorders in blood pressure control might have resulted from a variety of pathological causes but might all have been mediated by reduced blood volume or diminished cardiac preload in the upright posture.

7.4.1.3. Effects of Depletion and Excessive Repletion of Body Fluids

The volumes of the extracellular fluid and plasma compartments of the body can be acutely changed in either direction by rapid diuresis or rapid intravenous infusions of isotonic saline. If orthostatic blood pressure abnormalities are the consequence of diminished return of blood to the heart, they should be aggravated by acute diuresis and improved by rapid, large intravenous infusions of saline. We have tested this thesis in a number of persons with orthostatic blood pressure derangements of different types, with the following results.

a. Responses in a Patient with Orthostatic Systolic Hypotension. Figure 53 shows the blood pressure responses to diuresis and NaCl infusion, in a 35-year-old woman (patient #37, in Appendix II) whose systolic blood pressure had been previously shown to fall as low as 88 mm Hg, while her diastolic blood pressure did not fall, but rose in the upright posture (66–84 mm Hg), indicating the presence of orthostatic systolic hypotension. The study started at 7:45 a.m., when a butterfly needle was placed in a forearm vein and kept patent with dilute heparin solution for later use. Blood pressure was recorded automatically every 2 min with an Arteriosonde, while the patient lay quietly in bed for 1 hr; she then sat up with her legs dangling over the side of the bed for the next several hours, resuming recumbency for the final hour of the study. As shown in Figure 53, the average blood pressure fell from 107/72 to 87/64 when the patient changed to the sitting posture, confirming the previous findings of abnormal orthostatic reduction in systolic pressure, together with diastolic changes that were within the normal limits. Then, 1 hr later, furosemide, 40 mg, was injected intravenously through the heparinized needle, producing a brisk natriuresis and diuresis, particularly over the following 90 min, during which the blood pressure dropped further. An intravenous infusion of isotonic saline, 2 liters, was started shortly

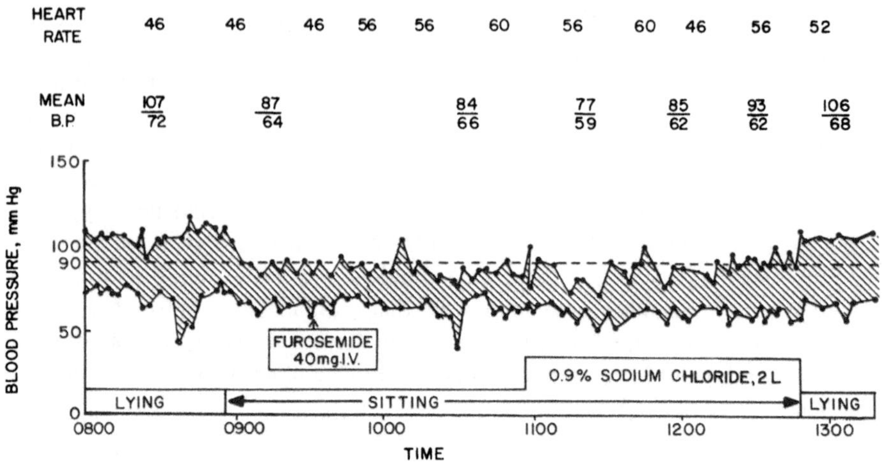

FIGURE 53. Blood pressure record in a patient with orthostatic systolic hypotension (even in the sitting position), showing that volume reduction by furosemide-induced diuresis aggravated orthostatic systolic hypotension, narrowed the pulse pressure into the abnormal range and resulted in pathological orthostatic diastolic hypotension. All these abnormalities were overcome by volume restoration with intravenous saline infusion.

before 11:00 a.m., at the beginning of which her average blood pressure was 77/59, while the heart rate had risen from 46 to 60 beats/min. Thereafter, the saline infusion induced a steady increase in mean systolic blood pressure to 85 and 93 mm Hg, which was associated with a widening of the pulse pressure from the subnormal value of 18 mm Hg, between 11:15 and 11:30 a.m., to 31 mm Hg at 12:30–12:45 p.m. When the recumbent position was resumed, the blood pressure returned to an average value (106/68) close to that at the start of the experiment. It is clear from Figure 53 that the furosemide-induced diuresis aggravated the orthostatic systolic hypotension, increased the orthostatic diastolic hypotension into the pathological range, and caused a shrinkage of the pulse pressure to a subnormal width, while the saline infusion increased systolic pressure and widened the pulse pressure into the normal ranges and even beyond the values present before the furosemide injection.

b. Responses in a Patient with Orthostatic Narrowing of the Pulse Pressure. The blood pressure responses to the same experimental protocol, of a patient known to have orthostatic narrowing of the pulse pressure (patient #104, Appendix II), are shown in Figure 54. When, after 1 hr in the supine position, this patient sat up, her average blood pressure changed from 117/83 to 108/84, less than the change to 102/88, which had been found in the standing posture (see Appendix II). The diuretic response to furosemide caused a further

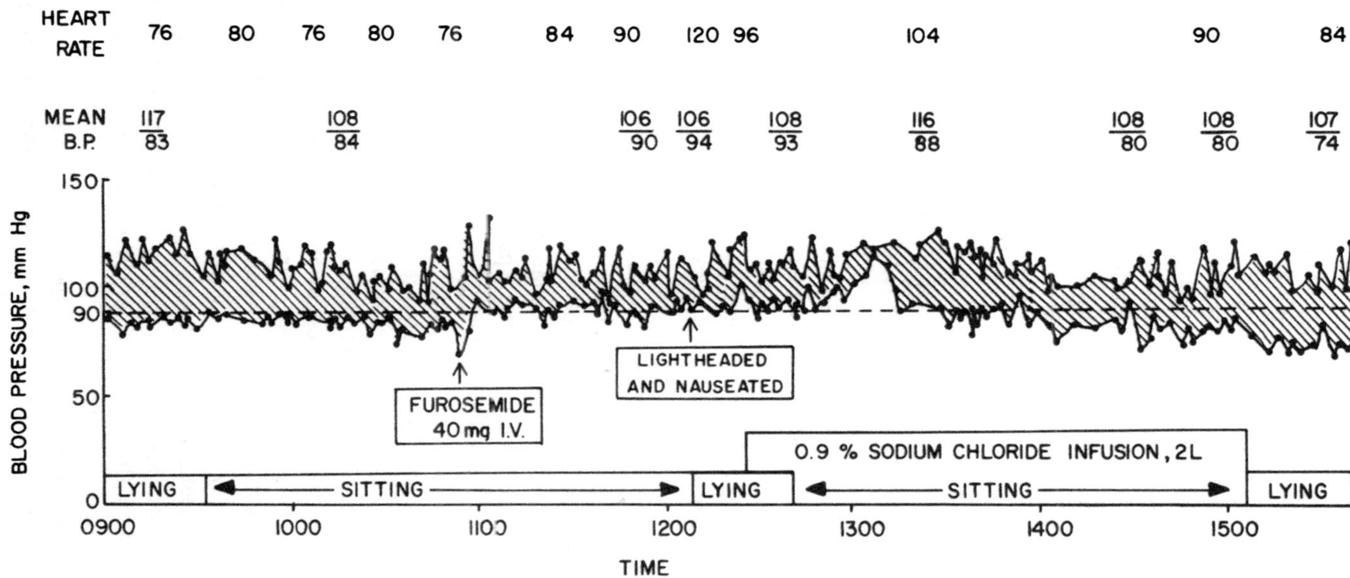

FIGURE 54. Record of a patient with excessive narrowing of the pulse pressure in the standing posture. When seated, her pulse pressure fell to 24 mm Hg, but furosemide-induced diuresis reduced mean pulse pressure further (to 16 and 12 mm Hg), predominantly by raising diastolic pressure, causing lightheadedness that required her to lie down. Saline infusion then restored seated blood pressure and pulse pressure to mean values (108/80 and 28 mm Hg resp) at least as good as those present before volume depletion.

shrinkage of pulse pressure into the clearly abnormal range (blood pressures 106/90, 106/94, 108/93), whereas the heart rate was increased transiently into the pathological range, reaching 120 beats/min in the sitting position. At this point, the patient experienced severe lightheadedness and nausea, two of the symptoms that had caused her to seek medical advice in the first instance. Because it appeared that she might faint, we allowed her to lie down; symptoms improved within a few minutes. The saline infusion that was then started enabled her to sit up again after 16 min and caused slowing of the heart rate and widening of the pulse pressure into the normal range, with blood pressures averaging 116/88 and 108/80 as the saline ran in.

c. *Responses in a Patient with Orthostatic Hypertension.* The response of a patient with orthostatic hypertension to the same procedure is shown in Figure 55. His blood pressure rose from 137/86 to 142/92 in the sitting posture and had risen into the pathological range (to 138/98) in the standing position (patient #84, in Appendix II). Volume depletion produced by the furosemide injection raised the diastolic blood pressure gradually to 98 and 100 mm Hg, while heart rate increased to 104 beats/min. Two liters of normal saline rapidly lowered the diastolic blood pressure to 82 mm Hg, widened the pulse pressure from 29 to 58 and 53 mm Hg, and slowed the heart rate from 104 to 88 beats/min in the sitting position.

It is evident from these three studies that acute fluid depletion aggravated and rapid repletion corrected the three orthostatic disorders previously documented in the standing posture in these patients: orthostatic systolic hypotension, orthostatic narrowing of the pulse pressure, and orthostatic diastolic hypertension. At their worst after vigorous diuresis, these patients all had narrowed pulse pressures and an accelerated heartbeat, whereas after saline administration all abnormalities were corrected.

To show that these are not isolated responses, Figure 56 depicts the results of the same experimental procedure in 13 patients with orthostatic hypertension whose blood pressures are compared with those of seven patients who had hypertension in all postures (persistent hypertension). It is of interest to note that recumbent pulse pressure was strikingly lower in the patients with orthostatic hypertension even in the reclining position (mean pulse pressure 45.7 mm Hg) than it was in the persistently hypertensive patients (mean pulse pressure 71.3 mm Hg). The general responses of the two groups of patients were similar, indicating that shrinkage of the pulse pressure with fluid depletion and widening of the pulse pressure with fluid repletion are not peculiar to patients with orthostatic disorders of the blood pressure.

In agreement with these findings, Campese *et al.* (1980) showed that furosemide-induced diuresis decreased the pulse pressure in the standing posture from 29 to 23 mm Hg in 11 normal subjects. Since the initial pulse pressure in

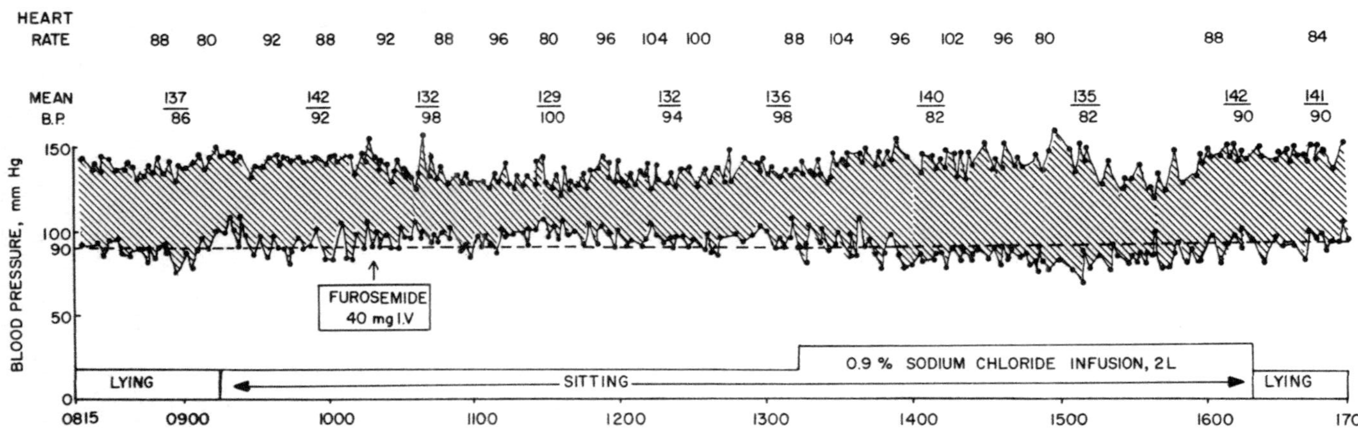

FIGURE 55. Blood pressure responses to volume depletion and repletion in a patient with diastolic hypertension in the standing posture. Diuresis raised seated diastolic pressure into the clearly abnormal range (98–100 mm Hg), whereas saline infusion lowered the diastolic pressure to 82 mm Hg, widened the seated pulse pressure, and slowed the heart rate from 104 to 80 beats/min.

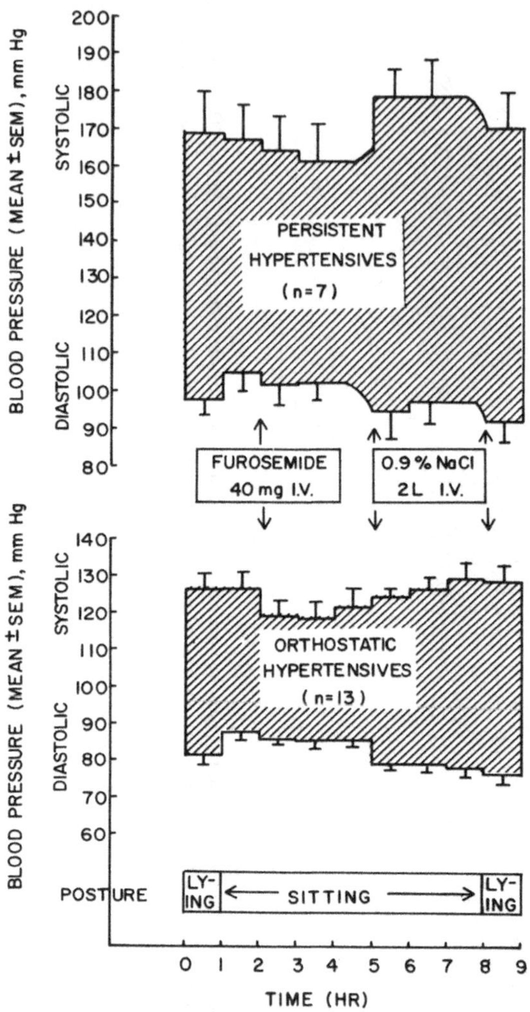

FIGURE 56. Mean of the blood pressure responses to diuresis and saline infusion in the seated posture, in 13 patients with orthostatic hypertension and seven patients with persistent hypertension. The narrower pulse pressures are shown in all circumstances in the patients with orthostatic hypertension; note the trend toward furosemide-induced reductions in systolic pressure and pulse pressure and increases in diastolic pressures in both groups of patients. Volume replenishment reversed all these trends.

our patients in the reclining posture was narrower in the group with orthostatic hypertension, the measurements more closely approached pathological levels after fluid depletion in these patients than in the persistently hypertensive group. It is worth noting that severe lightheadedness and unpleasant palpitations, requiring interruption of the study to permit the patient to lie down for several minutes, occurred in no fewer than four of the 13 patients with orthostatic blood pressure disorders after fluid depletion, while none of these symptoms was ever encountered in the patients with persistent hypertension. Thus, the thesis that diminution of the volume of blood in some part of the circulation (postulated to include the blood volume returning to the heart) is an important component of the pathogenetic mechanism of the described orthostatic derangements of blood pressure is supported by (1) the increased sensitivity to the adverse effects of fluid loss in patients with orthostatic blood pressure disorders, (2) the aggravation of their initial derangements by diuresis, and (3) the striking abolition of almost all measurable abnormalities after a 2-liter saline infusion.

7.4.2. *Evidence of Excessive Gravitational Pooling of Blood*

7.4.2.1. Effects of External Pressure

If the hypothesis is correct that excessive pooling of blood in the dependent parts of the body plays a role in the pathogenesis of orthostatic disorders of blood pressure control, it should be possible to correct the observed disorders by the application of external pressure to the lower limbs and the abdomen while subjects remain standing. In his classic experiments, performed almost 100 years ago, Hill (1895) showed that when rabbits, dogs, and other animals (but not monkeys) were suspended vertically (head up), the result was an immediate precipitous fall in blood pressure causing syncope because "the blood drains into the abdominal veins, the heart empties and the cerebral circulation ceases," all of which could be prevented by a tight abdominal bandage.

In an effort to investigate the possibility of preventing orthostatic blood pressure changes in man, we measured the changes in blood pressure and heart rate in patients with the described disorders, who were placed in antigravity suits that were initially deflated and then inflated. Using G-suits that had been worn by airmen in World War II, satisfactory results were obtained. However, since our patients were of all sizes and shapes, we were frequently unable to achieve adequate external compression even with the three suits of various sizes that we had on hand. For this reason, we have since used Military Anti-Shock Trousers (MAST suits, David Clark Co., Worcester, MA) for all our more recent studies, finding them more satisfactory for this purpose. In general, the patients have first had the suit applied over their underclothing and have remained lying down for blood pressure and heart rate measurements, either by sphygmomanometry and cardiac auscultation or by automatic equipment, such as the Arteriosonde (now no longer available) or the Dinamap (Critikon Co., Tampa, FL). When five or ten readings of blood pressure and heart rate had been obtained after 15 min in the supine position, the patients were asked (and helped!) to stand while blood pressure and heart rate measurements were continued for 5–10 min, with the arm on which the measurements were made held on a level with the sternal angle (see Section 6.1). The pressure suit was then inflated until the patient was aware of firm but not uncomfortable compression, either while the individual remained standing or after lying down again. Comparable results were obtained by either procedure, as inflation of the suit in recumbency made very little difference to the blood pressure in that posture.

7.4.2.2. Responses to the Inflated Pressure Suit

Figures 57 and 58 show the effects of inflating the pressure suit on the blood pressure of patients with orthostatic narrowing of the pulse pressure (patient #92, Appendix II), and orthostatic hypertension (patient #61, Appendix II). It is clearly evident that blood pressure in the upright posture was abnormal.

In the patient with excessive orthostatic narrowing of the pulse pressure (Fig. 57), inflation of the pressure suit immediately widened the pulse pressure into the normal range and relieved her severe lightheadedness, so that she was able to continue standing for 64 min without symptoms. Deflation of the suit at this point resulted in immediate convergence of the systolic and diastolic blood

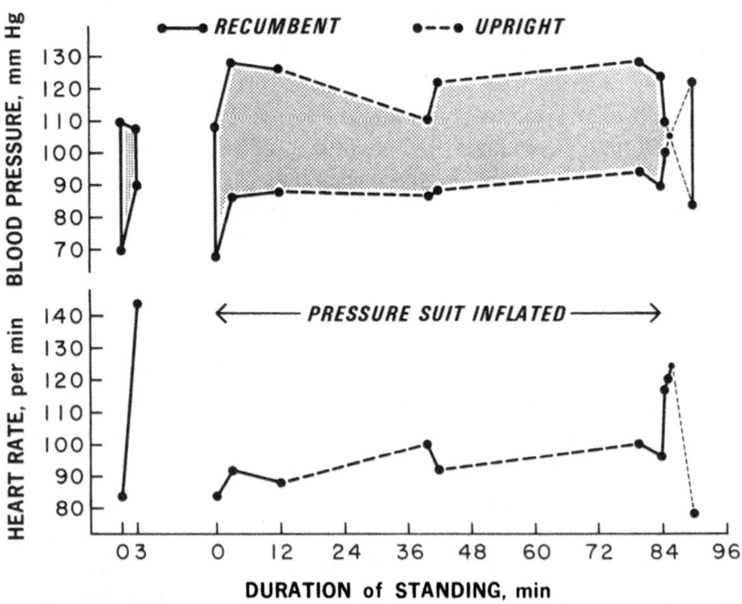

FIGURE 57. Effects of inflated antigravity suit on blood pressure in patient with excessive orthostatic narrowing of the pulse pressure. Blood pressure, pulse pressure, and heart rate were maintained within the normal ranges as long as the pressure suit was inflated, for 64 min. Deflation of the suit resulted in immediate shrinkage of the pulse pressure, acceleration of heart rate, and collapse, with rapid restoration of normal blood pressure and heart rate in recumbency.

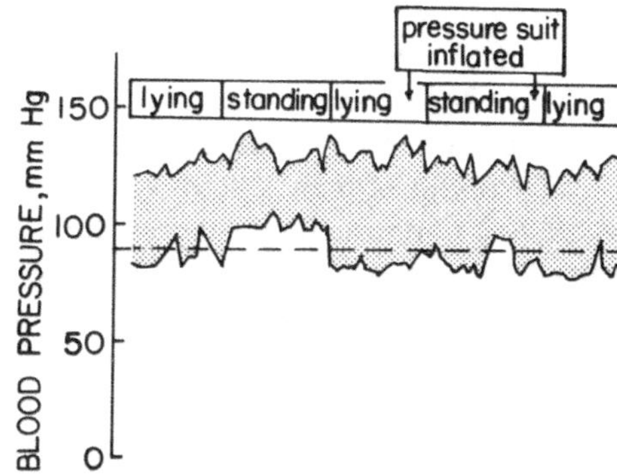

FIGURE 58. Correction of orthostatic diastolic hypertension by inflated pressure suit. With suit deflated, standing raised diastolic pressure from a mean of 83 mm Hg (recumbent) to 101 mm Hg (standing), but inflation of the suit lowered the mean standing diastolic blood pressure to 84 mm Hg. (From Streeten *et al.*, 1985.)

pressures, striking cardiac acceleration and impending syncope within 1 min, relieved by having the patient lie down immediately.

In the patient with orthostatic diastolic hypertension (Fig. 58), the diastolic blood pressure rose to 101 mm Hg (mean) in the upright posture; when the pressure suit was inflated, however, diastolic blood pressure was reduced again to 84 mm Hg. The consistent presence of orthostatic diastolic hypertension, even in the sitting posture in this patient, is shown in Figure 59. Within 1 min of changing from the lying to the sitting position, the diastolic blood pressure, recorded automatically on a Dinamap, rose above 98 mm Hg and stayed in the elevated range until its prompt fall to below 90 mm Hg when recumbency was resumed.

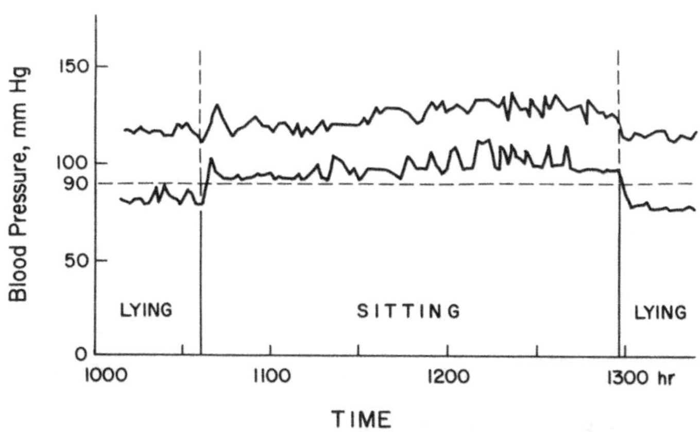

FIGURE 59. Automatic blood pressure measurements (by Dinamap) showing orthostatic diastolic hypertension in the sitting posture. (From Streeten *et al.*, 1985.)

In a patient with orthostatic systolic hypotension (patient #44, in Appendix II), the mean of several blood pressure determinations fell from 114/71 in recumbency to 92/62 in the standing posture, and the standing pressure was raised to 106/66 by use of the inflated pressure suit.

The results of these studies have been confirmed in a series of patients with each type of orthostatic blood pressure derangement. The observations in these patients have been compared with the effects of the inflated pressure suit on normal subjects and on six patients with orthostatic hypotension associated with autonomic insufficiency, in Figure 60. It is apparent that normal subjects showed no significant effect of the inflated pressure suit on the blood pressure, the orthostatic change in systolic pressure (expressed as a percentage) being 3.3 ± 19% (mean ± SEM) lower and the change in diastolic pressure 3.0 ± 1.7% lower in the inflated suit (both insignificant by Student's *t*-test for dependent

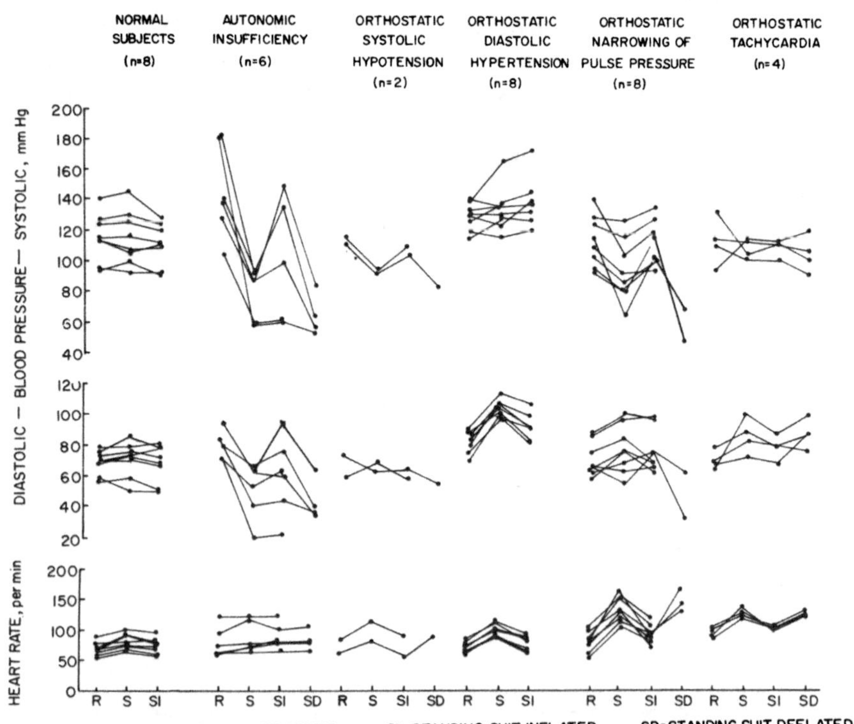

FIGURE 60. Blood pressures and heart rates recumbent (R), standing (S), in inflated (SI) and subsequently deflated (SD) antigravity suit in normal subjects and patients with orthostatic blood pressure derangements. Except in some of the patients with autonomic insufficiency, all orthostatic blood pressure and heart rate abnormalities were corrected with the inflated suit.

variables). The orthostatic change in pulse rate in the normal subjects, however, was reduced by 5.8 ± 2.2% ($p < 0.05$), in the inflated pressure suit. None of the patients with autonomic insufficiency showed a rise in heart rate in the upright posture, in spite of the large reductions in blood pressure shown in Figure 60. Inflation of the pressure suit restored the blood pressure to normal levels in four of the six patients with autonomic insufficiency but had no discernible effect in the remaining two patients. Correction of orthostatic hypotension in patients with autonomic insufficiency has also been accomplished by having the subjects stand in water up to the level of the heart (Stead and Ebert, 1941). In virtually every patient with the other types of orthostatic blood pressure disorder shown, the inflated pressure suit strikingly diminished the initial orthostatic derangement and in most cases corrected it completely. Statistical analysis showed that the inflated pressure suit significantly improved the presenting disorder in all groups (except in the group of two patients with orthostatic hypotension for whom data were not analyzed). Thus, (1) in the two patients with orthostatic systolic hypotension, the inflated pressure suit raised the systolic blood pressure in the upright posture from 94.0 to 107.5 mm Hg (mean); (2) in the eight patients with orthostatic diastolic hypertension, the pressure suit reduced the orthostatic change in diastolic blood pressure from +23.9 ± 3.4 to +12.6 ± 2.9% ($p < 0.001$); (3) in the eight patients with orthostatic narrowing of the pulse pressure, the orthostatic change in pulse pressure was reduced from −54.3 ± 10.8 to −13.7 ± 7.5% ($p < 0.001$) by the inflated pressure suit; and (4) in the four patients with orthostatic tachycardia, the inflated pressure suit reduced the orthostatic rise in heart rate from +36.0 ± 4.9 to +8.3 ± 4.0% ($p < 0.001$). In fact, the inflated pressure suit reduced the magnitude of orthostatic changes in diastolic blood pressure, pulse pressure, and heart rate from significantly excessive to nonsignificant changes within the normal ranges in all groups of patients.

These results lead to the conclusion that, whether orthostasis has caused excessive reduction in the systolic pressure alone, or an excessive rise in diastolic pressure, or excessive narrowing of the pulse pressure, or an excessive rise in heart rate alone or any combination of these abnormalities, inflation of the pressure suit in every case ameliorates or completely corrects the blood pressure disorder and simultaneously prevents the excessive orthostatic rise in heart rate in all the patients. This evidence indicates that reduction of orthostatic pooling in the capacitance vessels—which must surely be the main effect of an inflated pressure suit—corrects the various orthostatic disorders of blood pressure control. Bjure and Laurell (1927) and Laurell (1936) have previously described the reversal of orthostatic tachycardia and the fall in cardiac output, as well as correction of the associated headaches, lightheadedness, fatigue, and nausea in patients with "orthostatic arterial anemia," by having the patients stand immersed to the level of the sternum in a water bath or by applying external pressure to the abdomen with a girdle or corset. The obvious implication of these observations—that the disorders resulted from excessive orthostatic pooling in the capacitance vessels—is examined in the following section.

7.4.2.3. Direct Measurement of Orthostatic Vascular Pooling

We have devised and used a simple isotopic method for measurement of the orthostatic pooling of blood in the legs and orthostatic reduction of the blood content of the temporal region of the head. The subject's erythrocytes were first labeled with a small amount of technetium ([^{99m} Tc]pertechnetate), 2–3 mCi being used (approximately one-tenth the dose used for routine cardiac ventriculography). After an equilibration period of at least 20 min in recumbency, the γ emissions were counted through aluminum or polyethylene "ports," one of which was securely strapped to the lateral aspect of the right midcalf, while the other was glued into a hole in the side of a football helmet worn by the subject, in the area overlying the temporal region of the brain, as detailed by Streeten *et al.* (1985) (see Figs. 61 and 62). The "ports" were machined to fit snugly into the counting end of a scintillation detection probe, containing a $1\frac{1}{4}$-in.

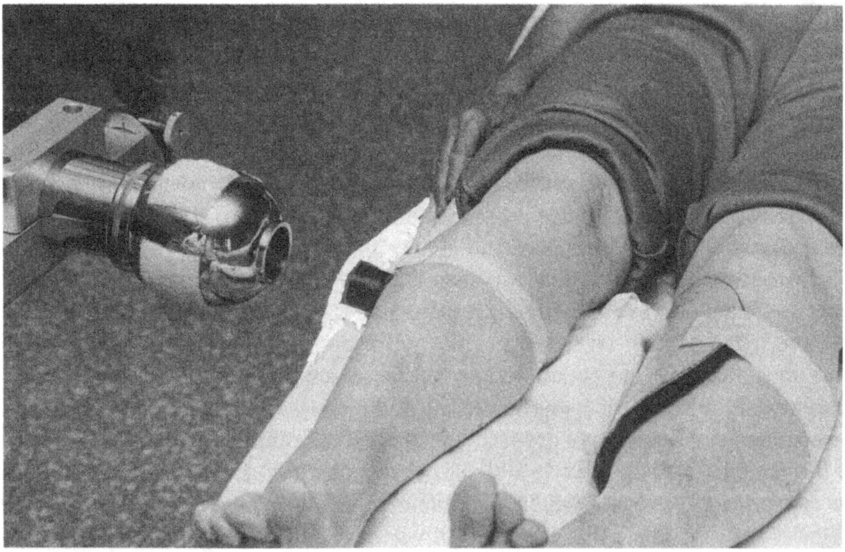

FIGURE 61. Measurement of orthostatic blood pooling in legs. After labeling patient's erythrocytes with [^{99m}Tc]pertechnetate, radioactivity is counted by engaging the port strapped to the leg with the scintillation probe, which is protected from radioactivity emanating from the other leg by the thin lead shield depicted. Repeated counts are made with the subject both recumbent and standing. (From Streeten *et al.*, 1985.)

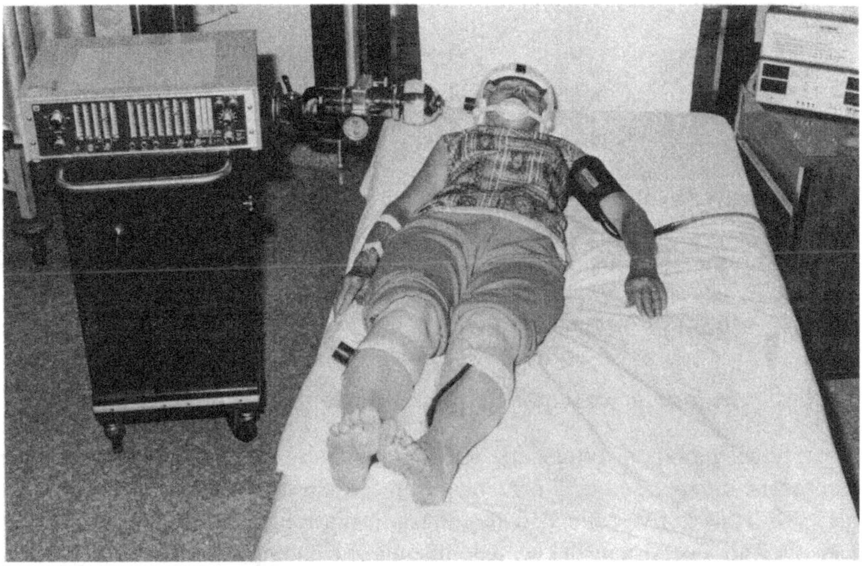

FIGURE 62. Measurement of orthostatic changes in blood content in the head. Counts are performed with the subject both recumbent and standing, through the port glued to the side of a football helmet strapped to the head. (From Streeten *et al.*, 1985.)

(32-mm) iodide crystal. Replicate counts after repeated re-engagements of the scintillation probe with the "ports" showed good reproducibility of the counts, reflected by coefficients of variation of 0.5–3.8% (mean 1.6) in repeated counts over the right calves of each of six subjects, and 0.8–3.4% (mean 1.5) in repeated counts over the right temporal region of the same six subjects. In each determination of gravitational vascular pooling, a series of counts of the radioactivity over the right calf and the right temporal region were made during a 15–20-min period in recumbency and again during about the same period of time in the standing position. The subject then lay down again, and counts were repeated over the calf and the temporal area in the supine posture. Since the isotope used ([^{99m}Tc]pertechnetate) was shown to be at least 94% bound to the erythrocytes, both at the beginning and at the end of the recumbent and the orthostatic measurements, the counts were direct indicators of the numbers of erythrocytes within the segments of the calf and head from which the γ emissions reached the scintillation probe in both postures.

After correcting for isotopic decay, the radioactivity in the leg and in the temporal area during orthostasis was compared with the mean of the radioactivity in these areas during the recumbent periods that preceded and followed the period of standing. The magnitude of orthostatic pooling was expressed as the ratio

$$\frac{\text{Counts in leg while standing}}{\text{Counts in leg while recumbent}} \times 100$$

The same ratio, applied to counts over the head, reflected the effects of gravitational pooling on the amounts of blood contained within the part of the head "seen" by the scintillation probe. Duplicate measurements of the orthostatic changes in blood content of the leg in 15 patients, made within 1 hr of one another, differed by (mean ± SEM) 3.7 ± 1.0%.

7.4.2.4. Orthostatic Vascular Pooling in Patients and Normal Subjects

The magnitude of orthostatic pooling (counts in standing posture/counts in recumbency, expressed as a percentage) in five normal subjects has been compared with that in five patients with orthostatic diastolic hypertension and in three patients with "persistent" (i.e., recumbent and standing) hypertension (Streeten *et al.*, 1985). The results indicated that in normal subjects, the amount of blood in the part of the calf monitored increased within 15 min in the upright posture to 227.4 ± 8.2% ($p < 0.001$) of the amount present in recumbency. This degree of orthostatic pooling was similar to that found in the three patients with "persistent" hypertension (mean 219.3%). In the five patients with orthostatic diastolic hypertension, however, orthostatic pooling was far greater (282.8 ± 14.2%) than in the normal subjects ($p < 0.01$).

These results have now been compared with findings in patients with other types of orthostatic derangements of blood pressure control. The results, depicted in Figure 63, show that the magnitude of orthostatic intravascular pooling (counts standing/counts recumbent, expressed as a percentage) was greater than in six normal subjects (226.0 ± 10.8%), not only in the patients with orthostatic diastolic hypertension, but also in the four patients with orthostatic narrowing of the pulse pressure (patients #76, 89, 117, and 122 in Appendix II), whose orthostatic pooling resulted in an increase in the blood content of the calf in the upright posture to 264.4 ± 11.8% of the recumbent value, a highly significantly greater degree of pooling than in the normal subjects ($p < 0.01$). In view of the described effects of the pressure suit, it was surprising that the degree of orthostatic intravascular pooling in the legs was always within the normal range in the five patients who were classified as having orthostatic tachycardia (mean pooling 232.8 ± 7.4%, not significantly different from the mean in the normal subjects). Whether this indicates that the pressure suit ameliorates orthostatic tachycardia by some mechanism other than reducing peripheral intravascular pooling or that there might be excessive pooling limited to the splanchnic (es-

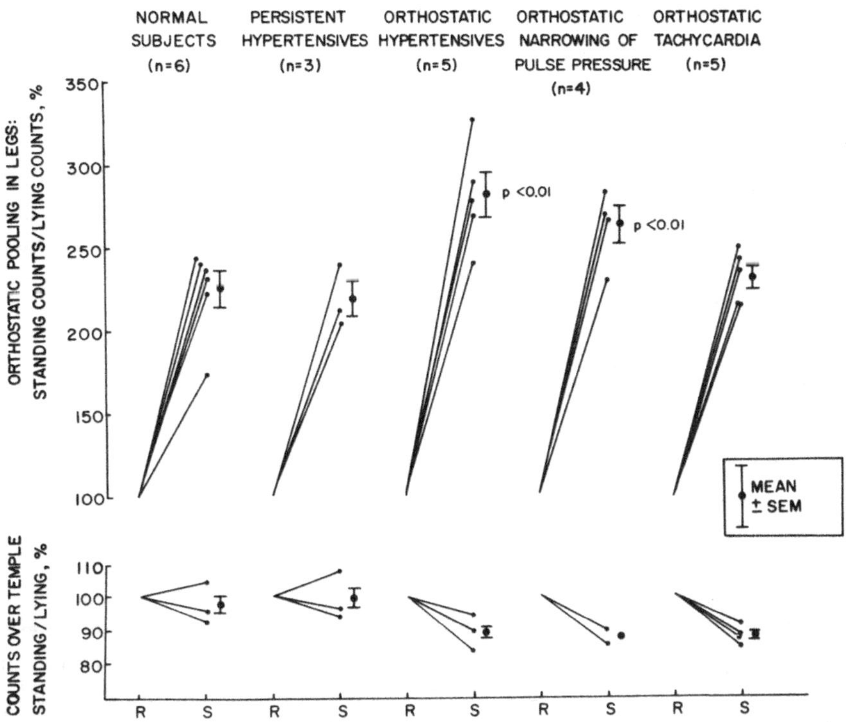

FIGURE 63. Effects of standing on magnitude of venous pooling in the legs and reduction of blood content in the head, in normal subjects and in patients with persistent hypertension, orthostatic hypertension, orthostatic narrowing of the pulse pressure, and orthostatic tachycardia.

pecially the hepatic) circulation in these patients (Hill, 1895; McCuskey, 1966), is unknown.

One patient with severe lightheadedness and other symptoms in the upright posture, but whose orthostatic blood pressure and heart rate changes were usually within the normal range, (patient #147, in Appendix II) had a degree of orthostatic pooling (264.2%) exceeding that in any of the normal subjects. The only patient with autonomic insufficiency we have yet been able to study by this technique showed orthostatic pooling (244%) as high as the highest value seen in our normal subjects (244.5%). This patient had experienced considerable symptomatic improvement and a reduction in the orthostatic fall in blood pressure while standing in an inflated pressure suit, suggesting that the borderline-excessive pooling in his capacitance vessels was contributing to his orthostatic hypotension.

Since venomotor as well as arteriolar responses to posture are lost in autonomic insufficiency (Page *et al.*, 1955; Sharpey-Schafer and Taylor, 1960), it is reasonable to expect that excessive venous pooling would occur in patients with autonomic insufficiency. In one such patient, Bannister *et al.* (1967) showed that lower body suction resulted in excessive increase in the volume of the lower limbs, indicating subnormal venous resistance to gravitational pooling. Weidinger *et al.* (1976) found that the "venous capacity" (i.e., the increase in leg volume induced by venous occlusion) is far larger in patients with "orthostatic dysregulation" than in normal subjects. These findings appear also to indicate the likelihood that the patients would have excessive venous pooling in the upright posture.

7.4.2.5. Correlation between Orthostatic Pooling and Rise in Diastolic Blood Pressure

If gravitational pooling of blood in the dependent parts has any role in the excessive postural rise in diastolic blood pressure seen in so many patients with orthostatic blood pressure derangements, there should be a correlation between these changes. It was previously shown (Streeten *et al.*, 1985) that there is a good correlation between the degree of pooling and the rise in diastolic blood pressure in the upright posture in normotensive individuals and patients with orthostatic hypertension. Figure 64 shows that there is also a highly significant correlation between the magnitude of orthostatic pooling and the rise in diastolic blood pressure, when the relationship between these variables is examined in normal subjects and in patients with orthostatic hypertension, orthostatic narrowing of the pulse pressure, and orthostatic tachycardia. This correlation supports the other evidence that excessive intravascular pooling is the primary abnormality that leads to orthostatic hypertension as well as to orthostatic narrowing of the pulse pressure in these patients.

7.4.2.6. Orthostatic Changes in Blood Contained within the Head

Unfortunately, only very few measurements are available of orthostatic changes in the blood content of the part of the head monitored. However, in the three normal subjects and the two patients with "persistent" hypertension who were studied there was always less than a 10% orthostatic reduction in blood content of the temporal area (mean 1.4 ± 2.3%), whereas two of three patients with orthostatic diastolic hypertension showed more than a 10% reduction (mean of the three patients, 11.5%). In contrast with these minimal and insignificant changes in normal and persistently hypertensive subjects, the patients who had orthostatic disorders of blood pressure control, considered as a single group (i.e., the patients with orthostatic diastolic hypertension, orthostatic narrowing of the

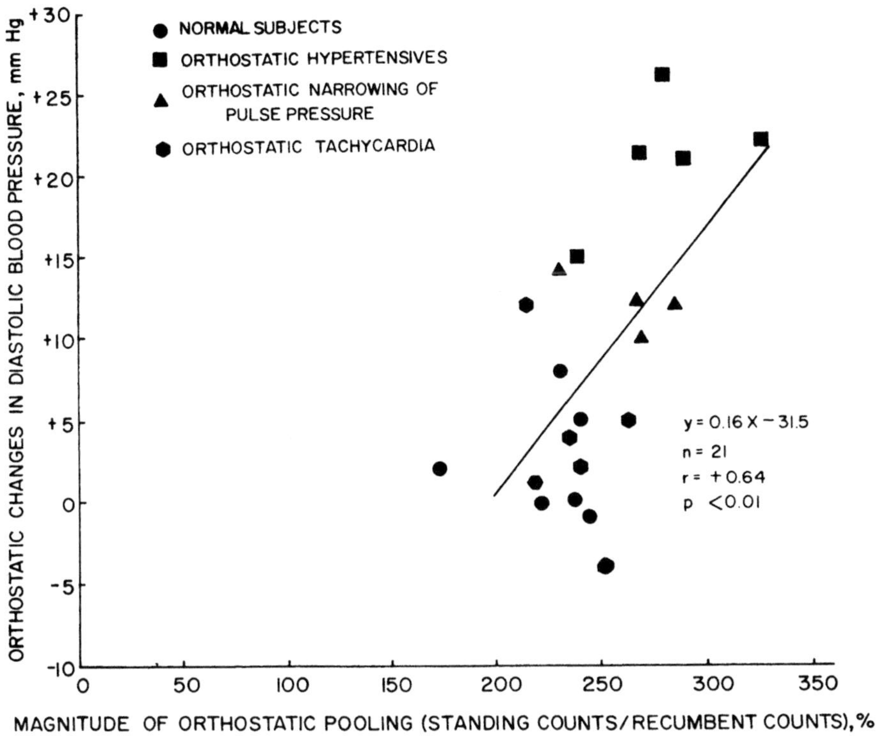

FIGURE 64. Correlation between magnitude of orthostatic blood pooling and orthostatic change in diastolic blood pressure in normal subjects and in patients with orthostatic hypertension, orthostatic narrowing of pulse pressure, and orthostatic tachycardia. The correlation ($r = +0.64$) was significant ($p < 0.01$).

pulse pressure and orthostatic tachycardia) had far greater orthostatic reduction of the blood in the temporal area of the head, *viz.* 12.1 ± 1.2% ($p < 0.01$). The effects of excessive pooling of blood in the capacitance vessels during orthostasis in these patients have been duplicated by the application of negative pressure to the lower body in normal subjects. Johnson *et al.* (1974) showed that as the pressure applied to the lower body became increasingly negative, at −20 to −50 mm Hg, there was a progressive fall in pulse pressure associated with systolic hypotension and/or diastolic hypertension (since mean aortic pressure remained unchanged) and a concomitant rise in heart rate. Thus the orthostatic abnormalities in our patients were reproduced in normal subjects by hypobarically-induced pooling of blood in the lower limbs.

7.4.2.7. Effects of Vasoactive Agents on Intravascular Pooling

After measuring the gravitational pooling of blood in the legs (expressed as standing counts × 100/recumbent counts), we have repeated these determinations during the intravenous infusion, or after the intravenous injection, of various vasoactive drugs in 10 patients with orthostatic derangements of blood pressure control. The results are shown in Figure 65. When infused at rates (4–16 μg/min) sufficient to raise diastolic blood pressure by 5–10 mm Hg in recumbency, norepinephrine reduced orthostatic intravascular pooling from 256.7 to 240.1% ($p < 0.02$), raised systolic blood pressure from 126.5 to 131.6 mm Hg ($p < 0.01$), changed diastolic pressure from 81.8 to 84.2 mm Hg (not significantly), and slowed the heart rate in the standing posture from 117.2 to 107.7 beats/min ($p < 0.02$), all comparisons being made by the *t*-test for paired variables. In spite of raising the standing systolic blood pressure as well, angiotensin II, infused at a rate sufficient to increase diastolic blood pressure (in recumbency) by 13 mm Hg (mean), failed to have significant effects on the diastolic blood pressure, heart rate, or degree of intravascular pooling in the upright posture. Dopamine, infused at 2 μg/kg per min, reduced orthostatic pooling to 244.6% ($p < 0.05$) but actually aggravated orthostatic tachycardia (*p*

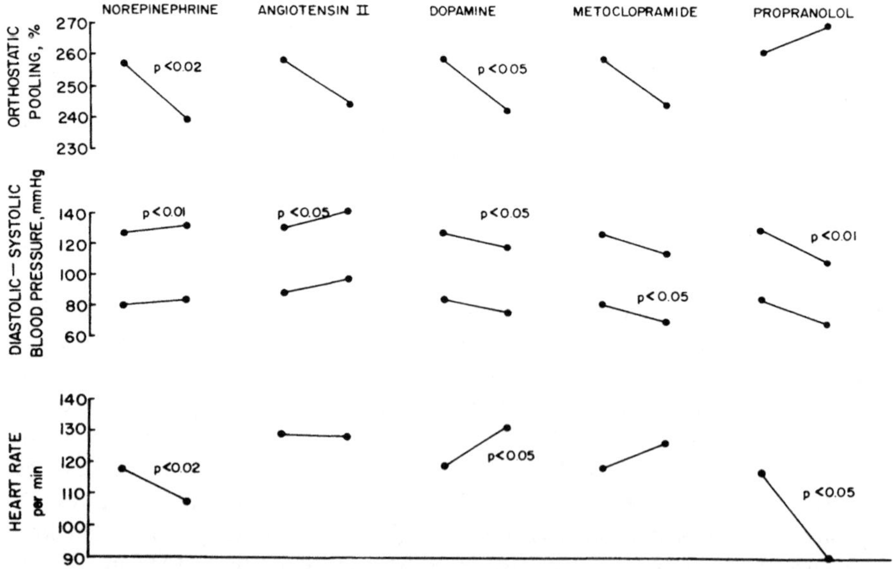

FIGURE 65. Effects of various vasoactive compounds on orthostatic blood pooling in the legs as well as on blood pressure and heart rate. Norepinephrine was the only compound tested that both reduced orthostatic pooling into the normal range and significantly reduced standing heart rate.

< 0.05). Metoclopramide, a dopamine receptor antagonist, had effects paradoxically similar to those of dopamine but not statistically significant. Propranolol reduced systolic blood pressure and heart rate in the upright posture but had no significant effect on pooling in the legs.

It is concluded from these studies that norepinephrine was the most effective agent in both reducing orthostatic intravascular pooling and ameliorating the effects of standing on heart rate, probably by inducing constriction of the veins of the lower limbs. However, none of the agents administered was effective in completely reversing the orthostatic blood pressure derangements. The observations recall the results of studies on forearm veins by Eckstein and Hamilton (1957), which have similar implications. These investigators used plethysmographic and venous pressure measurements to show in normal subjects that intravenous infusions of norepinephrine and (less) epinephrine decreased venous distensibility and increased venous pressure in forearm veins and caused large shifts of blood out of the veins when the forearms were dependent, 14 cm below the level of the atria. The venoconstriction action of infused norepinephrine on the hand veins of human subjects has also been well documented by Collier *et al.* (1972). Gauer and Thron (1962) and Sharpey-Schafer (1963) described venous constriction of the lower limbs in the upright posture, an apparently normal response to orthostasis. The potent vasoconstrictor action of norepinephrine infusion or sciatic nerve stimulation has been shown in the isolated, perfused hindlimb of the dog to result in translocation of 27.3% of the blood out of the hindlimb (Shadle *et al.*, 1958).

7.4.3. Effects of Posture on Cardiac Filling

Orthostatic reduction in cardiac size has long been inferred from observed changes in the radiological silhouette of the heart in both normal and affected subjects. In his early observations of physiological changes in heart size, Moritz (1904) clearly described and depicted the consistent reduction in the cardiac volume during standing. These observations were confirmed by Dietlen (1909), who demonstrated a correlation between orthostatic reduction in cardiac size and generally proportional degrees of tachycardia, reductions in systolic blood pressure, increases in both diastolic and mean blood pressure, and an inferred reduction in cardiac stroke volume. Since the orthostatic decrease in heart size and the increase in heart rate were both reduced by bandaging the legs, Dietlen concluded that pooling of blood (*überfüllung mit Blut*) in the blood vessels of the dependent parts was the probable cause of the orthostatic diminution in the size of the heart.

Laurell (1936) found that the usual normal orthostatic reduction of the roentgenographic silhouette of the heart was considerably exaggerated in patients with "orthostatic arterial anemia," a disorder thought to be associated with excessive reduction of cardiac output in the upright posture. Nylin and Levander (1948) calculated from simple chest radiographs that the volume of the heart of a patient with orthostatic hypotension decreased from 900 ml in recumbency to 640 ml in the standing position. More recently, radioactive tracer techniques have been used to confirm the reduction in thoracic blood volume and in heart size, in the upright posture (Weissler *et al.*, 1959; Holmgren and Ovenfors, 1960).

End-diastolic filling of the heart can now be visualized and quantitated more precisely by radionuclide ventriculography. After labeling autologous erythrocytes with [^{99m}Tc]pertechnetate, radioactivity can be measured over the heart with a scintillation camera. At our hospital, Dr. F. Deaver Thomas has made images and cumulative counts of radioactivity contained within the outline of the left ventricle during end-diastolic and end-systolic phases of every heartbeat, in consecutive 10-min periods both in the reclining and in the standing posture (for technical details, see Streeten *et al.*, 1985).

In a normotensive subject (Table VI), changing from the lying to the standing position caused only slight alterations in end-diastolic volume, stroke volume (expressed as the mean difference between radioactivity in the left ventricle immediately before and after systole, averaged over the 10-min periods of lying and standing) and cardiac output. By contrast, a subject with orthostatic hypertension was found to experience profound orthostatic reductions in cardiac filling (end-diastolic counts integrated over 10 min) and consequently in cardiac output (which fell to 56% of the recumbent value) in the standing posture. The end-diastolic left ventricular volumes during orthostasis in five normotensive patients, calculated by these methods, are compared with those in five patients with

TABLE VI. Effects of Posture on Relative Volume of Left Ventricle in a Patient with Orthostatic Hypertension and a Normal Subject[a]

Posture	Diastolic BP (mm Hg)	End-systolic counts	End-systolic counts	Stroke counts	Stroke counts × heart rate
Orthostatic hypertensive					
Supine	88	21,761	10,210	11,552	716,224
Standing	110	8,544	4,692	3,852	400,608
Standing/Supine (%)	125	39	46	33	56
Normal					
Supine	78	16,281	3,465	12,817	871,556
Standing	80	15,814	2,710	13,105	1,061,505
Standing/Supine (%)	103	97	78	102	122

[a]The [^{99m}Tc]pertechnetate counts over the left ventricle reflect the relative volume of the ventricle at end-diastole and end-systole, from which relative stroke volume and cardiac output, supine and standing, have been calculated.

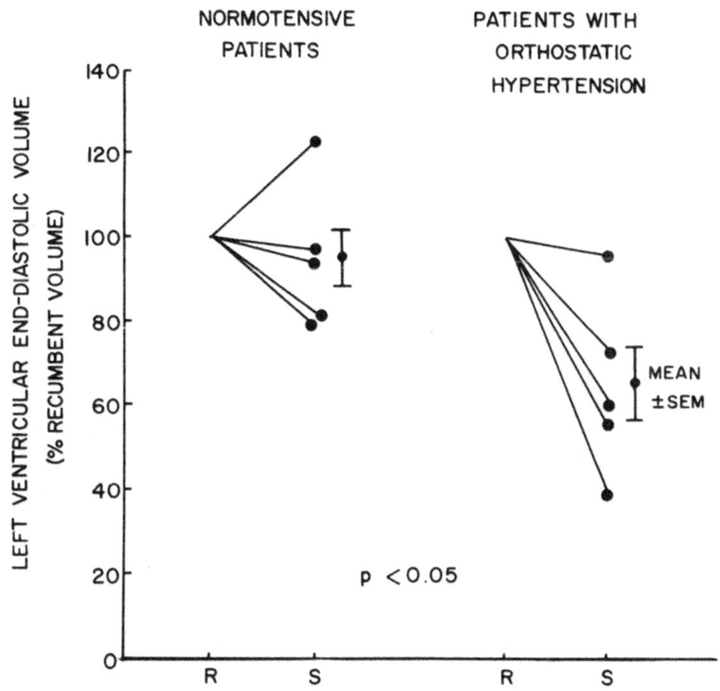

FIGURE 66. Orthostatic change in left ventricular end-diastolic filling is shown in five normal subjects and five patients with orthostatic hypertension.

orthostatic hypertension, in Figure 66. It is evident in the normotensive individuals that mean left ventricular filling was reduced during standing to 95.0 ± 7.0% of the mean recumbent level of filling, while the orthostatic fall in cardiac filling in four out of five patients with orthostatic hypertension was considerably greater, the mean for the entire group being 65.0 ± 8.4% of recumbent values ($p < 0.05$). This evidence indicates that in patients with orthostatic hypertension, cardiac filling is greatly reduced in the upright posture—presumably because of excessive venous pooling—and this abnormality appears to result in an excessive orthostatic fall in cardiac output.

7.4.4. Effects of Posture on Cardiac Output

The implication of the above isotopic data—that in patients with orthostatic hypertension the cardiac output fell excessively in the standing posture—was further explored with the use of a noninvasive respiratory technique of measuring cardiac output (Farhi *et al.*, 1976), by Dr. J. Howland Auchincloss, Jr. With this rebreathing method (described in detail by Streeten *et al.*, 1985), at least five determinations of cardiac output were made with the subject reclining, followed by an approximately equal number of determinations made in the standing position. The cardiac output was found to stabilize after less than 5 min of standing and to change very little thereafter as standing continued for the next 15–30 min. Cardiac output was measured yet another five or six times while the patient stood in an inflated pressure suit.

In the eight normal subjects studied, cardiac output changed very little from the recumbent levels during 15–30 min of standing, provided that the subjects were allowed to move their feet from time to time, as they desired. In the normal subjects, the mean change in cardiac output in the standing posture was a fall of 13.3 ± 3.7% (see Fig. 67), a change very similar to the orthostatic fall of 16% reported by Clements *et al.* (1984) but smaller than the 13–40% mean reduction observed when the beneficial effects of muscular contraction were absent in normal subjects, passively tilted to 60–90° on a tilt table (Naimark and Wasserman, 1962; Matalon and Farhi, 1979; Payen *et al.*, 1982). By contrast, in patients with orthostatic hypertension, orthostatic fall in cardiac output was far greater (mean 27.3 ± 2.9%, $p < 0.01$).

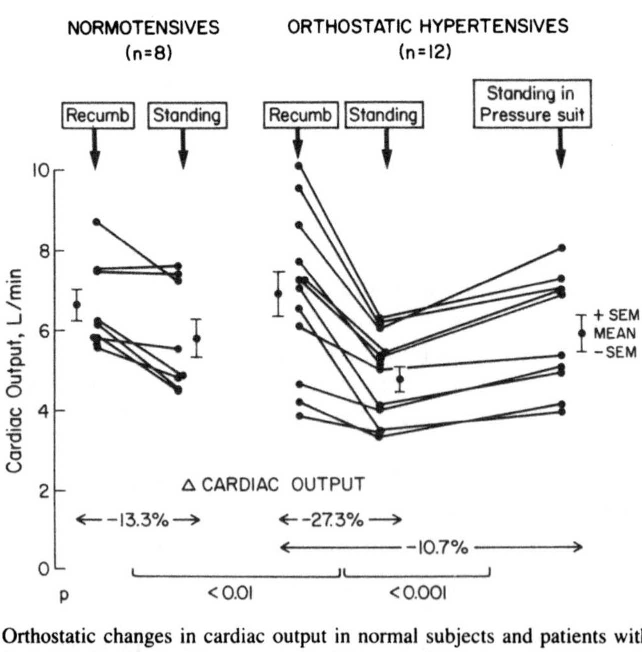

FIGURE 67. Orthostatic changes in cardiac output in normal subjects and patients with orthostatic hypertension (in deflated and inflated pressure suit). The excessive orthostatic fall in cardiac output in the patients with orthostatic hypertension was corrected to within the normal range by inflation of the suit. (From Streeten *et al.*, 1985.)

In the 10 patients in whom cardiac output was measured again while standing in the inflated pressure suit, cardiac output was found to be only 10.7 ± 4.3% below initial recumbent levels. Since this change was now no longer significantly different from the orthostatic change in the normal subjects, it was concluded that the abnormally large fall in cardiac output in the upright posture in patients with orthostatic hypertension resulted from a disorder that could be completely overcome with external compression—presumably excessive intravascular pooling of blood in the dependent parts. This conclusion is in good agreement with the demonstration by Naimark and Wasserman (1962) in normal subjects that orthostatic reduction in stroke volume and cardiac output during tilting (head up) to 60°, could be prevented by minimizing the associated shifts of blood volume into the lower limbs. Excessive reduction of cardiac output in the upright posture has been described previously in patients with orthostatic arterial anemia (Bjure and Laurell, 1927), in two patients with orthostatic hypotension (Brehm, 1955), in a group of patients with persistent hypertension, yet with an excessive rise in diastolic pressure during head-up tilt (Frohlich *et al.*, 1967), in three patients with orthostatic hypotension of the "sympathicotonic" type (Glezer *et al.*, 1972), and in four patients with Shy–Drager syndrome (Chokroverty *et al.*, 1969). Saline infusion substantially reduced the orthostatic reduction in cardiac output in the patients with autonomic insufficiency (Chokroverty *et al.*, 1969). The possibility that orthostatic reduction in cardiac output might be the result (and not the cause) of the increased diastolic blood pressure seems unlikely both because this mechanism is far less potent than reduced venous return in decreasing cardiac output (Guyton *et al.*, 1959), and because the beneficial effect of the pressure suit would be hard to interpret as being mediated by reduction in afterload rather than by increase in preload.

The correlation between the orthostatic fall in cardiac output and the orthostatic rise in diastolic pressure in the group of normal subjects and patients with orthostatic hypertension studied ($r = -0.52$) fell just short of accepted levels of statistical significance ($0.1 < p > 0.05$). Unfortunately, we have measured the changes in cardiac output in only four patients with other orthostatic derangements of blood pressure control. In these patients, cardiac output showed an orthostatic fall of 21.8 ± 6.8%, which was reduced to 5.0 ± 8.6% when the measurements were repeated while the patients were standing in an inflated pressure suit. Thus, the responses of these patients to the upright posture were very similar to those of the patients with orthostatic hypertension.

7.4.5. Postural Changes in Plasma Norepinephrine Concentration

The combination of excessive orthostatic increases in diastolic blood pressure and heart rate in patients with most of the orthostatic blood pressure disorders we have been discussing suggested the likelihood that an unusually marked stimulation of the sympathetic nervous system was taking place when these patients were on their feet. Although plasma concentrations of norepinephrine are not an infallible guide to the presence or severity of a sympathetic discharge, there is little doubt that an acute increase in plasma norepinephrine concentration usually accompanies and results from increased activation of the sympathetic nervous system in man. Moreover, the change from recumbency to standing is well known to be associated invariably with an increase in plasma norepinephrine concentration in healthy persons, and the magnitude of this normal change has been defined by several investigators (Eide *et al.*, 1978) (see also Chapter 1). We therefore measured plasma norepinephrine concentrations in our patients both after they had been lying down for at least 30–45 min and after standing for 5, 10, 15, 30, and 60 min. We have reported (Streeten *et al.*, 1985) that the orthostatic rise in plasma norepinephrine concentration at these times is significantly greater in patients with orthostatic hypertension than in normal subjects (Fig. 68).

We have subsequently found that the orthostatic rise in plasma norepinephrine concentration was significantly greater than the normal rise in patients with orthostatic narrowing of the pulse pressure, orthostatic systolic hypotension and orthostatic tachycardia, as well as in patients with orthostatic hypertension. This excessive catecholamine discharge appeared to be a specific response to the gravitational stimulus, since, at least in the patients with orthostatic hypertension, the responses to such other physiological stimuli to the sympathetic nervous system as sustained, isometric muscle contraction and the cold pressor test were not exaggerated (Streeten *et al.*, 1985). It therefore seems likely that the excessive sympathetic discharge that follows assumption and maintenance of the upright posture in these patients with orthostatic blood pressure disorders, results from an appropriate response to an excessively strong orthostatic stimulus rather than from a nonspecific or a primary overresponse of the sympathetic nervous system. To establish the correctness of this interpretation, however, will require demonstration that overcoming the abnormally large orthostatic pooling by means of external pressure will also reduce the rise in plasma norepinephrine concentration into or below the normal range. These studies are in progress.

The finding of excessive orthostatic increases in plasma norepinephrine concentration in patients with the described orthostatic disorders is in good agreement with the observations of Rosen and Cryer (1982), who reported a supranormal orthostatic rise in plasma norepinephrine concentration in a patient with orthostatic tachycardia, orthostatic systolic hypotension, and orthostatic narrowing of the pulse pressure. Rosen and Cryer expressed the opinion, and we would agree, that their patient was similar to our patients with hyperbradykininism (Streeten *et al.*, 1972).

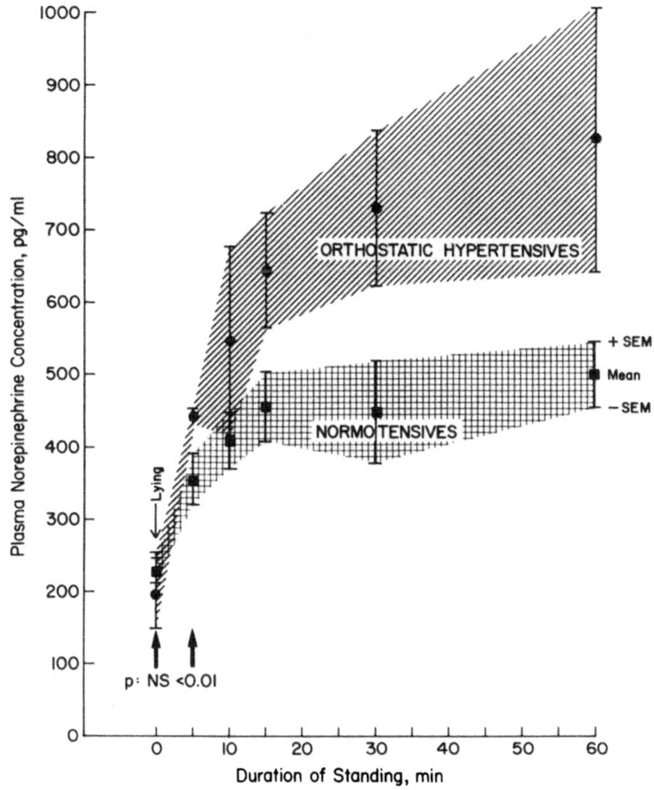

FIGURE 68. Plasma norepinephrine concentrations both recumbent and after standing for up to 60 min, in groups of normotensive and orthostatic hypertensive individuals. The differences between the two groups was significant ($p < 0.01$) from the first 5 min of standing. (From Streeten *et al.*, 1985.)

7.4.6. Blood Kinin Concentration

In 1972, we described the syndrome of hyperbradykininism (Streeten *et al.*, 1972) in five patients who presented with orthostatic lightheadedness, purple discoloration of the legs in the upright posture, a tendency to facial erythema or flushes, especially in recumbency, and characteristic orthostatic blood pressure and heart rate changes, which included an excessive fall in pulse pressure and rise in heart rate (Fig. 69). The role of bradykinin was supported by the findings that (1) blood concentrations of bioassayable bradykinin were frequently, but not invariably, elevated (Fig. 70), and (2) a significant correlation existed between the blood bradykinin concentration and the severity of the orthostatic tachycardia

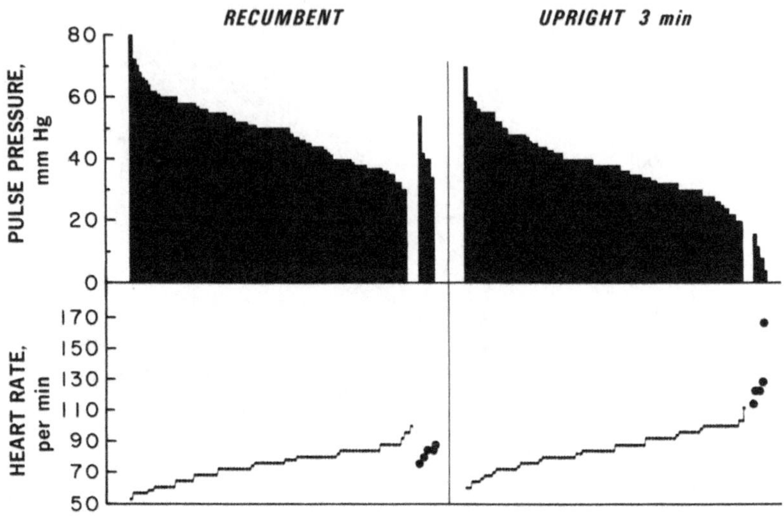

FIGURE 69. Orthostatic changes in pulse pressure and heart rate in five patients with hyperbradykininism compared with measurements in 92 normal subjects.

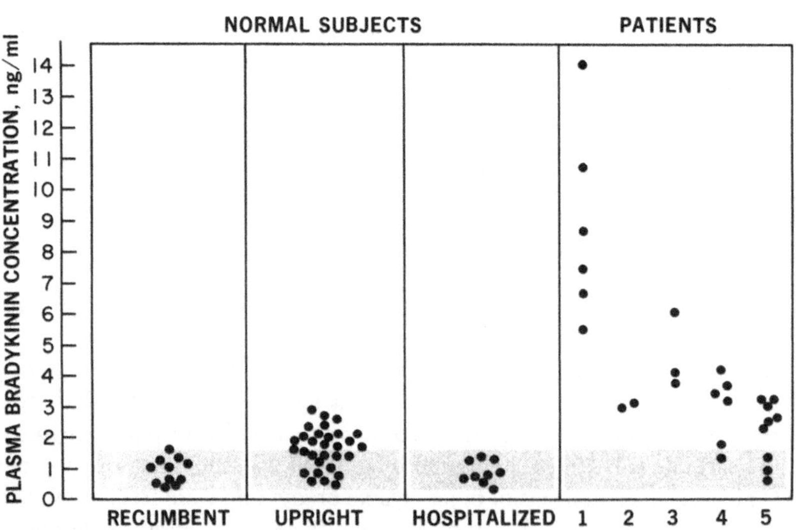

FIGURE 70. Blood bradykinin concentration, measured by bioassay, in normal subjects, hospital controls, and patients with hyperbradykininism. (From Streeten *et al.*, 1972.)

and shrinkage in pulse pressure, as measured at the time of the blood sampling (Fig. 71). The elevated levels of bradykinin in the blood appeared to result from subnormal concentrations of circulating bradykininase I, which were found to be present (Fig. 72), at least in the members of one of the families in whom the disorder was detected (Fig. 73).

Bradykininase I was measured by its esterolytic action on hippuryl-L-lysine. The bradykininase I deficiency detected by this method was confirmed by finding a subnormal rate of degradation, *in vitro,* of authentic bradykinin by plasma obtained from two of the patients, in comparison with the action of plasma from two normal subjects. Since plasma kallikreinogen concentrations were normal in all patients studied, it was thought unlikely that excessive production was as important as subnormal degradation of endogenous bradykinin in the pathogenesis of the disorder. In a subsequent article, (Streeten, 1976) elevated blood bradykinin concentrations were reported in another 10 patients who also presented with the symptoms of hyperbradykininism.

During the intervening years, thanks to the development by Dr. Theodore Dalakos of an antibody to bradykinin, we have been able to use RIA for the study of patients with hyperbradykininism, as well as of several patients with the

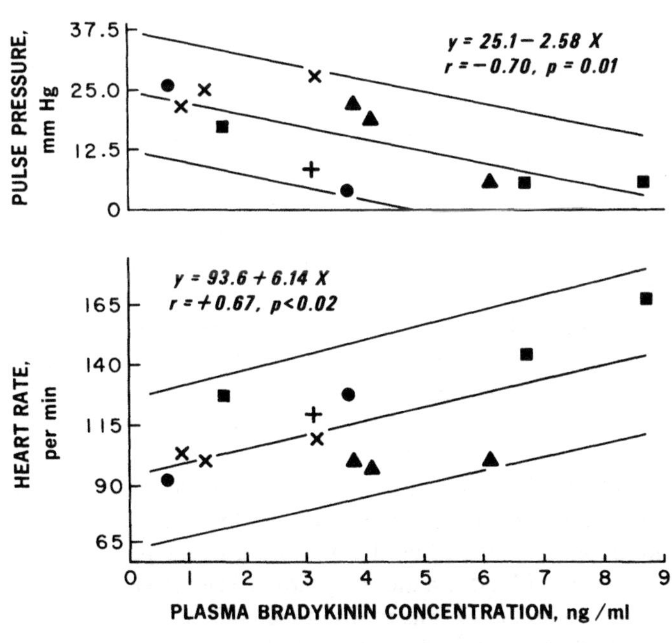

FIGURE 71. Correlations between plasma bradykinin concentrations and pulse pressures and heart rates in five patients with hyperbradykininism while standing. Both regressions are shown together with their 95% confidence limits. (From Streeten *et al.*, 1972.)

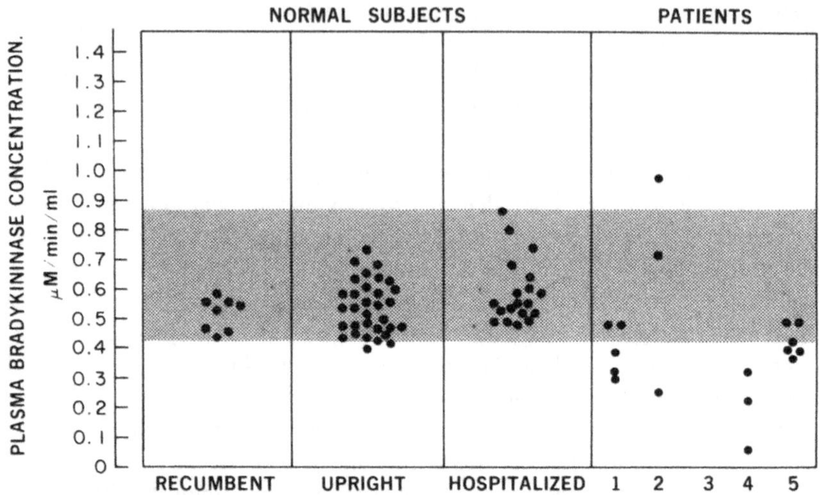

FIGURE 72. Plasma bradykininase I concentrations in normal subjects, hospital controls, and four patients with hyperbradykininism. The stippled area encloses the range of values in the normal and hospitalized control subjects. (From Streeten *et al.*, 1972.)

different varieties of the pooling syndrome described in this chapter. Since the antibody has been found to have 100% cross-reactivity with kallidin, our RIA results should correctly be described as measurements of blood kinin concentrations. We have found that several of the patients displaying clinical features of hyperbradykininism have had elevated blood concentrations of kinins by RIA. These findings appear to provide strong support for the evidence derived from entirely independent bioassay measurements, that blood concentrations of bradykinin and/or kallidin are raised in many cases. At least one, and frequently several, elevated blood kinin concentrations have been found in many patients who presented with the described variants of the venous pooling syndrome. Thus, as can be seen in Appendix II, blood kinin concentration was raised above the upper limits of normal (i.e., above 0.5 ng/ml) and/or plasma bradykininase I concentration was low (below 0.4 μmoles/ml-min) in seven of the 19 patients with orthostatic systolic hypotension who did not have hypoaldosteronism, in two of the 24 patients with orthostatic diastolic hypertension, in 25 of the 50 patients who presented with orthostatic narrowing of the pulse pressure, and in six of the 15 patients with orthostatic tachycardia. The blood kinin measurements by RIA in patients with the various forms of the pooling syndrome are compared with those in 12 subjects who had no demonstrable abnormality of blood pressure control in the erect posture, in Figure 74. Kinin assays could not be performed on all patients. It is evident, however, that elevated blood kinin levels and/or subnormal bradykininase I concentrations have been common findings among the patients with the various forms of the pooling syndrome. This evidence further strengthens the view that all these patients may represent variations of a common pooling disorder, in the pathogenesis of which excessive blood levels of kinin may play an important role, perhaps by stimulating prostaglandin formation (Roscher *et al.*, 1984). Unfortunately, no specific antagonist of the kinins is available for clinical study or therapeutic use. It is therefore impossible to demonstrate conclusively that kinin excess is the cause of the pooling in many of these patients, and impossible to investigate the potential effectiveness of treatment with such an antagonist in the patients.

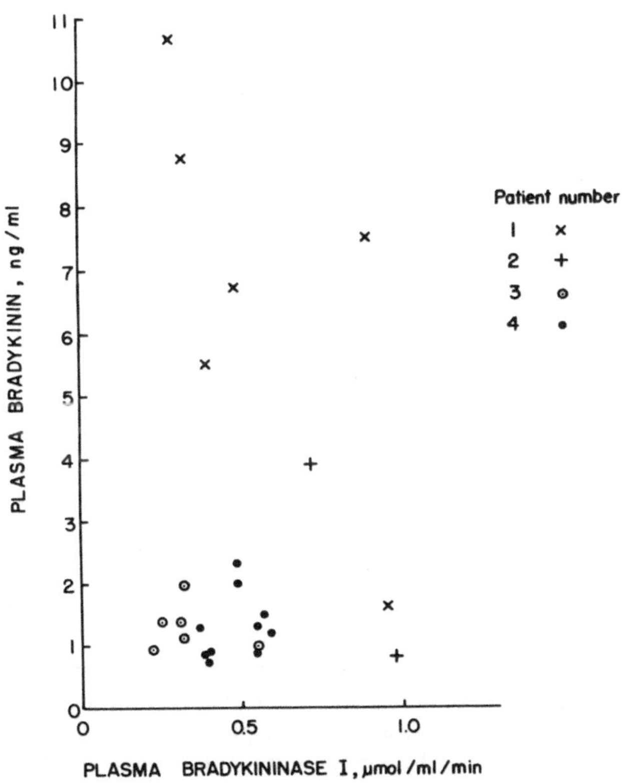

FIGURE 73. Relationship between plasma bradykininase and bioassayable bradykinin concentrations in four patients with hyperbradykininism. An inverse correlation between these variables in two members of the same family (mother and daughter, data depicted by × and +) implied the likelihood of a causal relationship between these variables. (From Streeten *et al.*, 1972.)

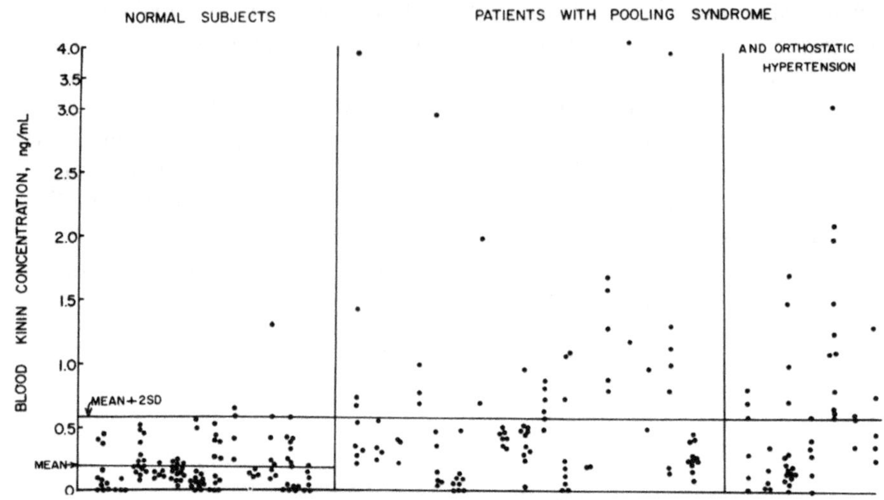

FIGURE 74. Blood kinin concentrations measured on several occasions by radioimmunoassay in patients with various forms of the pooling syndrome and in 12 control subjects without blood pressure abnormalities.

7.4.7. Potential Role of Insulin

Miles and Hayter (1968) showed that insulin administration, even before it causes a measurable fall in plasma glucose concentration, results in orthostatic hypotension and tachycardia, both of which are greatly exaggerated in the presence of reflex baroreceptor failure. Whether excessive endogenous release of insulin might contribute to orthostatic hypotension in some patients is unknown.

7.5. CONCLUSIONS

1. *Failure of the autonomic nervous reflex:* At some or several sites this is almost always responsible for the consistent drop in diastolic blood pressure when it is associated with failure of the heart rate to rise in the standing (or sitting) posture. This can be confirmed without difficulty by demonstrating that the plasma norepinephrine concentration fails to increase appropriately in the upright posture. The many possible types and sites of lesions that might cause such autonomic insufficiency have been described.
2. *Idiopathic orthostatic hypotension:* This may be the problem in patients whose diastolic blood pressure consistently falls by 10 mm Hg or more

in the upright posture but whose heart rate rises appropriately; it may conceivably be due to a defect limited to the efferent sympathetic supply to the peripheral arterioles and without involvement of cardiac innervation.

3. *Orthostatic diastolic hypertension:* Although this may have several possible causes, including excessive sympathetic nervous system responses to a variety of stimuli (Sapru *et al.*, 1979) and nephroptosis (McCann *et al.*, 1940; Clorius *et al.*, 1978), sometimes with excessive orthostatic renin release (Takada *et al.*, 1984), there is little doubt that it frequently results from excessive intravascular pooling in the upright posture.
4. *Orthostatic systolic hypotension:* This can probably result from hypovolemia in hypoaldosteronism and states of sodium depletion. When it is idiopathic, however, it appears to represent another form of response to excessive orthostatic pooling and reduced venous return (see MacLean *et al.*, 1944), with or without the associated abnormalities described in 3, 5, or 6.
5. *Orthostatic narrowing of the pulse pressure:* When not caused by plasma hypovolemia or hypocortisolism, this is the end result of a pathogenetic sequence that begins with excessive gravitational pooling; it is very similar to changes that lead either to orthostatic hypertension or to orthostatic systolic hypotension.
6. *Orthostatic tachycardia:* This usually accompanies 3, 4, and 5, but it may occur alone. It, too, may represent a response to hypovolemia, to hypocortisolism or, as MacLean *et al.* (1940, 1944) recognized, to excessive intravascular pooling in the upright posture.

Thus, although disorders 3–6 may have other causes and pathogenetic mechanisms, there is strong evidence that they may coexist in the same patient at the same time or at different times and may all result from excessive pooling of blood within the capacitance vessels, in the upright posture. It might be reasonable, therefore, to refer to disorders 3–6 as *venous pooling syndromes,* when they have been shown not to result from low blood volume or deficiency of cortisol or aldosterone. The excessive gravitational pooling appears to reflect abnormal dilatation or diminished contractility of the veins or venules. This, in turn, might result from an intrinsic or neurogenic disorder of venous function or from the effects of a circulating vasodilator. The evidence implicating hyperbradykininism has been described above, but it is likely that other vasodilators such as histamine and some of the prostaglandins may be responsible for the venous dilatation and excessive intravascular pooling in at least some of these patients. These possibilities are supported by the observations reported by Åkesson (1946), who showed that histamine injections in normal subjects result in orthostatic reduction in systolic blood pressure, elevation in diastolic pressure, and narrowing of pulse pressure, together with orthostatic tachycardia and palpitations. Roberts and colleagues at Vanderbilt University showed that excessive amounts of vasodilators (probably histamine and prostaglandin D_2) released from the mast cells in systemic mastocytosis may give rise to a similar group of symptoms (Roberts *et al.*, 1982; Turk *et al.*, 1983; Roberts, 1984). These are clearly very important findings. However, much work is needed before the cause of the excessive vasodilatation can be precisely identified in all these patients.

Since excessive gravitational pooling has been shown to reduce end-diastolic filling of the left ventricle, it is likely to decrease filling of the atria as well. This possibility is supported by the experiments of Johnson *et al.* (1974) showing that pooling of blood in the lower parts of the body, induced by negative pressure, does indeed reduce atrial pressure in normal subjects. Reduced distention of the atria would be expected, through decreased firing of the type B volume receptors in the atria (Coleridge *et al.*, 1963, 1964; Pelletier *et al.*, 1973) and in the pulmonary circulation (Ledsome and Linden, 1964, 1967; Kappagoda *et al.*, 1972; Linden, 1973) to initiate excessive sympathetic activity *via* the vagal afferent and sympathetic efferent fibers mediating this reflex. Intravascular blood pooling in the lower limbs, induced by the application of negative pressure (−40 mm Hg) to the lower parts of the body, has been shown to induce arteriolar constriction and reduced blood flow to the arms, without a fall in systemic blood pressure, through sympathetic stimulation mediated by the same cardiopulmonary low-pressure receptors (Zoller *et al.*, 1972; Rowell *et al.*, 1973). In patients with borderline hypertension (with blood pressures intermittently above 150/90 in the recumbent or the upright posture, on three separate occasions, Mark and Kerber (1982) showed that lower-body negative pressure increased forearm vascular resistance more than in normal subjects. Since their borderline hypertensive and normotensive subjects showed identical responses to the cold pressor test, these investigators concluded that there was an excessive tonic inhibitory influence of the cardiopulmonary baroreceptors in the borderline hypertensive patients.

It is evident that the pathophysiology of borderline hypertension and of orthostatic hypertension is strikingly alike, and we wonder whether the blood pressure elevations in some patients with borderline hypertension might be predominantly or exclusively orthostatic. This conclusion is strongly supported by the work of Hull *et al.* (1977), who showed that the only feature that consistently separated their findings in patients with borderline hypertension from those in normotensive subjects was that diastolic blood pressure rose significantly more (13 vs. 6 mm Hg, $p < 0.01$) at 70° tilt or on static standing, and exceeded 90 mm Hg during tilting in 15 of 21 borderline hypertensive subjects and in none of the normotensive individuals. Safar *et al.* (1973) found in borderline hypertensive patients, that peripheral vascular resistance was abnormally elevated only during upright tilt and exercise in patients with high cardiac index. Lower-body suction also causes splanchnic vasoconstriction mediated either by the same cardiopulmonary receptors (Johnson *et al.*, 1974) or by the high-pressure carotid baroreceptors (Abboud *et al.*, 1979).

Hemodynamic abnormalities were reported by Brehm (1955) to be very similar to those described above in patients with various types of orthostatic lability. In three patients who conform, respectively, to our definitions of orthostatic hypertension (with orthostatic tachycardia), idiopathic orthostatic diastolic hypotension (with orthostatic tachycardia), and autonomic insufficiency resulting from lumbosacral sympathectomy (also with orthostatic tachycardia), there was always a striking reduction in stroke volume and cardiac output (per minute), associated (in the first two patients) with a tremendous orthostatic rise

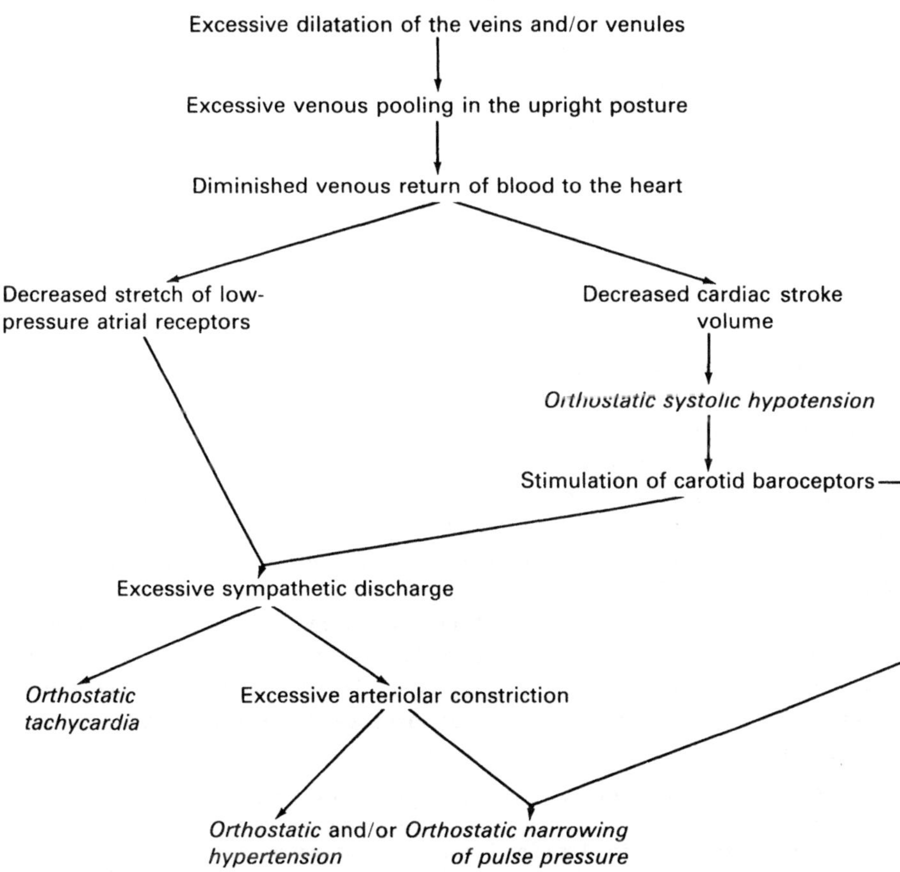

FIGURE 75. Pathogenesis of the venous pooling system.

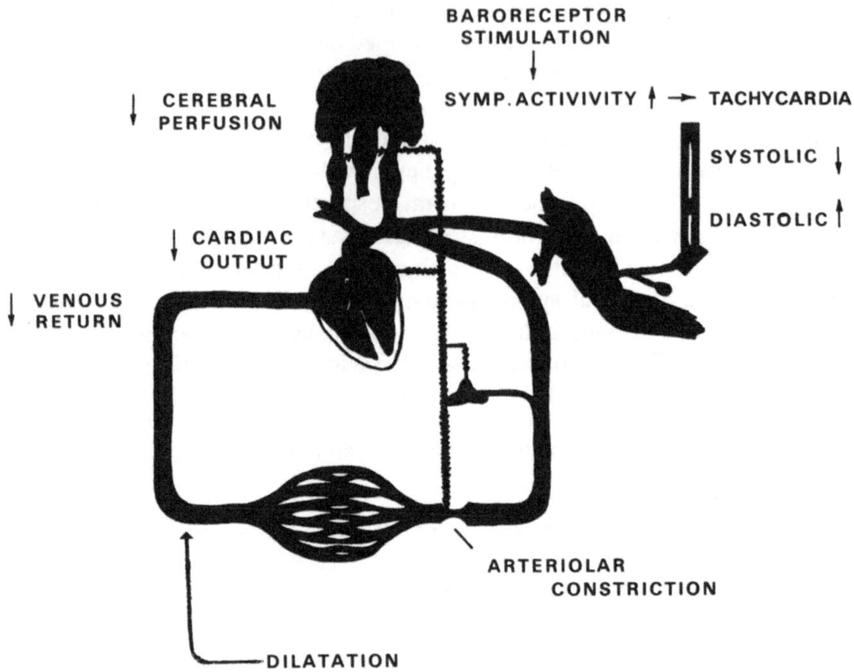

FIGURE 76. Schematic depiction of the apparent pathogenesis of the venous pooling syndrome.

in systemic vascular resistance. Brehm attributed the orthostatic abnormalities in all three patients to venous pooling and subnormal venous return of blood to the heart "*Die Ursache ist vielmehr in einem verringerten venösen Blutangebot zum Herzen zu suchen.*" Brehm concluded that the three patients all had "orthostatic circulatory weakness" with differing degrees of severity. The results derived from our data accord very well with Brehm's view.

The pathogenesis of the venous pooling syndromes is summarized in Figure 75 (see also Figure 76).

It is of some interest to note that these syndromes appear to result from a pathologically excessive venous pooling that induces appropriately excessive physiological responses of the normal type. These conclusions were foreshadowed as long ago as 1905, when Erlanger and Hooker concluded that, in normal subjects

> The changes of the circulatory conditions when the erect posture is assumed are induced mainly by the action of gravity . . . [and are probably elicited by] bleeding into the lower extremities. The effect is compensated presumably by peripheral constriction and by an increase in the energy of the heart. Immersion of the body in the erect posture in water of a comfortable temperature and compression of the legs while

in the standing posture result in the production of circulatory conditions that resemble those that obtain when the body is in the recumbent posture.

7.6. SUMMARY

The known causes and pathogenetic mechanisms of autonomic insufficiency are described. The many other disorders that may give rise to abnormal orthostatic blood pressure changes of the types described in Chapter 6 include pheochromocytoma, hypocortisolism, hypovolemia from blood loss or dehydration, cardiac dysfunction of various types, debility and inactivity, transient increases in intrathoracic pressure, excessive orthostatic pooling of blood in the dependent parts of the body, and idiopathic causes. Evidence from the literature shows that as blood volume was progressively reduced by venesection in normal human subjects, orthostasis resulted in gradual increases in heart rate and diastolic blood pressure, together with decreases in systolic pressure and pulse pressure. However, when the volume of blood removed exceeded 14 ml/kg, there was a precipitous fall in systolic and diastolic blood pressures in the upright posture. Thus, as the magnitude of induced hypovolemia increased, the subjects experienced orthostatic tachycardia, orthostatic systolic hypotension, orthostatic narrowing of the pulse pressure, and a tendency toward orthostatic diastolic hypertension, before severe hypovolemia caused profound orthostatic systolic and diastolic hypotension.

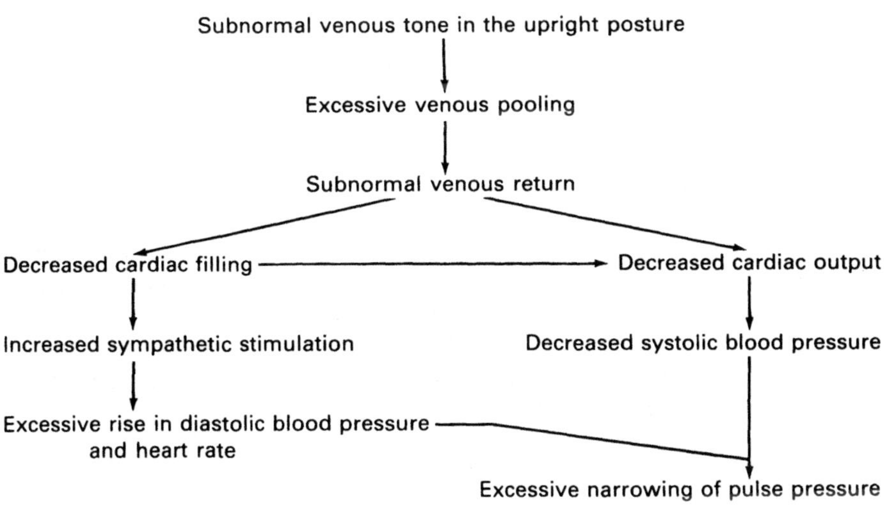

FIGURE 77. Summary of the pathogenesis of the venous pooling syndrome.

In several of our patients with spontaneous orthostatic disorders of blood pressure control, we have measured the effects of acute hypovolemia resulting from furosemide-induced diuresis, followed by acute hypervolemia induced by rapid intravenous saline infusions in the sitting position. In general, the diuresis resulted in a fall in systolic blood pressure, a rise in diastolic pressure, narrowing of the pulse pressure, and acceleration of the heartbeat, whereas the saline infusion reversed all these changes. To determine whether excessive orthostatic pooling of blood in the lower limbs, by reducing venous return of blood to the heart, might be responsible for the spontaneous orthostatic abnormalities seen in these patients, the responses to external pressure have been tested by means of a pressure suit (MAST suit). In all types of orthostatic blood pressure disorders, the inflated MAST suit ameliorated or completely corrected the orthostatic abnormalities.

The magnitude of orthostatic pooling has been measured by direct external counting of [^{99m}Tc]pertechnetate-labeled autologous blood, in groups of patients with orthostatic blood pressure disorders. Except in patients who had only orthostatic tachycardia, orthostatic blood pooling has been shown to be excessive in all groups of patients and to be significantly correlated with the orthostatic rise in diastolic blood pressure.

Norepinephrine infusions were found to reduce the orthostatic pooling toward the normal range in these patients. In some of the same subjects, scintillation counting over the heart showed that orthostasis led to an excessive reduction in the amount of blood within the left ventricle. This was presumably the reason for the significant drop in cardiac output in the upright posture, a change largely corrected by the inflated MAST suit in these patients. Excessive orthostatic reduction in atrial distention resulting from decreased venous return presumably triggered the excessive orthostatic rise in plasma norepinephrine concentration *via* low-pressure volume receptors in the heart. Since all groups of patients responded similarly to these procedures, it seems likely that they all represent slightly different forms of abnormal blood pressure and heart rate responses to excessive orthostatic pooling of blood.

It is concluded that the pathogenesis of these various forms of the venous pooling syndrome is as shown in Figure 77. Why venous tone is apparently subnormal in these patients is still unknown. Whether their veins are inadequately provided with α_2-adrenergic receptors to respond to the norepinephrine released into their blood or whether the dilatation of their capacitance vessels results from the excess of circulating kinins often shown in our assays to be present is still unclear and awaits further study.

8

ORTHOSTATIC DISORDERS OF BLOOD PRESSURE CONTROL

Clinical Features

8.1. FREQUENCY OF MAIN SYMPTOMS

Almost all the symptoms and signs attributable to the orthostatic disorders of blood pressure control appear to be the consequence of reduced cerebral blood flow. Blood flow to the brain is presumably reduced by the excessive orthostatic fall in blood pressure or diminution of cardiac output and the inadequacy of compensatory cerebral autoregulation. The chief symptoms reported by 159 patients are listed among the details of each subject in Appendix II. The frequency with which each of the main symptoms was elicited is shown in Table VII.

Additional symptoms and signs, not listed in Table VII, include dull chest pain that occurs usually in the upright posture (8.0%), mitral valve prolapse diagnosed clinically and confirmed by echocardiography (8.0%), diabetes mellitus (6.0%), dyspnea in the erect posture (5.3%), and severe sleepiness (4%); smaller numbers of patients (almost all with autonomic insufficiency) had features of parkinsonism (4.7%) as well as impotence (3.3%) and incontinence (2.7%).

8.2. INTRACRANIAL FEATURES

8.2.1. Lightheadedness and Blurred Vision

Lightheadedness was the presenting symptom in most patients in all groups, except among those with orthostatic hypertension, a large number of whom were

TABLE VII. Frequency of Primary Symptoms in Patients with Orthostatic Blood Pressure Disturbances

Symptom/sign	Prevalence (%)			
	Autonomic insufficiency (N = 19)	Idiopathic orthostatic hypotension (N = 9)	"Pooling syndrome" (N = 123)	Total prevalence (N = 151)
Lightheadedness	100	78	77	80.7
Headaches	5	44	41	37.3
Weakness	26	22	37	35.3
Fatigue	5	0	39	32.7
Syncope	58	11	29	32.0
Palpitations	0	0	23	18.7
Blurred vision	16	22	14	14.7
Flushing	0	11	16	14.0
Excessive sweating	0	22	15	13.3
Nausea	0	0	14	11.1
Aggravation by heat	5	0	13	11.1
Edema	21	0	10	10.7
Impaired thinking	0	11	11	10.0

referred because of the finding of a blood pressure over 90 mm Hg, invariably measured in the sitting position, by their own physicians.

Lightheadedness was variously described as giddiness, dizziness, "wooziness," and a feeling of an impending fainting spell. Further inquiry almost always revealed limitation of these symptoms to times when the patient was sitting or, more commonly, standing, especially if the individual was required to stand still for more than a few minutes, as in church services, standing in line for admission to movies or to pay for purchases in supermarkets, and standing at attention in parades. A sense of rotation or true vertigo seldom occurred. Blurring of vision, "graying out" and a sense of impending syncope were common. Many of our patients were also greatly troubled by impaired mental capacity and of consequent inability to think clearly and to do work adequately in the upright posture. For example, one young man had a frustrating inability to obtain a passing grade in his chemistry laboratory courses in spite of consistent A grades in theoretical chemistry.

8.2.1.1. Transient Lightheadedness

In questioning patients about lightheadedness it is important to rule out those symptoms that are limited to a momentary sensation of giddiness during the first few seconds after changing from the supine or sitting position to the standing posture. Such symptoms presumably result from the very brief fall in blood pressure that has been shown by continuous intra-arterial recordings of the blood pressure to occur in healthy subjects immediately after assuming the standing position (Green *et al.*, 1948; Borst *et al.*, 1984) (see Chapter 6). These transient blood pressure changes and the symptoms they cause probably result from the time lag between sudden changes in posture and effective arteriolar constriction *via* the baroceptor reflex. The symptoms are so common as to be considered a "normal" phenomenon. In contrast to these "normal" symptoms, complaints in patients with orthostatic derangements of blood pressure control become gradually or rapidly more severe as the patients continue to stand still.

a. *Effects of Exercise on Lightheadedness.* Walking about will frequently tend to diminish the lightheadedness in those in whom the disorder is mild but makes little difference in many patients who are more severely affected. Some patients, especially those with autonomic insufficiency, report that exercise, particularly strenuous physical labor or sporting activity, aggravates their symptoms considerably (Stead and Ebert, 1941).

Bannister (1983) characterized the orthostatic symptoms of patients with autonomic insufficiency; his excellent description applies equally to the complaints of many patients with other orthostatic disorders of blood pressure control:

> The postural attacks may be 'drop' attacks resembling sudden brainstem vascular dysfunction, but more commonly there is a gradual fading of consciousness over half a minute or so while the patient is standing or walking. A neckache radiating to the occipital region of the skull and shoulders, often precedes actual loss of consciousness. Sometimes there are transient visual disturbances, scotomata, positive hallucinations, or tunnel vision, suggesting occipital lobe ischemia. The patient may then fall to his knees but experience teaches him that after lying flat, recovery and loss of all symptoms, including the neckache, will occur within a few minutes.

It might be added that after experiencing many episodes of the same kind, most patients learn roughly how long they are able to stay on their feet, as well as when it is essential that they sit or lie down to avoid syncope.

8.2.1.2. Diurnal Variations

All groups of these patients find that symptoms tend to be most severe in the early morning; symptoms may become mild enough as the day progresses to enable such patients to spend longer periods of time attending to their daily affairs with fewer or no symptoms in the afternoon and evening (MacLean and Allen, 1940). These diurnal variations in the severity of the symptoms result from greater abnormalities in the orthostatic blood pressure changes during the early morning (Stead and Ebert, 1941; Bannister *et al.*, 1969). We have repeatedly confirmed this finding in the various types of orthostatic blood pressure disorders. Mann *et al.* (1983) have documented this phenomenon in patients with autonomic failure, by continuous intra-arterial blood pressure measurements with Oxford blood pressure monitoring equipment. The phenomenon probably results from the tendency of the plasma volume to fall overnight by 150–200 ml normally and even by as much as 500 ml in some patients, such as those receiving ganglion-blocking drugs (Cranston and Brown, 1963; Bannister *et al.*, 1969). It might also be related to the progressive slowing of the heart rate from morning to evening known to occur in normal subjects (Knox, 1815).

Recumbent blood pressure measurements in one of our patients with autonomic insufficiency who illustrated this phenomenon are shown in Figure 78. This patient's reclining blood pressure was normal during the early morning (124/78), at which time there was a striking orthostatic fall (not depicted) to 60–70/50–56. Recumbent pressures gradually rose during the morning to hypertensive levels in the afternoon, reaching values as high as 212/130 in the late afternoon, at which time standing reduced the pressure to levels (±150/110) that caused no symptoms and permitted him to continue working as a laborer.

The orthostatic rise in heart rate in patients with the pooling syndrome is also most severe in the morning, becoming gradually less severe as the day progresses. This phenomenon is even evident in healthy subjects, as Knox found in 1815. Knox reported an orthostatic increase in heart rate of 15–20 beats/min in the morning, 10 beats/min at midday, and 4–6 beats/min in the evening.

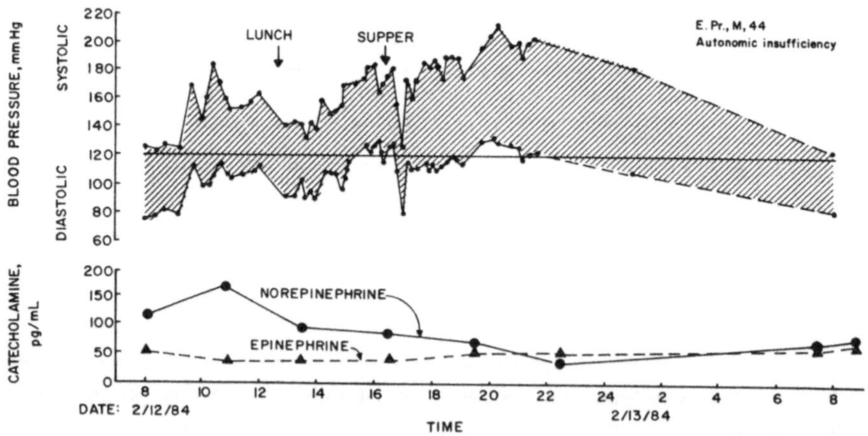

FIGURE 78. Diurnal variation in recumbent blood pressures of a patient with autonomic insufficiency, showing the characteristic rise from morning to evening.

8.2.2. Syncope

When it occurs, syncope is short lived, not usually associated with incontinence, and followed after less than 1 min by return of consciousness. Complete recovery invariably follows, presumably unless a cerebrovascular accident (CVA) has occurred during syncope, which we have never seen happen. However, some patients with autonomic insufficiency die after apparently having been on their feet, as suggested by the fact that they have been found on the floor of their homes. It must therefore be concluded that cerebral or cardiac ischemia might be so severe in some patients with autonomic failure as to cause death if they are unable to lie down rapidly enough at the start of the episode of orthostatic syncope. In contrast to these typical experiences in patients who have autonomic insufficiency, we know of no patients with other types of orthostatic blood pressure derangements who have died as a result of functional cerebral or cardiac ischemia. However, head injuries, fractured bones, and other complications of falling are not uncommon, especially in the elderly, in whom falls are more frequent. Syncope, at least during vasovagal attacks in subjects with intact autonomic function, is followed by oliguria brought on by the effects of vasopressin released during the hypotensive episode (Wiggins *et al.*, 1977).

8.2.3. Convulsive Seizures

Seizures may occur after orthostasis (Bradbury and Eggleston, 1925) but, with isolated exceptions (Su *et al.*, 1977), these virtually never take the form of generalized grand mal convulsions. However, Meyer *et al.* (1956) reported a focal seizure in a patient with unilateral carotid artery occlusion in whom a fall in blood pressure was induced by head-up tilting to 70°. And T. L. Riley and Friedman (1981) described a patient who had had an antecedent cerebral infarction and in whom the subsequent development of orthostatic hypotension caused orthostatic focal seizures or hemiplegic attacks. We have seen one patient whose symptoms strikingly exemplify this phenomenon. A brief summary of his findings follows.

8.2.4. Orthostatic Hemiplegia

An 85-year-old man, previously in good health, was admitted to the neurosurgical ward of the SUNY Health Science Center, in Syracuse, New York, because of frequent lightheadedness and blurring of vision, together with less frequent episodes of numbness, weakness, and jerking movements in the right arm and leg, accompanied by transient motor aphasia. These episodes had taken place at intervals of several months for the previous 9 years but had begun to occur once or twice daily for the 3 weeks before his admission. The patient had noticed that the attacks took place only when he attempted to walk about in his home and that they stopped upon lying down. He knew of no previous CVAs and had been well enough, after the death of his wife, to remarry at the age of 80. Examination revealed a blood pressure of 156/58 in the supine posture, gradually falling during 10 min in the standing position to 120/52, 126/54, 102/50, 112/52, 112/54, 96/56, 110/52, 100/52, and 96/52, whereas the heart rate, which had been 60 beats/min in recumbency, changed only to 72 beats/min in all six determinations over the 10-min period. After standing for 5 min, he began to complain of numbness in the right leg, and jerking muscular contractions started in the right arm and leg. Between 8 and 10 min after the onset of standing, his speech became slow and hesitant, and by the end of 10 min he was unable to talk, although consciousness was unimpaired. The jerky movements of the right arm and leg continued while he remained on his feet but ceased immediately upon his return to bed. His hand grip, measured with a dynamometer, was 130 arbitrary units when he lay in bed and fell to 80 units when the jerking movements started in the standing position (normal for adult males > 350 arbitrary units). Neurological findings in recumbency were normal. The patient showed no blood pressure or heart rate response to the cold pressor test but did show an increase in heart rate from 72 to 96 beats/min, in response to atropine (1 mg by the IV route). Twelve days later, aphasia and right-sided jerky movements were again observed when the patient was on his feet. When he was dressed in a MAST suit, and the suit was inflated, however, the blood pressure was 142/70 in the reclining position, changing only slightly in the standing posture to 116/58, 128/68, 144/66, 148/68, 148/62, 142/64, and 142/64, while the heart rate was 72 beats/min supine and 78 beats/min standing. In the pressure suit he was asymptomatic and able to walk about his hospital room and to talk normally. Fludrocortisone therapy was initiated (0.1 mg/day), and the patient was able to lead as active a life as he desired, with blood pressures of 160–192/62–86 recumbent and 162–186/78–86 in the standing posture, without further spells of orthostatic hemiplegia and aphasia, until shortly before death in his sleep, 3 years later, at the age of 88. Although no autopsy was allowed, we concluded that this patient had had a previous partial obstruction of a branch of the left middle cerebral artery and that the transient hemiplegic and aphasic symptoms resulted from orthostatic reduction in blood flow through the partially obstructed vessel when his blood pressure fell in the upright posture.

In a case reported by Riley and Friedman (1981), jacksonian seizures starting in the left arm first occurred 8 months after a stroke that had left the patient with mild left-sided hemiparesis. The seizures were found to occur only in the upright posture, in which position his blood pressure fell from recumbent levels of 150/105 to 70/0 mm Hg.

8.2.5. Headaches

Although headaches were uncommon in our 19 patients with autonomic insufficiency, they were common in the other patients with orthostatic blood pressure disorders, occurring in more than 40% of cases. Most commonly, the headaches were occipital, precipitated by prolonged standing, relieved by lying down, and sometimes associated with an aching sensation in the back of the neck.

A few patients were bothered by pain in one or other shoulder, and 8% complained of dull chest pain, seldom related to exercise, in the midline or on one or both sides of the chest, similar to the complaints of some patients with mitral valve prolapse. Some of these patients actually did have prolapse of the mitral valve demonstrable on echocardiography; it is important to recall that mitral valve prolapse has been shown often to be associated with orthostatic hypotension (Malcolm *et al.*, 1976; Santos *et al.*, 1981; Depace *et al.*, 1981). Several patients had severe frontal or supraorbital headaches, often immediately above one eye. This type of headache was usually unilateral, sometimes associated with scintillating scotomata and other features typical of migraine, and relieved by bed rest and sleep. These features were most commonly seen in patients with severe narrowing of the pulse pressure in the upright posture, associated with the highest blood kinin concentrations.

8.2.5.1. Effects of Exercise

Severe occipital headaches after vigorous muscular exercise were the presenting symptoms in a few young males (e.g., patients #25, 32, 33, 46, and 53, in Appendix II). Typically, these patients found that very severe headaches would start during a game of football or basketball or after competitive running, making it impossible for them to continue with their sporting activities. Such headaches were relieved by lying down. Since in most of these patients lightheadedness was either absent or overshadowed by the headaches, the existence of orthostatic hypotension or orthostatic narrowing of the pulse pressure was not suspected, and the physician who first saw the patients had not measured the blood pressure in the upright posture.

8.2.6. Symptoms of Carotid or Basilar Artery Insufficiency

Meyer *et al.* (1956) showed that the EEG abnormalities and the symptoms found in a large number of patients with carotid and/or basilar artery insufficiency are associated with cerebral ischemia aggravated by the fall in systolic blood pressure that occurs during head-up tilt or while standing. Thus, orthostatic hypotension due to autonomic failure commonly seen in elderly subjects or due to the pooling syndrome may have a predominant role in the symptomatology of these common cerebrovascular occlusive diseases.

8.3. OTHER CLINICAL FEATURES

8.3.1. Fatigue and Weakness

The major complaints of about one-third of patients were fatigue and weakness, often overshadowing lightheadedness, which was not even mentioned until its presence was specifically inquired into. Because fatigue and "weakness" are such common, relatively nonspecific symptoms that do not lead physicians to suspect the presence of orthostatic hypotension, few of these patients had previously had their blood pressures measured while they were standing. Many had gone through extensive laboratory tests with entirely negative results, leading to an erroneous diagnosis of psychoneurosis.

8.3.2. Nausea

Although nausea was seldom the chief complaint, it did occur together with lightheadedness and/or headaches in 14% of patients with various forms of the pooling syndrome. In no case was vomiting associated with nausea.

8.3.3. Palpitations, Flushing Spells, and Excessive Sweating

These problems occurred in 13–18.7% of the patients, although never in patients with autonomic insufficiency. These symptoms had led some of the patients and their physicians to suspect the presence of hypoglycemia, for which no evidence could be found. The great difficulty in differentiating the symptoms of hypoglycemia from those of orthostatic hypotension or the pooling syndrome has been observed on many occasions, even in diabetic patients who have been taking insulin for several years (Miles and Hayter, 1968; Page *et al.*, 1976). In some patients, visible facial erythema, especially in recumbency, raised the possibility of the carcinoid syndrome, but no other evidence of this disease could be found. These symptoms also raised the possibility of thyrotoxicosis; two of our patients (#100 and #146, Appendix II) were shown to have overactive thyroid function, which, when corrected, reduced but failed to cure the orthostatic derangements of blood pressure control. It should be mentioned that several of our patients with autonomic insufficiency noticed sweating in the face, especially after meals, as has been described in diabetics with autonomic neuropathy (Watkins, 1973; Page and Watkins, 1976). Most patients with autonomic insufficiency, including those with parkinsonism, were also found to have a greasy sebaceous secretion visible and palpable exclusively over the face.

8.3.4. Nocturia

A frequent symptom is nocturia. It appears to result from retention of urine in the sitting or standing posture during the daytime. Diuresis occurs at night, as this reversal of the normal excretory pattern is overcome when patients spend a day in the reclining position (Bradbury and Eggleston, 1925).

8.3.5. Aggravation by Heat

High environmental temperatures dilate the blood vessels and usually aggravate both the measurable orthostatic changes in blood pressure and the symptoms associated with these disorders. This direct vasodilatory effect of heat was noted by 11% of our patients. Since at least two of our patients with autonomic insufficiency died on exceptionally hot days, this effect of high temperatures is certainly of more than academic interest.

8.3.6. Edema

The pathogenesis both of orthostatic edema and of the pooling syndrome involves excessive orthostatic pooling of blood in the dependent parts, albeit probably in different segments of the microvasculature (see Fig. 2). Since renal excretion of sodium and water is greatly reduced in patients with orthostatic hypotension while standing (Bachman and Youmans, 1953), we were surprised to find that orthostatic edema occurred infrequently (in only 10 of 123 cases) among patients with the pooling syndrome. Equally surprising, since it has received scant attention in the literature, was the finding that no fewer than one-fifth of our patients with autonomic insufficiency had readily demonstrable pitting edema; this problem sometimes became very troublesome when fludrocortisone and other sodium-retaining drugs were used in the therapy of their orthostatic hypotension.

The occurrence of severe peripheral edema in some diabetic patients with autonomic neuropathy and normal serum creatinine concentrations was described by Edmonds *et al.* (1983). A peculiar brawny edema was seen in one of our original patients with hyperbradykininism. This 37-year-old woman was bedridden for several years because of orthostatic hypotension and tachycardia. Occasionally her blood pressure fell even in recumbency. When this happened, she was given intravenous infusions of saline followed by rapidly developing edema, reminiscent of the capillary leak syndrome. On one such occasion, her wedding ring had to be sawn off to avoid ischemic damage to the finger. The indentation left by the ring was clearly visible 2 days later (Fig. 79) and remained visible for at least 6 weeks.

8.3.7. Cyanosis of the Legs

Careful comparison of the legs of patients with the pooling syndrome with those of normal subjects often revealed a mild but definite purplish hue below the knees in the upright posture. This color change probably resulted from excessive orthostatic pooling of blood, of which there is much collateral evidence. It might occasionally even have diagnostic value but cannot be relied on unless the patient's legs can be compared in a good light with those of an individual who has no orthostatic derangements. Occasionally, in patients with very severe orthostatic pooling, with or without autonomic insufficiency, deep cyanosis of the dependent legs has been evident when the patients have been standing or sitting (Fig. 80).

8.3.8. Changes in Blood Pressure and Heart Rate

As has been described in detail in Chapter 6, blood pressure and heart rate responses to standing should be considered abnormal when they exceed the changes that have been observed in healthy subjects, in one or more of several respects:

1. *Orthostatic diastolic hypotension:* Diastolic pressure falls by 10 mm Hg or more, with or without a fall in systolic pressure. Especially when caused by autonomic insufficiency, orthostatic hypotension is often accompanied by recumbent hypertension (Bradbury and Eggleston, 1925; Stead and Ebert, 1941).
2. *Orthostatic systolic hypotension:* Systolic pressure alone falls by 20 mm Hg or more, or to below 94 mm Hg. This disorder is particularly common in the elderly (Caird *et al.*, 1973).
3. *Orthostatic hypertension:* Diastolic pressure is 90 mm Hg or less in recumbency and rises to 98 mm Hg or more in the standing posture.
4. *Orthostatic narrowing of pulse pressure:* Pulse pressure falls to less than 20 mm Hg in the upright posture.
5. *Orthostatic tachycardia:* Heart rate increases by 28 beats/min or more or rises to 110 beats/min or more in the upright posture without abnormal blood pressure changes.

Conditions 2–5 constitute different manifestations of the venous pooling syndrome, which may coexist at the same time or at different times in the same patient.

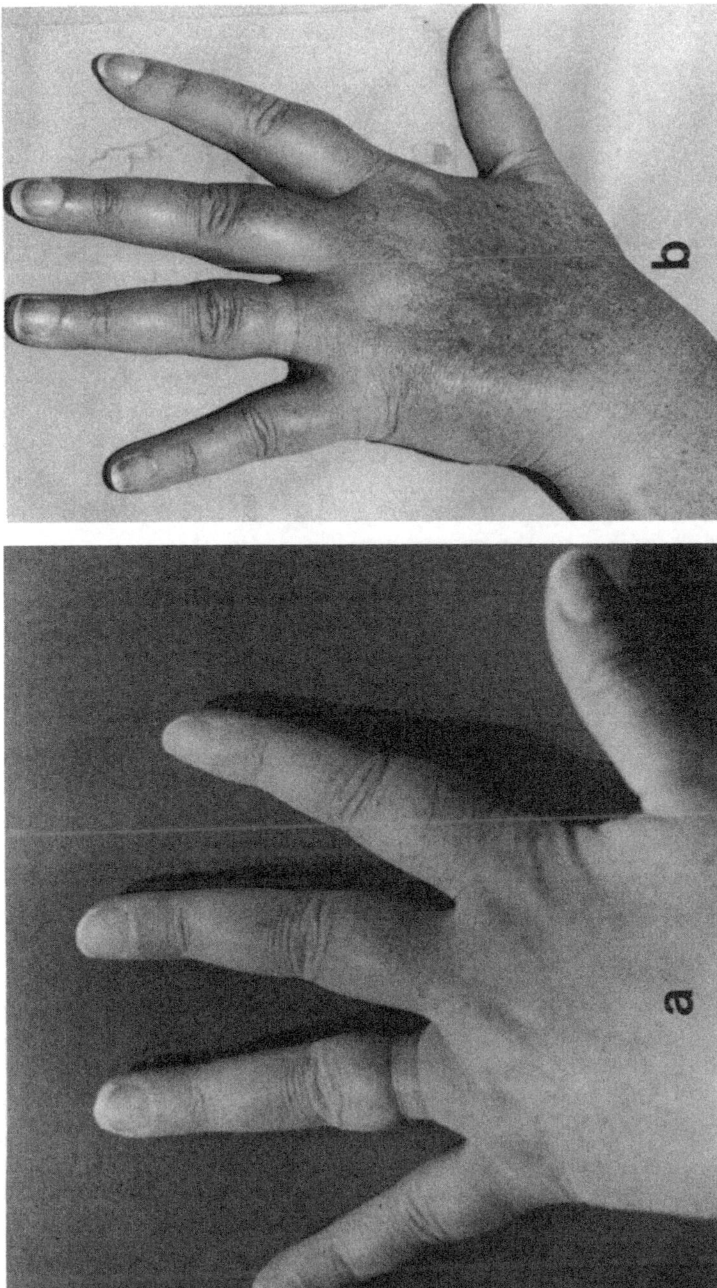

FIGURE 79. Acutely developing brawny edema of the fingers (especially proximal phalanges) in hyperbradykininism. Note the resultant indentation under the wedding ring of this patient, which was strikingly evident 50 hr after the ring had been removed (a) and was still clearly visible 6 weeks later (b). The sudden leakage of a protein-rich fluid from the capillaries seems likely to have occurred during an exacerbation of her hypotension, which coincided with the edema formation.

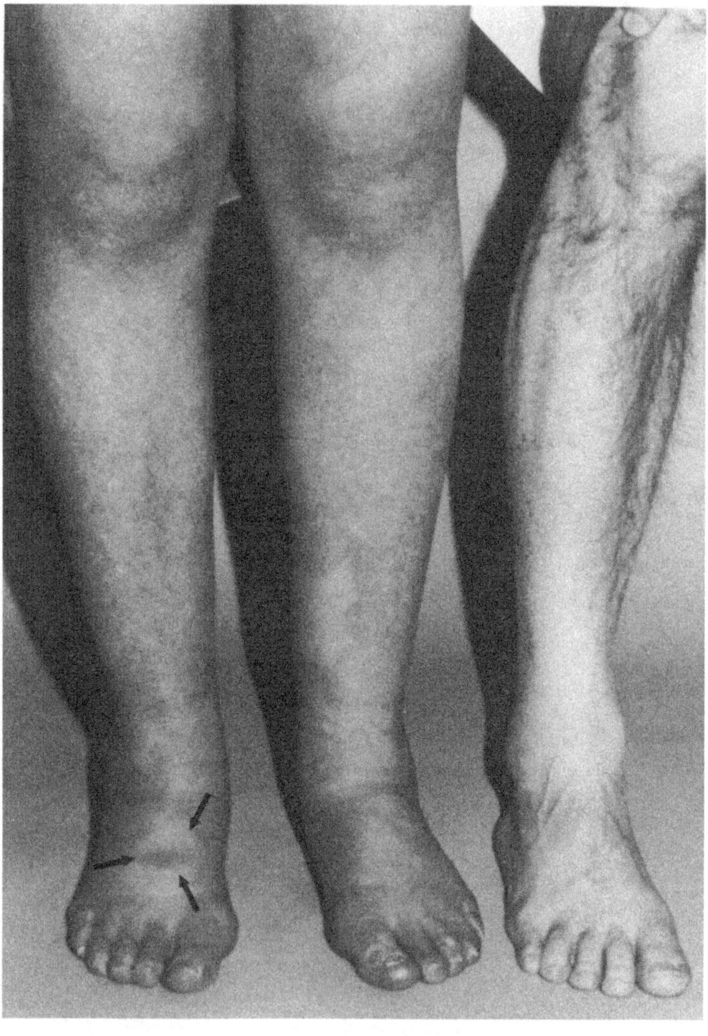

FIGURE 80. Orthostatic cyanosis in the legs of a patient (left) who had hyperbradykininism associated with orthostatic systolic and diastolic hypotension, orthostatic tachycardia, excessive orthostatic shrinkage of pulse pressure, and orthostatic edema (pitting demarcated with arrows), compared with the leg of a normal subject (right).

Although the orthostatic changes in blood pressure and heart rate have been described as abnormal, such changes may be seen in persons who are largely or completely asymptomatic. Thus, among 2000 healthy U.S. airmen, shortly after World War I, Schneider and Truesdell (1922) reported that in the upright posture systolic blood pressure fell below 100 mm Hg in 5%, diastolic blood pressure rose above 100 mm Hg in 0.6%, and heart rate increased by at least 30 beats/min in 12.6%. Similarly, among 1000 apparently healthy persons, Currens (1948) found orthostatic diastolic hypertension present in 4.1% of subjects.

In diabetic patients with autonomic insufficiency, orthostatic hypotension may be dramatically aggravated while the blood glucose concentration is falling for 3 hr or more after each insulin injection, apparently due to insulin-induced vasodilatation (Page and Watkins, 1976), which reduces venous return, right atrial pressure, and cardiac output (Miles and Hayter, 1968). In some diabetic patients with autonomic failure, we have found that poor control of hyperglycemia, by inducing osmotic diuresis and hypovolemia, severely aggravates orthostatic hypotension.

8.3.9. Cardiac Disorders

8.3.9.1. Mitral Valve Prolapse

This disorder was shown to be present in 8% of our patients (designated by a Y in Appendix II), including 10% of those with the pooling syndrome, but none with autonomic insufficiency. The incidence of mitral valve prolapse in patients with the pooling syndrome is probably much higher than 10%, since we were neither familiar with the physical signs of this disorder nor able to perform echocardiography at the time that many of the patients were studied. Patients with hyperbradykininism appeared to have mitral valve prolapse even more commonly than the others (*viz.* in 22% of these patients). In four families with hyperbradykininism, at least two members of different generations were shown to have mitral valve prolapse (#40, 61; 46, 93, 142, 143; 102, 103; and 104–106). Mitral valve prolapse has been associated with syncopal attacks in 14% of patients (Malcolm *et al.*, 1976) and with orthostatic systolic hypotension and tachycardia in 12 of 86 patients (Santos *et al.*, 1981) and in two patients described by Depace *et al.* (1981).

8.3.9.2. Premature Ventricular Contractions

PVCs have been found to be present either exclusively or predominantly in the upright posture in four of our patients with the pooling syndrome (#32, 118, 123, and 147). It is possible that more severe ventricular tachyarrhythmias occurred intermittently and caused the lightheadedness and syncope experienced by these patients, but such dysrhythmias have never been found. Echocardiography and blood kinin measurements were not performed in these patients, so we do not know whether their dysrhythmias might have been associated with mitral valve prolapse, as has been reported by Malcolm *et al.* (1976) and Winkle *et al.* (1976), or with hyperbradykininism.

8.3.9.3. Recumbent Tachycardia

Autonomic insufficiency is associated with recumbent tachycardia (Clarke and Ewing, 1982) and with slow left ventricular ejection, subnormal stroke volume, and reduced cardiac output, all of which contribute to the orthostatic fall in blood pressure, together with an elevated systemic vascular resistance in recumbency that remains unchanged in the standing position (Magrini *et al.*, 1976).

8.3.9.4. Angina Pectoris

This symptom complex may occur especially but not exclusively in patients with associated coronary occlusive disease, because of impaired myocardial perfusion at the subnormal blood pressures present in the upright posture.

8.3.9.5. Electrocardiographic Changes

Several Scandinavian physicians have reported the occurrence of orthostatic lowering of the ST segments and inversion of the T waves in leads II and III of the ECG in patients with orthostatic arterial anemia (Åkesson, 1936, 1946; Nordenfelt, 1941; Hammarström, 1947), probably identical with what has been referred to in this book as the venous pooling syndrome.

8.3.10. Plasma Volume Changes

Plasma volume was subnormal in eight patients with autonomic insufficiency (Ibrahim *et al.*, 1975). Later measurements of plasma volume in five patients with autonomic failure were found not to be significantly lower than in five carefully matched controls (Wilcox *et al.*, 1984). In response to a restricted sodium intake, these patients lost more weight than the healthy controls, probably because of hyporeninemic hypoaldosteronism, which is known to occur in most patients with severe autonomic insufficiency (Gordon *et al.*, 1967). Sodium deprivation reduced the plasma volumes of these patients to an extent that was very close to being statistically significant ($t = 2.2$) compared with the normal controls. Barraclough and Sharpey-Schafer showed in 1963 that, when circulatory reflexes are absent, even slight reductions in venous return may decrease cardiac output and blood pressure severely. Plasma volume is not only reduced but translocated out of the thorax in patients with autonomic insufficiency (Magrini *et al.*, 1976), probably because of the decreased venous tone in the periphery (Page *et al.*, 1955; Sharpey-Schafer and Taylor, 1960).

8.3.11. Other Features of Autonomic Failure

Impotence is a frequent early symptom of autonomic insufficiency in males. Reduced thermal sweating occurs in about one-third of patients (Spingarn and Hitzig, 1942) and is often associated with exaggerated facial sweating after meals. Urinary and (later) fecal incontinence supervene as autonomic function worsens. Constipation is common and probably reflects parasympathetic insufficiency. Gastric dilatation and stasis frequently occur as the autonomic failure progresses, particularly in diabetic patients. The greater prevalence and earlier onset of the symptoms of parasympathetic (as opposed to sympathetic) damage in diabetic patients were pointed out by Tifft and Chobanian (1982).

Associated neurological abnormalities in patients with the central type of autonomic failure include the well-known features of Parkinson's disease or of multiple system atrophy. According to Bannister (1983), these abnormalities may present as:

1. *Striatonigral degeneration:* severe rigidity, slight tremor, loss of facial expression, leg weakness, slurred speech
2. *Olivopontocerebellar atrophy:* impaired gait, trunkal ataxia, slurred speech
3. *Pyramidal lesions:* described by Bannister (1983)

Occasional clinical manifestations of the pooling syndrome, seen mainly in adolescents and children, include subconscious fidgeting of the legs and virtual inability to keep the legs still in the upright posture. These features appear to constitute the patients' subconscious response to the fact that their symptoms are aggravated by loss of the facilitating effect of muscular movements on venous return of the blood to the heart.

8.4. SUMMARY

Symptoms resulting from orthostatic cerebral ischemia were present and predominant in patients with autonomic insufficiency (lightheadedness, 100%; syncope, 58%; blurred vision, 16%), as well as in patients with idiopathic orthostatic hypotension (78%, 11%, and 22%, respectively) and in patients with the pooling syndrome (77%, 29%, and 14%, respectively). Nevertheless, some patients in each group presented with symptoms that appeared to be nonspecific in type and did not suggest the presence of reduced cerebral blood flow in the upright posture: headaches, weakness, fatigue, and malaise. Only by compulsively measuring the blood pressure and heart rate in the recumbent and the upright posture in every patient can the risk of overlooking these syndromes be overcome. Differences in the frequency of various symptoms in the three groups of patients are listed (Table VII).

Most symptoms were worst in the mornings, diminishing in intensity as the day progressed. It was common, for instance, for orthostatic hypotension and symptoms of orthostatic cerebral ischemia to be severe in the early morning and to become less severe as recumbent hypertension supervened in the afternoon and evening in many patients with autonomic insufficiency. Rarely, orthostatic hypotension might induce focal symptoms because of a previous unknown local vascular obstruction; in one of our patients, it caused a striking syndrome of orthostatic hemiplegia, jacksonian seizures, and motor aphasia, all of which could be totally prevented by overcoming orthostatic hypotension with fludrocortisone therapy. Headaches were often severe after sporting events, especially in young adult and adolescent males. Orthostatic palpitations, flushing spells, and excessive sweating were frequently complained of in patients with the pooling syndrome but were never present in patients with autonomic insufficiency. Because of the vasodilatory effect of environmental heat, virtually all patients appeared to be adversely affected by hot weather. Among the many other clinical findings, it might be mentioned that edema occurred in 21% of patients with autonomic insufficiency, mitral valve prolapse in at least 10% of patients with the pooling syndrome and 22% of those with demonstrable hyperbradykininism, and PVCs exclusively in the upright posture in four patients.

9

ORTHOSTATIC DISORDERS OF BLOOD PRESSURE CONTROL

Prevalence and Diagnosis

9.1. PREVALENCE

Unfortunately, there is no scientific basis for an accurate estimate of the prevalence of any of the disorders described in this chapter. Orthostatic hypotension due to autonomic insufficiency is a rare disorder, except in two groups of individuals: the elderly, in whom autonomic insufficiency is often associated with other CNS derangements, such as parkinsonism, and long-term diabetic patients, whose neuropathy usually involves somatic as well as autonomic nerves and is accompanied by other degenerative complications of diabetes mellitus.

The various forms of pooling syndrome are far more common than would be believed by physicians who do not measure blood pressure both in the recumbent posture and after standing for at least 3 min, as part of their routine physical examination. Since we have been able, by chance and not by design, to study comparable numbers of patients with the pooling syndrome and with orthostatic edema, during the past 25 years, the two types of disorder are probably of comparable prevalence. We do have some indication that orthostatic hypertension is very common, however. Among 1800 patients referred to our hypertension program in a 7-year period for evaluation of the pathogenesis of their (usually) refractory hypertension, 181 were found to have diastolic blood pressures below 90 mm Hg in the reclining posture and above 90 mm Hg when standing and, when it was measured, in the seated position as well. Almost all their referring physicians, on excellent authority (Kirkendall *et al.*, 1980; Joint National Committee on Detection, Evaluation and Treatment of High Blood Pressure, 1980), had measured the blood pressure in the sitting position. Whether 90 mm Hg is or is not an appropriate, practical cutoff point for the diagnosis of hypertension in seated individuals, or whether it should be 98 mm

Hg, as we now think would be more appropriate, may be debatable. However, if 90 mm Hg is the best lower limit of the normal blood pressure in the sitting position, one would have to conclude that orthostatic hypertension is a disorder of immense proportions, accounting as it did for 10% of our group of referred hypertensive patients. Orthostatic hypertension is often recognizable among patients described as having mild hypertension, borderline hypertension, or labile hypertension, at least half of some series of borderline hypertensive patients having been shown to exhibit an excessive orthostatic rise in diastolic blood pressure (Payen *et al.*, 1982; Safar *et al.*, 1973).

Since such milder forms of hypertension are generally thought to be far more common among the population at large, who are not referred for consultation, than among patients with refractory hypertension, who are frequently referred for consultation, it seems quite likely that the prevalence of orthostatic hypertension might be considerably higher than 10% of the entire hypertensive population. If hypertension afflicts about 25% of the American population, as some have estimated (Hypertension Detection and Follow-up Program Cooperative Group, 1977; Joint National Committee on Detection, Evaluation and Treatment of High Blood Pressure, 1985), 2.5% of the entire U.S. population, or more than 5 million individuals, might be expected to have the variant of hypertension described as orthostatic hypertension.

We do not really know whether all patients with orthostatic hypertension owe their disorder to excessive pooling of blood in the dependent parts of the body, as our present information would tend to imply. Moreover, a large number of patients with orthostatic hypertension lack the symptom complex seen in most other patients with the pooling syndrome. It may not be valid, therefore, to consider orthostatic hypertension as being always pathogenetically related to the other types of the pooling syndrome, in spite of all the evidence cited earlier, which strongly implies that orthostatic hypertension does often result from excessive orthostatic pooling. If orthostatic hypertension and the other forms of the pooling syndrome are indeed pathogenetically related, the other forms of the orthostatic pooling syndrome are probably of comparable prevalence.

Occasional lightheadedness and fainting spells are common in the general population. When antigravity muscle activity is minimal, such as in head-up tilt-table studies, 22% of healthy young men (aged 18–28 years) will faint within 20 min (Allen *et al.*, 1945). In the study cited, the subjects who fainted were generally found to have more rapid mean heart rates, lower systolic and diastolic blood pressures, and narrower pulse pressures than did those who did not faint, the orthostatic pulse pressures being significantly lower in the "fainters" than in the "nonfainters" ($p < 0.02$). Since fainting could be prevented in these subjects by bandaging the legs, it is evident that 22% of these normal males may be considered, under the very demanding conditions of this study, to have had a condition similar to or identical with the venous pooling syndrome. Such a "disorder" would be expected to give rise to fainting spells when the individuals' occupations required standing still for several hours at a time, or standing still after acute exhausting exercise (Taylor and Allen, 1941), or standing at attention in a military parade on a hot day. Thus, the frequency with which the venous pooling syndrome becomes clinically manifest is probably dependent on the occupation of the population studied.

9.2. SEX INCIDENCE AND AGE OF ONSET

Table VIII shows the sex incidence and age of onset (mean and range) of the 159 patients whose orthostatic blood pressure disorders we have studied. It is readily apparent from Table VIII that autonomic insufficiency is predominantly a disorder of old men, although women and some middle-aged individuals (mainly but not exclusively patients with diabetic neuropathy) are less frequently affected. The frequent occurrence of orthostatic systolic hypotension in the elderly has been described by Caird *et al.* (1973), who found it present in 24% of 494 people aged 65 years or more. In striking contrast to the findings in patients with autonomic insufficiency, the pooling syndrome affects women and young girls more frequently than men, and is generally a young person's disorder, the mean age of onset (25.8 years) reflecting the large numbers of individuals in whom symptoms clearly go back to childhood or in whom the derangement is actually discovered during childhood or adolescence. Being aware of these disorders, my pediatric colleague, Dr. Robert Richman, has found and kindly referred for study no fewer than five children with orthostatic blood pressure disorders due to excessive gravitational pooling, during the past 6 years. Idiopathic orthostatic hypotension has an approximately equal sex incidence among the small number of patients we have studied, and the mean age of onset is 40.8 years, although both extremes of the age range are represented in this group of patients.

TABLE VIII. Sex Incidence and Age Distribution of Patients with Orthostatic Blood Pressure Disorders

Disorder	M/F ratio (%)	Age of onset (in years)	
		Mean	Range
Autonomic insufficiency	79 : 21	60.0	43–81
Idiopathic orthostatic hypotension	44 : 56	40.8	11–73
Pooling syndrome	30 : 70	25.8	9–74

9.3. HEREDITARY FACTOR

There is no evidence that orthostatic hypotension either due to autonomic insufficiency or of the idiopathic type is an hereditary disorder. However, the high familial prevalence of chronic neurocirculatory asthenia, which is associated with symptoms and signs strongly suggestive of the pooling syndrome, was clearly shown by Cohen *et al.* (1951), who concluded that the disorder was inherited as a mendelian dominant. The occurrence of the pooling syndrome in multiple members of the same family was reported in the original description of hyperbradykininism (Streeten *et al.*, 1972) and has been confirmed in many instances, in the subsequent years. Thus, Appendix II reports the findings in no fewer than four individuals with the venous pooling syndrome in whose families at least one other member had been found to have the same syndrome. In two families we have been able to show that the pooling syndrome was present in three successive generations, implying dominant mendelian inheritance, with slightly increased penetrance among females.

9.4. DIAGNOSIS OF ORTHOSTATIC BLOOD PRESSURE DERANGEMENTS

The recognition and classification of the various types of orthostatic derangements of blood pressure control are simple and straightforward. In the first place, because of the diversity of symptoms that may result from abnormalities of the blood pressure in the upright posture, it is essential that measurements of blood pressure and heart rate both in the supine position and after 3 min of standing become an integral part of the routine physical examination. If this is done on more than one visit, and preferably on repeated occasions (Ibrahim *et al.*, 1975), in patients whose symptoms are suggestive of impaired cerebral blood flow in the upright posture and if the procedures described in Chapter 6 are followed, there can be little difficulty in diagnosing the several types of orthostatic blood pressure abnormalities:

1. *Orthostatic hypotension:* Characterized by persistent and reproducible fall in diastolic blood pressure by 10 mm Hg or more in the upright posture
2. *Pooling syndrome:* associated with one or more of several orthostatic changes in blood pressure or heart rate:
   a. Fall in systolic pressure by ≥20 mm Hg
   b. Rise in diastolic pressure from ≤90 mm Hg to ≥98 mm Hg

c. Narrowing of pulse pressure to <20 mm Hg
d. Rise in heart rate by ⩾28 beats/min or to ⩾110 beats/min

9.4.1. *Orthostatic Hypotension*

If orthostatic hypotension is found to be present, the cause should be sought:

9.4.1.1. Drugs

Many agents in widespread use may cause postural hypotension. It is therefore important to determine whether any of these drugs have been prescribed by another physician or are being taken surreptitiously by the patient. Drugs most likely to cause orthostatic hypotension include α-adrenergic receptor blockers (e.g., phentolamine, phenoxybenzamine, and prazosin), catecholamine-depleting agents (e.g., guanethidine, reserpine), α_2-agonists (e.g., clonidine, guanabenz, and methyldopa), ganglionic-blocking agents (e.g., pentolinium), potent diuretics of all types, psychotropic agents, inhibitors of cortisol production (e.g., metyrapone), and many others.

9.4.1.2. Autonomic Insufficiency

The possibility of an underlying autonomic insufficiency should be strongly suspected, if, in the face of orthostatic hypotension, the heart rate fails to increase by more than 20 beats/min in the upright posture. The coexistence of parkinsonism, diabetic neuropathy, or any of the noncirculatory manifestations of autonomic insufficiency (impotence, incontinence, absence of thermal sweating) would greatly increase the suspicion of autonomic insufficiency.

Autonomic insufficiency can be diagnosed with some certainty, at this point, by showing that plasma norepinephrine concentration fails to rise normally above recumbent levels after the patient has remained standing for at least 2 min and preferably for 5 or 10 min (Cryer and Weiss, 1976). There is a rather wide range of normal plasma concentrations of norepinephrine in the supine posture (90–320, mean 211.4 ± SEM 18.6 pg/ml in our laboratory), which does not always exceed the concentrations found in autonomic failure (Sever, 1983). However, standing for 2–5 min or more usually results in an approximate doubling of the plasma norepinephrine concentration in healthy subjects, to above 300 pg/ml (mean at 5 min 341.5 ± 28.1 and at 10 min 416.8 ± 25.0 pg/ml). Failure of the plasma norepinephrine concentration to rise to this extent provides the best confirmation currently available of the presence of autonomic insufficiency. It is important to try to identify the cause of autonomic insufficiency when this is found to be present.

9.4.2. Differentiation of Central from Peripheral Autonomic Failure

1. The association of a low recumbent plasma norepinephrine concentration with its failure to rise upon standing has been described as an indication that the autonomic insufficiency is of the peripheral type (Hickler *et al.*, 1960; Ziegler *et al.*, 1977). This is still controversial, however, since some investigators have found that the two types of plasma norepinephrine abnormalities do not consistently differentiate central and peripheral types of autonomic failure (Bannister *et al.*, 1977; Cryer, 1979; Sever, 1983).
2. Kopin *et al.* (1983) recently found that peripheral autonomic failure, in which total norepinephrine production is strikingly decreased, is associated with subnormal excretion of vanillyl mandelic acid (VMA), normetanephrine, and 3-methoxy-4-hydroxyphenylglycol (MHPG). On the other hand, in central autonomic failure or multiple-system atrophy, total norepinephrine production is normal, but there is disproportionate reduction of excretion of normetanephrine, which reflects O-methylation of norepinephrine released from sympathetic nerve endings.
3. Plasma norepinephrine concentrations tend to be lower in the peripheral than in the central types of autonomic failure (Bannister *et al.*, 1979; Polinsky *et al.*, 1981).
4. The degree of supersensitivity to infused norepinephrine or isoproterenol (Cannon and Rosenblueth, 1949) is greater in peripheral than in central autonomic neuropathy (Bannister *et al.*, 1979; Polinsky *et al.*, 1981).
5. Responses to tyramine are different in these two forms of autonomic failure, patients with the central type showing a normal rise in blood pressure and those with the peripheral type showing no blood pressure response (Ziegler *et al.*, 1977).
6. A rise in heart rate in response to the partial β-adrenergic agonist, pindolol, indicates low occupancy and/or increased number of β-receptors, facilitating the manifestation of the β-agonist action of the drug, and indicating the presence of peripheral autonomic failure (Man in 't Veld and Schalekamp, 1981).
7. Tilting the patient initially to 60° and eventually to 90° for 10 min elicits a normal rise in plasma vasopressin concentration in patients with peripheral autonomic neuropathy but no change in patients with afferent or central lesions (Zerbe *et al.*, 1983).

Even if heart rate does increase in the upright posture, as was found to be the case in three of our 19 patients with autonomic insufficiency (see patients #2, 12, and 13 in Appendix II), plasma norepinephrine concentration should be measured in the supine and standing positions, to establish as conclusively as possible whether autonomic insufficiency is present. Other functional tests to confirm the presence of autonomic failure include the responses to the Valsalva maneuver, variations in the ECG RR interval during deep respiration (Pfeiffer *et al.*, 1984) and 30–15 sec after changing from recumbency to the standing posture (Ewing *et al.*, 1985), and pupillometry (Pfeiffer *et al.*, 1984). If autonomic insufficiency is not present, amyloid disease should be ruled out by means of a rectal or gingival biopsy.

9.4.2.1. Volume Contraction

This may result from diuretic action, excessive losses of sodium and water in the urine, diarrheal stools, or in profuse vomiting, prolonged bed rest, pregnancy, and diabetes mellitus.

9.4.2.2. Adrenal Diseases

In patients whose heart rate rises appropriately in response to orthostatic diastolic hypotension, the possible presence of adrenal disease, involving deficiency of cortisol and/or aldosterone production, or the presence of a pheochromocytoma should be ruled out.

1. *Cortisol deficiency:* May best be diagnosed by using the metyrapone test or the insulin tolerance test (see Streeten *et al.*, 1984), and/or an ACTH test, to determine whether the hypocortisolism is primary, due to adrenocortical dysfunction, or secondary to ACTH deficiency.
2. *Aldosterone deficiency:* Best diagnosed by measurement of plasma renin activity and plasma aldosterone concentration 3 hr after an intravenous injection of furosemide, 40 mg. During the second and third hours after the furosemide injection, patients are requested to stand or sit, if symptoms and the level of blood pressure permit. After these potent stimuli to the renin-angiotensin-aldosterone system, normal subjects show an increase in plasma renin activity to 1.7–8.5 ng/ml per hr and in plasma aldosterone concentration to 18–50 ng/dl. Failure of the plasma aldosterone concentration to rise to the normal extent strongly suggests aldosterone deficiency, the presence of which can be confirmed by finding a subnormal rise in plasma aldosterone concentration after 4 and 8 hr of an intravenous infusion of cosyntropin (Cortrosyn R), 0.25 mg in 500 ml 5% dextrose solution over 8 hr, preferably preceded by furosemide, 40 mg IV. If a subnormal aldosterone response to either or both stimuli is found, it may be attributed to primary failure of the adrenocortical zona glomerulosa (if plasma renin activity rose normally or excessively in response to furosemide and standing) or to deficient renin release and

hyporeninemic hypoaldosteronism (if plasma renin activity failed to increase normally after the stimulus of the furosemide injection and standing for 2 hr).

3. *Pheochromocytoma:* May be suspected by the finding of excessive urinary excretion of VMA, metanephrines, and catecholamines or by the finding of elevated plasma catecholamine concentrations (Bravo *et al.*, 1979). An adrenal tumor is evidenced by CT scanning of the adrenals, and abnormal failure of the plasma norepinephrine concentration to fall 3 hr after an oral dose of clonidine, 0.3 mg (Bravo *et al.*, 1981), is a sensitive and specific test for pheochromocytoma.

9.4.2.3. Idiopathic

If orthostatic hypotension is associated with normal plasma norepinephrine responses to standing, normal cortisol and aldosterone responses to their specific stimuli, and no evidence of pheochromocytoma or amyloid disease, the disorder is presently considered idiopathic.

9.4.3. Venous Pooling Syndrome

The pooling syndrome is diagnosed primarily by repeated demonstration of the described abnormalities in the blood pressure and/or heart rate responses to the standing posture. Since the heart rate rises normally or excessively in the upright posture in these patients, the plasma norepinephrine response to standing is not needed for the diagnosis; if it is measured, plasma norepinephrine concentration is found to rise excessively, usually to above 700 pg/ml, a level reached only occasionally in healthy subjects. In diagnosing the pooling syndrome, it is important to rule out the presence of hypovolemia. This may result from anemia (detected by a blood count), low plasma volume due to hypoalbuminemia, and low extracellular fluid volume caused by excessive sodium losses in the urine (e.g., due to renal tubular disease, diuretic administration, adrenocortical insufficiency), the stools (due to diarrhea of any type), the vomitus (due to any of the innumerable causes of vomiting), or the skin (e.g., due to excessive thermal sweating, cystic fibrosis).

Most of these disorders can be ruled out by clinical findings, but specific laboratory measurements are required to demonstrate the presence or absence of low blood, plasma, or extracellular fluid volumes and to eliminate the possible presence of adrenocortical deficiency of cortisol or aldosterone production. If these known potential causes of the pooling syndrome are shown to be absent, the syndrome is considered idiopathic, unless blood kinin determinations can be performed. When the blood kinin concentration is found to be elevated (above 0.6 ng/ml), the diagnosis of *hyperbradykininism* may be made.

9.5. SUMMARY

The prevalence of these disorders cannot be determined, but recognition of the pooling syndrome is certainly not uncommon if one measures the blood pressure in both the supine and standing position in all patients. Whereas autonomic insufficiency is predominantly a disorder of old men (M : F = 79 : 21; mean age of onset, 60 years), the pooling syndrome is more common among young women (M : F = 30 : 70; mean age at onset, 25.8 years) and is often inherited as a mendelian dominant.

Diagnosis depends heavily on frequent measurements of blood pressure and heart rate both recumbent and standing. Consistent orthostatic diastolic hypotension with little or no orthostatic tachycardia strongly suggests autonomic insufficiency. The absence of an increase in plasma norepinephrine concentration after 2–10 min of standing establishes the diagnosis. If recumbent norepinephrine concentration is below 90 pg/ml, the autonomic insufficiency is likely to be of the peripheral type. A variety of additional tests, including heart rate responses to the Valsalva maneuver, blood pressure, and heart rate responses to the cold pressor test, sweat tests, and responses to atropine, can be used to confirm the presence of, and to characterize, the autonomic insufficiency. When orthostatic tachycardia is present, it is most important to exclude, by appropriate tests, the presence of hypocortisolism, hypoaldosteronism, pheochromocytoma, and hypovolemia (from anemia or fluid losses) before diagnosing the pooling syndrome.

10

ORTHOSTATIC DISORDERS OF BLOOD PRESSURE CONTROL

Treatment and Prognosis

10.1. TREATMENT

Surprisingly, it has been found that orthostatic hypotension due to autonomic insufficiency and most other causes, as well as the various forms of the pooling syndrome, all appear to respond to similar forms of treatment. This finding provides further indirect support for the view that these derangements are all consequences of similar pathogenetic mechanisms. The one important group of exceptions to these generalities is that hypocortisolism, hypoaldosteronism, pheochromocytoma, drug-induced disorders, and other derangements of known etiology should obviously be treated, whenever possible, by correction or removal of the cause and frequently without the need for the therapeutic measures described in this chapter.

In general, the forms of available treatment may be divided into the following categories:

1. Physical compression of the lower limbs and abdomen
2. Vasoconstricting drugs, especially α-adrenergic agonists
3. Inhibitors of vasodilators, including β-adrenergic blockers
4. Volume expanders, especially salt-retaining drugs
5. Prostaglandin inhibitors
6. Vasopressin
7. Atrial pacemakers
8. Other measures

10.1.1. Physical Compression of the Lower Limbs and Abdomen

The simplest form of this type of treatment, helpful only in patients whose disorder is mild, is to use elastic stockings, as closely fitted to the individual limbs as possible. The best forms of such garments are custom-made by the Jobst Company and other manufacturers, on the basis of measurements of the limb circumference at intervals of approximately 1 inch up the limbs, as well as pelvic and abdominal measurements to permit the use of waist-high fitted garments. For mild or even severe forms of orthostatic hypotension and the pooling syndrome, such waist-high garments, designed to apply external pressure of about 50–60 mm Hg, are frequently helpful to these patients, sometimes producing only slight but worthwhile improvement and in other instances dramatically enabling bed-ridden patients to be restored to an active, productive lifestyle (Levin *et al.*, 1964; Sheps, 1976; Thomas *et al.*, 1981). Although one can never be certain that these pressure garments are going to be of significant, lasting value, and despite their high cost because of the need for individual construction of each garment, most patients whose symptoms are severe should be fitted with one of them, if possible. For emergency use or for patients who are found to experience no benefit from elastic garments, MAST suits (made by the David Clark Company, Worcester, MA), G-suits of World War II vintage (Sieker *et al.*, 1956), available in some Army and Navy surplus stores, or similar antigravity suits may be of temporary value. Although most antigravity suits are both unsightly and cumbersome, some patients have derived continued benefit from their use for several years (Rosenhamer *et al.*, 1973).

10.1.2. Vasoconstricting Drugs

Despite the fact that intravenous infusions of norepinephrine at rates sufficient to raise recumbent blood pressure fail to prevent orthostatic hypotension (Chokroverty *et al.*, 1969; Streeten, unpublished), a large variety of α-adrenergic drugs and other types of vasoconstrictors have been tried as forms of treatment for orthostatic hypotension and the pooling syndrome. These have included

10.1.2.1. α_1-Adrenergic Agonists

These agents include phenylephrine, midodrine, and norepinephrine. Phenylephrine and midodrine (2.5–5 mg 3 times daily) have value in some patients with autonomic insufficiency (Schirger *et al.*, 1981), but are generally disappointing in that, when used in doses high enough to reduce orthostatic hypotension, they tend to cause recumbent hypertension (Davies *et al.*, 1978). Itskovitz and Wartenburg (1983) reported a good response to phenylephrine (10–15 mg every 4–6 hr) together with tranylcypromine (10 mg twice daily) in a patient with autonomic failure whose condition was not improved by fludrocortisone, indomethacin, or elastic stockings. Hickler *et al.* (1959*b*) found in a patient with autonomic failure that the blood pressure could be maintained in the upright posture by an intravenous infusion of norepinephrine. An ingenious electromechanical device for the delivery of norepinephrine has been used experimentally in two patients with autonomic insufficiency by Polinsky *et al.* (1983). The equipment comprises an intra-arterial blood pressure sensor linked by an electromechanical interface with a pump from which norepinephrine is infused intravenously at rates sufficient to maintain the mean blood pressure close to a predetermined setpoint. The device closely simulated the responses of the normal baroreceptor reflex, maintaining blood pressure at the preset level with a standard error of less than 2 mm Hg while the patients were tilted to 85° and while they changed from the recumbent to the sitting and standing postures for 4 hr.

10.1.2.2. Releasers of Norepinephrine

Releasers at the sympathetic nerve endings include ephedrine, methylphenidate (Ritalin), and amphetamines. These drugs are occasionally of therapeutic value in patients whose autonomic denervation spares the postganglionic fibers, where these drugs act. More often than not, however, these compounds are of only slight value and in spite of sometimes raising recumbent blood pressure somewhat, they bring about little if any improvement in orthostatic hypotension. They are seldom of value in the venous pooling syndrome. The general lack of usefulness of these therapeutic agents is in striking contrast with their efficacy and value in patients with orthostatic edema.

10.1.2.3. Epinephrine Injections

Although seldom if ever used nowadays, epinephrine injections given subcutaneously raised the systolic blood pressure and increased the heart rate, with mildly beneficial clinical responses to standing, in the three patients with autonomic insufficiency reported by Bradbury and Eggleston (1925).

10.1.2.4. Drugs that Enhance Norepinephrine Release and Retard Its Reuptake

These drugs have been used by Seller (1969), Diamond *et al.* (1970), Lewis *et al.* (1972), and Nanda *et al.* (1976), with or without a monoamine oxidase inhibitor, such as tranylcypromine (Parnate, 10–20 mg tid) or phenelzine (Nardil). Although some benefit has resulted, these forms of treatment tend to cause severe recumbent hypertension, usually with disappointingly slight improvement in the orthostatic hypotension (Davies *et al.*, 1978).

10.1.2.5. α_2-Agonists

Drugs such as clonidine and presumably other drugs of the same type (e.g., guanabenz, methyldopa) have recently been shown to be dramatically effective in a small group of patients with severe, perhaps almost complete sympathetic nerve degeneration (Robertson *et al.*, 1983). In these patients, the central α_2-agonistic action of the drugs on the cardiovascular center located in the medulla of the brain, which is the basis of their action as inhibitors of sympathetic nervous system function and consequently as hypotensive agents, is lost because of the absence of any effect *via* the nonfunctional sympathetic nervous system on peripheral arterioles. The peripheral α_2-agonistic effect, presumably exerted directly on the α_2-receptors, especially in the veins (DeMey and Vanhoutte, 1980), however, is preserved; consequently, these drugs bring about constriction of the veins, reduction of the pooling resulting from lack of venous tone, and improved return of venous blood to the heart. Thus, the orthostatic fall in blood pressure will be reduced, presumably to the extent that this results in the first place from subnormal venous tone and pooling of blood in the veins. When used in such patients, clonidine is first administered in very small doses, such as 0.05 mg (because one can never be certain that the central action of the drug might not lower blood pressure further). The dosage is then gradually increased, as tolerated by the patient, until optimal maintenance of blood pressure in the upright posture is accomplished. Doses as high as 0.4 mg twice daily have been required in a few patients reported by Robertson *et al.* (1983). Unfortunately, the potent central action of most currently available α_2-agonists, which are their most valuable attribute in the treatment of hypertension, reduces their potential value considerably in the treatment of orthostatic hypotension and results in their actually aggravating orthostatic hypotension both in patients with selective baroreceptor dysfunction (Robertson *et al.*, 1983) and in at least some patients with the venous pooling syndrome. If and when an α_2-agonist becomes available that does not penetrate the blood–brain barrier or for some other reason lacks the central action of the present drugs in this group, it would probably be useful in patients with orthostatic hypertension and with the pooling syndrome. In a few patients who have presented with orthostatic hypertension, clonidine therapy has restored the diastolic blood pressure in the upright posture to normal (Fig. 81).

10.1.2.6. Dopamine Antagonists

Kuchel *et al.* (1980) found that the dopamine antagonist metoclopramide improved orthostatic hypotension in a patient who had undergone sympathec-

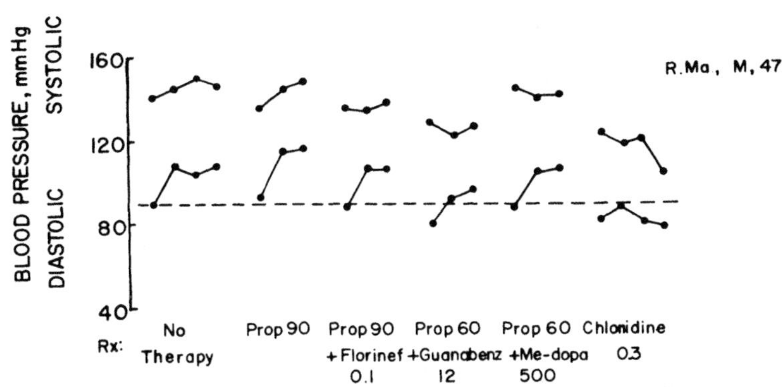

FIGURE 81. Effects of drug treatment in a patient with orthostatic hypertension. In this patient propranolol (prop), with or without fludrocortisone (Florinef R) and methyldopa (Me-dopa), was ineffective but propranolol with guanabenz or clonidine alone reduced orthostatic hypertension. Daily doses of medications (in mg) are shown.

tomy. Beretta-Piccoli and Weidmann (1982) confirmed the efficacy of metoclopramide (10 mg tid), with or without concomitant treatment with a nonsteroidal anti-inflammatory agent (flurbiprofen 100 mg/day), in two diabetic patients with autonomic neuropathy. Increase of exchangeable body sodium was observed in one patient, but plasma volume was not increased by the drugs in either patient. We have found consistently elevated plasma free dopamine concentrations in one patient with autonomic insufficiency (patient #1, in Appendix II). Since intravenous infusions of dopamine at 2 μg/kg per min appear to aggravate orthostatic tachycardia (Streeten *et al.*, unpublished observations), it is conceivable that metoclopramide might be helpful in patients with raised plasma dopamine concentrations.

10.1.2.7. Other Vasoconstrictors

The vasoconstrictor action of the ergot alkaloids has been known for many years and held responsible for the gangrene that may result from the administration of these alkaloids in excessive doses. Recently, this vasoconstrictive effect of the ergot derivative, dihydroergotamine, has been put to therapeutic use in the treatment of orthostatic hypotension (Benowitz *et al.*, 1970; Jennings *et al.*, 1979). The intramuscular administration of dihydroergotamine in divided doses of up to 10 mg/day or oral doses of 10–20 mg/day (not yet available in the United States) is reportedly useful in reducing orthostatic hypotension in some patients with this disorder. Although this drug is certainly no panacea for orthostatic hypotension, in our very limited experience it does appear to have some clinical value and is probably worthy of trial when other drugs that are easier to administer have failed.

In patients with autonomic insufficiency, Wagner and Braunwald (1956) showed that vasopressin injections (Pitressin tannate in oil) raised recumbent blood pressure and reduced orthostatic hypotension. Lysine vasopressin nasal spray is sometimes helpful in decreasing excessive orthostatic reductions in blood pressure (Chobanian *et al.*, 1977). Dramatic correction of orthostatic hypotension and of the excessive fall in cardiac output associated with it has been reported (Brehm, 1955) following the therapeutic administration of Peripherin (1 ml), which is marketed in West Germany by the Homburg Company. The recommended dose contains ephedrine 21.4 mg, theophylline 43.4 mg, and a theophylline analogue, etofyllin, 65 mg (Oelkers, personal communication). These findings do not appear to have been confirmed.

10.1.3. β-Adrenergic Antagonists

The first recognition of the existence of β-adrenergic receptors was based on the vasodilatory action of epinephrine when its vasoconstrictor effects were blocked (Alquist, 1948). This action of β-adrenergic agonists on their receptors in vascular tissue may be viewed, in a sense, as antagonistic to the vasoconstrictor action of α-adrenergic agonists on the same blood vessels.

Since the mechanisms of the orthostatic hypotension present in autonomic insufficiency include lack of vasoconstrictor action on the arterioles (and probably on other segments of the microvasculature) and perhaps an active vasodilatation (Diamond *et al.*, 1970), it was reasonable to explore the possible efficacy and usefulness of β-blocking drugs in the therapy of orthostatic hypotension (see Chobanian *et al.*, 1977). Chobanian and co-workers first reported that propranolol had some effect on, and some value in the treatment of, the postural hypotension of patients with peripheral autonomic failure. Unfortunately, the therapeutic benefit from this effect of propranolol is usually modest and sometimes negligible, in our experience. Nonetheless, the treatment of orthostatic hypotension in autonomic insufficiency is still so unsatisfactory that a trial of propranolol in doses of 40–160 mg/day is certainly worthwhile in patients who respond inadequately or adversely to fludrocortisone treatment. Based on the same rationale of trying to inhibit vasodilator influences on the microvasculature, we have used propranolol with some effectiveness in the treatment of patients with the pooling syndrome resulting from hyperbradykininism (Streeten *et al.*, 1972). The beneficial effects of propranolol on the orthostatic narrowing of the pulse pressure and on the severe orthostatic tachycardia in patients with the pooling syndrome are shown in Figure 82. Again, the drug should be started in small doses, such as 10 mg three times daily, and increased until the best individual result is accomplished, often at doses of 40 mg three times daily, with

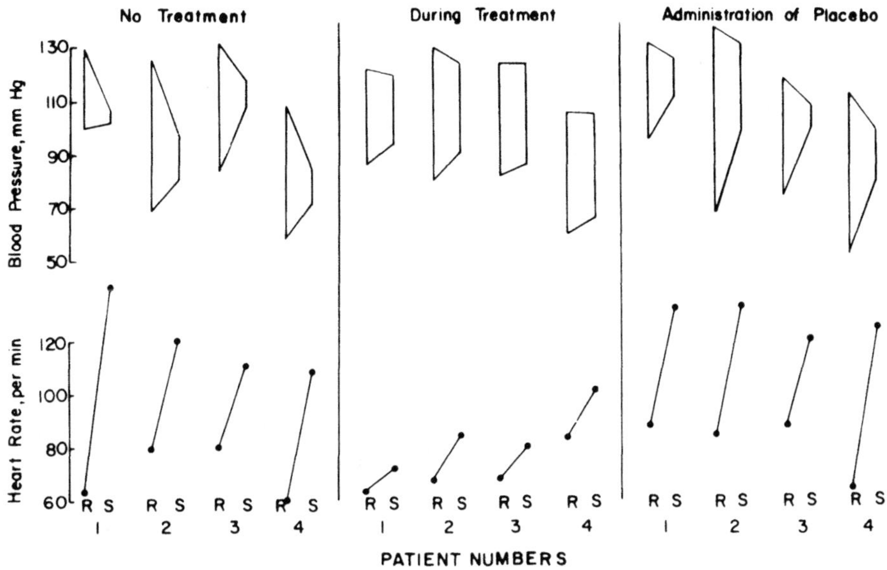

FIGURE 82. Effects of treatment for patients with hyperbradykininism using propranolol (patients 1–3) or fludrocortisone (patient 4), in comparison with placebo. (From Streeten *et al.*, 1972.)

or without concomitant administration of fludrocortisone. Whether the desired actions of propranolol result from its β_1- or its β_2-blocking action has not been determined; for this reason, it is difficult to know whether specific β_1- or β_2-blockers might be preferable to drugs such as propranolol, which block both types of receptor. In our limited experience, the relatively specific β_1-blocker, atenolol, seems to be at least as effective as propranolol; it also has the advantage of a far longer biological half-life, so that it can be administered once daily, with good effect. If congestive heart failure or hyperkalemia accompanies the orthostatic hypotension (as in some diabetic patients, particularly) β-blockers should not be used, in view of the tendency of these agents to aggravate both heart failure (Conway *et al.*, 1968) and hyperkalemia (Rosa *et al.*, 1980).

It was recently shown (Man in 't Veld *et al.*, 1981, 1982; Robson, 1981) that pindolol, through its partial β-agonistic action, has dramatically beneficial effects on orthostatic hypotension resulting from peripheral autonomic insufficiency but aggravates the orthostatic drop in blood pressure in patients with the central type of autonomic failure, in Shy–Drager syndrome (Davies *et al.*, 1981). It is therefore important to determine whether autonomic failure is of the central or peripheral type (see Chapter 9) and to use pindolol (in doses of 5 mg tid) only in patients with peripheral autonomic insufficiency. A simple test of whether pindolol is likely to be useful or harmful in a given patient involves evaluation of the effect of pindolol administration on heart rate: An increase in heart rate most likely indicates the presence of a peripheral neuropathy (Man in 't Veld, 1982). After 4 weeks' treatment with pindolol, there was a striking reduction of the supersensitivity of cardiovascular beta receptors, both to the nonselective agonist isoproterenol, and to the β_2-agonist, salbutamol (Man in 't Veld *et al.*, 1982).

10.1.4. Fludrocortisone and Other Volume Expanders

The useful therapeutic effects of injections or subcutaneous pellets of deoxycorticosterone acetate (DOCA) on the orthostatic fall in blood pressure seen in Addison's disease and in tabes dorsalis were first reported by Spingarn and Hitzig (1942). The dramatically beneficial effects of fludrocortisone on the orthostatic hypotension associated with adrenal insufficiency treated with hydrocortisone alone were recognized and used by many endocrinologists, including Stefan S. Fajans and other investigators at the University of Michigan, soon after this agent first became available for clinical use, in about 1957. Its application in the treatment of orthostatic hypotension resulting from autonomic insufficiency may be viewed as replacement therapy for the greatly reduced aldosterone secretion that occurs in autonomic failure (Slaton and Biglieri, 1967). Hickler *et al.* (1959*a*) were the first to report the effectiveness of fludrocortisone in patients with autonomic insufficiency, and their findings have been abundantly confirmed (Schneider, 1962; Schirger *et al.*, 1962; Schatz *et al.*, 1963; Bannister *et al.*, 1969; Campbell *et al.*, 1976).

Fludrocortisone should be started in doses of 0.1 mg/day and increased, if necessary, to 0.1 mg twice daily or even larger doses. Some physicians have used doses as high as 1.0 mg/day, and occasionally such high doses are significantly more effective than 0.2 or 0.3 mg/day in divided doses. At high dose levels, the hypokalemic action of fludrocortisone becomes troublesome. The therapeutic effect of fludrocortisone depends on its sodium-retaining action, and the drug is of no value if sodium intake is inadequate. Its action is generally considered to result from expansion of the initially normal or slightly increased plasma volume (Bannister *et al.*, 1969) in these patients. However, the steroid also increases the responses of the arterioles to intravenously infused norepinephrine in normal subjects (Schmid *et al.*, 1966) and restores some active vasoconstriction during orthostasis (Bannister *et al.*, 1969). Fludrocortisone is the most effective agent, not only for orthostatic hypotension but for most forms of the pooling syndrome as well. We have used this drug very frequently, ever since we reported its efficacy in some of the first five patients with hyperbradykininism (Streeten *et al.*, 1972) (see Fig. 81). It is evident from the data in Appendix II that fludrocortisone was effective in the treatment of four of the 18 patients with autonomic insufficiency, as well as in four of 10 patients with idiopathic diastolic hypotension and in 31 of 113 patients with the various forms of the venous pooling syndrome (excluding those with hypocortisolism). Thus, fludrocortisone, in the doses administered, was therapeutically useful in almost one-third of patients. Nevertheless, it certainly did not always restore orthostatic blood pressure abnormalities entirely to normal, even in these patients, and the drug was sometimes of little value. As shown in Table IX, fludrocortisone was found to lower the diastolic blood pressure very effectively in the four patients with orthostatic hypertension to whom it was administered for 2–4 weeks.

Recumbent hypertension is probably the commonest side effect of fludrocortisone therapy in patients with autonomic insufficiency. Hypokalemia, sometimes associated with metabolic alkalosis, which may be severe (Burns *et al.*, 1983), is another common side effect of large doses of fludrocortisone but is seldom seen with a dosage of 0.1 or 0.15 mg/day. The other main side effects of this drug in patients with orthostatic blood pressure disorders are aggravation or induction of edema and, very exceptionally, precipitation of congestive heart failure. These complications can usually be avoided or minimized by reducing the dose of fludrocortisone to 0.05 mg (a half-tablet) twice daily, once daily, or once every second day, as required.

Fludrocortisone expands the plasma volume (Chokroverty *et al.*, 1969) by 265 ml (mean) and presumably increases cardiac output during the first 10 days of its administration (Chobanian *et al.*, 1979). In patients in whom recumbent hypertension develops after several months of treatment with large doses of fludrocortisone (0.5–1.0 mg/day) plasma volume and cardiac output return to control levels, while the drug-induced recumbent hypertension is sustained by increased peripheral resistance (Chobanian *et al.*, 1979). When oral intake of drugs is not possible for any reason, intramuscular injections of deoxycor-

TABLE IX. Blood Pressure Response to Fludrocortisone Therapy (0.1 mg/day) in Patients with Orthostatic Hypertension[a]

	Recumbent position[b]			Standing[b]		
Patient no.	Without therapy	With therapy	Δ	Without therapy	With therapy	Δ
1	118/80	128/86	+10/+6	122/108	124/94	+2/−14
2	144/76	130/80	−14/+4	132/102	130/92	−2/−10
3	134/72	138/86	+4/+14	164/106	146/94	−18/−12
4	144/90	140/88	−4/−2	148/110	150/94	+2/−16
5	162/90	136/82	−26/−8	158/104	120/84	−38/−20
Mean	140.4/82.0	134.4/84.4	−5.6/+2.4	144.8/106.0	134.0/91.6	−10.8/−14.4
SEM	7.2/3.9	2.3/1.5		7.9/1.4	6.0/2.0	

[a]Blood pressure measurements (in mm Hg) were made before and after at least 1 week of treatment with fludrocortisone.
[b]Blood pressure readings are shown with and without fludrocortisone therapy.

ticosterone acetate (Gregory, 1945) can be used, either in doses of 2.5–5.0 mg/day, or in injections of the long-acting deoxycorticosterone trimethylacetate, 100–200 mg every 2–4 weeks.

When administering these or other sodium-retaining medications, such as 2-methyl, 9α-fluorohydrocortisone (Wagner, 1957), in these patients, it is essential to monitor serum potassium concentration (especially if large doses of the drug are used) and to evaluate for excessive fluid accumulation, inordinate weight gain, or any of the features of congestive heart failure at followup. Occasionally a dietary regimen of high salt intake alone will overcome orthostatic hypotension (Shear, 1963). The combination of fludrocortisone (0.6 mg) and of L-dopa (1.5 g/day) has been found superior to either drug alone in the treatment of Shy–Drager syndrome (Steiner *et al.*, 1974).

10.1.5. Prostaglandin Synthetase Antagonists

Drugs that reduce the synthesis of prostaglandins might theoretically be helpful in orthostatic hypotension and in the pooling syndrome because some prostaglandins are vasodilators and because prostaglandin inhibition tends to cause sodium retention. Indomethacin (75–150 mg/day) and various nonsteroidal anti-inflammatory agents have been used in the treatment of orthostatic hypotension (Kochar *et al.*, 1978; Abate *et al.*, 1979) and of the venous pooling syndrome, with beneficial effects in some patients. Further assessment of the clinical value of these drugs is needed. An enhanced response to the cold-pressor test and improved orthostatic reduction in forearm blood flow suggest that indomethacin ameliorates the disordered autonomic reflex vasoconstriction in these patients (Abate *et al.*, 1979).

10.1.6. Vasopressin

Vasopressin has occasionally been used with benefit in patients with autonomic failure (Hickler *et al.*, 1959*a;* Wagner and Braunwald, 1956; Chobanian *et al.*, 1977), but its use is not recommended because of hyponatremia, which is likely to result. Whether intranasal or subcutaneous use of dDAVP would be beneficial is unknown but is not likely, since this synthetic compound acts mainly on the renal V2 receptors and has little or no action at the vascular V1 receptors.

10.1.7. Atrial Pacemakers

The beneficial effects of atrial tachypacing in orthostatic hypotension associated with autonomic insufficiency was first reported by Moss *et al.* (1980) but was not confirmed by Tifft and Chobanian (1982). The tendency to nocturnal hypertension in patients treated with atrial pacing has been overcome by maintaining the heart rate at 95 beats/min during the day and at 55 beats/min at night (Kristinsson, 1983). This method of using the cardiac pacemaker was shown to raise systolic and diastolic blood pressure as well as cardiac output in the upright posture and to abolish the symptoms of orthostatic hypotension over the 9-month period of investigation. In the two patients studied, this type of atrial pacing proved superior to the other therapeutic modalities previously used.

10.1.8. Other Measures

10.1.8.1. Cool Environment

The vasodilatory action of high environmental temperatures tends to aggravate all manifestations of orthostatic hypotension and of the pooling syndrome. In hot weather, syncopal attacks become more frequent. For these reasons, we have found it helpful to recommend the use of air conditioning, at least in the room used by patients for most of the day, and to suggest avoidance of exposure to high temperatures.

10.1.8.2. Elevation of Head of Bed

MacLean and co-workers were the first to recommend that patients with autonomic insufficiency sleep with the head of the bed elevated about 40 cm, on two kitchen chairs, in order to reduce the abnormal nocturnal loss of intravascular fluid and fall in plasma volume which was thought to cause the early morning aggravation of postural hypotension (MacLean and Allen, 1940; MacLean *et al.*, 1944). These investigators also showed that the same simple form of treatment was helpful in 16 of 19 patients (84%) who appear to have had the venous pooling syndrome manifested by orthostatic tachycardia with or without orthostatic hypotension.

The beneficial effects of sleeping in the sitting position were confirmed by Corcoran *et al.* (1942) and by Stead and Ebert (1941). Bannister (1983) still considers this a useful therapeutic adjuvant, both in order to avoid diuresis and to lower the blood pressure at night in those patients with autonomic insufficiency whose orthostatic hypotension is associated with recumbent hypertension.

10.1.8.3. Improvement of Skeletal Muscle Tone

Improvement of skeletal muscle tone in the abdominal wall and the lower limbs by gymnastics and light forms of sport has been recommended by Laurell (1938).

10.1.9. Treatment of Orthostatic Hypertension

Since this disorder was previously recognized only infrequently as a distinct form of hypertension, it has been treated by most physicians as if it were persistent hypertension, and usually without appreciation of the fact that the blood pressure was often well below 90 mm Hg, or even below 80 mm Hg, in the recumbent posture. Treatment with a diuretic, which is usually the first type of drug administered in the currently popular "stepped-care" therapeutic regimen, may aggravate or induce lightheadedness and the other symptoms of the venous pooling syndrome. Diuretics may actually exaggerate the orthostatic rise in diastolic blood pressure in these patients, leading to the mistaken conclusion that the hypertension is refractory to therapy.

It is reasonable to question whether orthostatic hypertension, when asymptomatic and mild (e.g., 122/76 in recumbency and 126/100 standing), should be treated at all. When the pressure is more severely elevated (e.g., 144/88 in recumbency and 142/116 standing), one would be far more inclined to prescribe treatment, since the long-term effects and complications, if any, of orthostatic hypertension have not been investigated.

Although fludrocortisone does reduce orthostatic hypertension (see Fig. 75), we have not yet used this drug for the long-term management of more than occasional cases of orthostatic hypertension. We do not know whether orthostatic hypertension is (1) a "nondisease"; (b) a form of mild hypertension with complications similar to those of persistent hypertension; or (3) a precursor of more severe, persistent hypertension, as suggested by the work of Eide *et al.* (1978) and Payen *et al.* (1982). Because of this uncertainty, it is probably wise to adopt the following approach:

1. Not to treat patients whose diastolic blood pressure is <80 mm Hg in recumbency and 90–100 mm Hg standing. This is because most of the therapeutic trials in hypertensive patients (Veterans Administration Cooperative Study Group, 1970; Management Committee, 1980; Helgeland, 1980; Kaplan, 1982) have led to the conclusion that the beneficial effects of treating such mild degrees of diastolic pressure elevation continue to be equivocal.
2. To treat patients whose diastolic blood pressures are 85–90 mm Hg in recumbency and >100 mm Hg in the sitting or standing posture, using either of the following agents:
   a. A very small dose of an α_2-adrenergic agonist, such as clonidine (0.05 mg/day), guanabenz (4 mg/day), or methyldopa (250 mg/day) (see Fig. 81), and gradually increasing the dosage to tolerance and until orthostatic diastolic blood pressure is below 90 mm Hg
   b. A β-blocker, such as propranolol (10 mg bid), atenolol (50 mg/day),

or metoprolol (50 mg bid), with subsequent increase in dosage, as required.
If these drugs are ineffective or poorly tolerated, other agents should be tried.

10.2. PROGNOSIS

Orthostatic hypotension due to autonomic insufficiency has serious prognostic implications, especially when it is of the central type, associated with parkinsonism (Hughes *et al.*, 1970; Schirger and Thomas, 1976) or (even worse) with multiple system atrophy (Bannister, 1983). Of 52 patients with multiple system atrophy and severe orthostatic hypotension followed up by Thomas and Schirger (1970), less than 20% were alive after 75 months. Death occurred within 7–8 years of the onset of symptoms. However, 18 of the 52 patients (35%) reported by the same investigators were still alive after 3–33 years (mean 8 years). Five of our 18 patients died within 18 months of their first visit. Others, especially patients with peripheral autonomic failure, have remained substantially unchanged for several years. Spontaneous improvement is seldom seen, and progressive deterioration with eventual incapacitation is common. The prognosis for patients with diabetes mellitus in whom autonomic insufficiency develops is also generally poor. Ewing *et al.* (1980) reported that 53% of such patients died within 5 years, either from renal failure or from sudden or unexpected causes probably related to their autonomic neuropathy.

Patients with orthostatic hypotension not due to autonomic insufficiency and those with the pooling syndrome have an entirely different prognosis. There is no evidence that these disorders shorten life. Complications of syncopal attacks, such as bone fractures, head injuries, and automobile accidents (when syncope has occurred while driving a car), are the most serious hazards; but these can usually be avoided by alteration of life-style. However, long-term orthostatic lightheadedness and other consequences of orthostatic cerebral ischemia may have important effects on the life-style of these patients if their responses to therapy are inadequate. The learning capacity of schoolchildren or young adults may be impaired because of their inability to concentrate during prolonged teaching sessions and sometimes because of the need for more than an average duration of sleep at night. In those patients whose symptoms are severely aggravated by strenuous physical exertion or by high environmental temperatures, career choices may need to be changed appropriately. A tendency to faint may create special hazards in patients who work on ladders or with heavy machinery. Occupations such as nursing or working as sales personnel in stores, which require standing for prolonged periods, may become impossible for these persons. Some patients have had to retire from their previous occupations because of inadequate therapeutic relief of their severe lightheadedness, fatigue, or tendency to syncope.

Although we have followed several patients with orthostatic hypertension for more than 10 years, during which none has shown any tendency to progression or any serious complications, the prognosis of orthostatic hypertension remains unknown.

It is important to appreciate that the prognosis of patients who have syncopal attacks because of the venous pooling syndrome is benign. None of our patients has died, as far as we are aware, during a followup period of 3–25 years. This excellent prognosis for life is to be compared with the mortality of 30 ± 6.7% in 12 months in 53 patients who had syncope due to cardiovascular disease, most commonly ventricular tachycardia or the sick sinus syndrome (Kapoor *et al.*, 1983).

10.3. SUMMARY

It is essential, as far as possible, first to correct any cause of orthostatic dysfunction that may be discovered, such as anemia, dehydration from chronic diarrhea or diuresis, and use of sympatholytic drugs. When this has been accomplished, fludrocortisone therapy, starting with 0.1 mg/day, is far and away the most effective and useful form of treatment available both for autonomic insufficiency and for the pooling syndrome. When results are suboptimal, many other modalities of treatment should be considered, including the use of elastic stockings or Jobst-type, waist-high, custom-fitted garments; vasoconstricting drugs of which midodrine appears to be the most promising (although it has not yet been approved for use in the United States by the FDA); β-adrenergic blocking drugs such as propranolol, atenolol, and pindolol (the last-mentioned in patients with peripheral autonomic insufficiency only); prostaglandin synthetase inhibitors; use of a home air-conditioner in the summer; and sleeping with the head of the bed elevated. Avoidance of diuretic therapy, exposure to heat, and unnecessary physical exertion is recommended.

Treatment often produces improvement—sometimes dramatic rehabilitation. The prognosis depends on the disorder being treated. The pooling syndrome is a form of chronic ill health that seldom reduces longevity. Autonomic insufficiency, on the other hand, carries a poor prognosis, with 80% of patients with multiple system atrophy failing to survive more than 6 years. The peripheral form of autonomic insufficiency is far less lethal, being compatible with longer survival.

APPENDIX I

Clinical and Laboratory Data Obtained in 169 Patients with Orthostatic and Nonorthostatic Edema

CLASSIFICATION

Patients have been classified, by the criteria to be described, into five groups:

1. *Orthostatic sodium retainers:* Urinary sodium excretion in the upright posture subnormal, either by the "posture test" (standing/recumbent Na ratio <34%) or during the first day of orthostasis for 12 hr on a 200-mEq Na diet (urinary Na <106 mEq/day)
2. *Orthostatic water retainers:* Na excretion normal but water excretion subnormal in upright posture, either <55% of a standard water load (20 ml/kg) being excreted in 4 hr or urinary osmolality in the "posture test" being above normal (i.e., >390 mOsm/kg) in the upright posture
3. *Orthostatic sodium and water retainers:* Showing both of the above orthostatic abnormalities
4. *Nonorthostatic edema:* Patients with normal Na excretion and normal urinary osmolality in the "posture test," as well as (when known) normal excretion of the water load in the upright posture, and normal increase in leg volume and body weight during 2 hr of standing, in the balance study
5. *Others*

KEY TO COLUMNS

Ages: (in years). Ht: height (in cm). Wt: weight (in kg) when first seen off therapy. Comp: percentage difference in weight compared with Metropolitan Life Insurance Company standards (overweight: +, underweight: −). Blood pressure: (in mm Hg) before treatment, recumbent and standing 3 min. Heart rates: (per min) before treatment, recumbent and standing. Symptoms: A: chest pain; Ax: subtotal adrenalectomy in past; B: cold intolerance; C: carpal tunnel syndrome; Cd: chronic obstructive airways disease; Co: carpal tunnel syndrome treated surgically; D: discomfort in legs; Dm: diabetes mellitus; E: flushes; F: fatigue; G: thyromegaly; H: headaches; Ha: edema aggravated by heat; Hi: hives; I: impaired mental concentration; Ir: irritability; J: joint pains; Jb: backache; K: hypoglycemic symptoms; L: lightheadedness; M: menstrual aggravation of edema; N: nocturia; Na: nausea; O: edema aggravated by oral contraceptives; P: onset of edema in pregnancy; Pa: paresthesias; Pe: periorbital edema only; Prx: psychotherapy in progress; Ps: pseudotumor cerebri; Q: palpitations; R: heat intolerance; S: dyspnea; S: sleepiness; Sw: excessive sweating; Sx: sympathectomized; Sy: syncope; T: excessive thirst; Th: hyperthyroidism; T1: hypothyroidism; U: brawny edema; V: varicose veins; Vo: varicose veins operated upon; W: weakness; X: lethargy; Y: mitral valve prolapse present; Z: mental depression.

ORTHOSTATIC CHANGES

Effects of orthostasis on (1) excretion of sodium expressed as standing Na excretion/recumbent Na excretion in "posture test," or, when underlined, percentage of Na intake excreted within 24 hr in balance study on 200-mEq Na diet; (2) urinary osmolality (Osm) in mOsm/kg, during orthostasis for 2 hr, in "posture test"; and (3) water excretion, expressed as percentage of 20 ml/kg water load excreted while standing for 4 hr; (4) change in leg volume (Leg vol) (in ml); and (5) changes in weight (Wt) in kg, from 8:00 a.m. to 8:00 p.m. in balance study (Bal), or at home from time of rising to time of sleep (ID: intra diem i.e., from morning to bedtime), without treatment (sRx); and (6) with the treatment indicated (cRx).

THERAPY

Effects on changes in morning weight, in kg (ΔWt a.m.; i.e., total change in morning wt during therapy) of a course of therapy with the drugs indicated: A: amiloride; C: chlorthalidone; D: dextroamphetamine; Des: desoxyn; Dex: dexamethasone; Dig: digoxin, digitoxin; E: ephedrine; F: furosemide; H: hydrochlorothiazide and chlorothiazide; M: midodrine; P: propyl thiouracil; S: spironolactone; and others, as indicated.

APPENDIX I

	Age					Blood pressure		Heart Rate		
#	When seen	Edema onset	Ht (cm)	Wt (kg)	Comp wt (%)	Rec. (mm Hg)	Standing (mm Hg)	Rec. (per min)	Stand (per min)	Symptoms
1. Orthostatic Sodium Retainers										
1	36	16	155	47	−20	100/70		100		HT
2	25	21	163	64	−2	104/76	100/68	72	88	HM
3	57	43	156	70	+19	144/78	122/70	76	88	HJLM
4	47	46	151	85	+49	144/82		76		HJM
5	45	43	162	66	+2	168/96	174/102	88	92	
6	44	29	152	60	+3	120/80	114/82	80	92	CoDEHaMSw
7	38	28	155	100	+67	125/80		65		DJb
8	32	27	166	73	+7	110/58	108/74	84	104	HO
9	38	32	163	59	−9	120/90	116/80	90	108	Tl
10	41	38				140/80	136/84	80	84	P
11	26	19	160	115	+67	148/78	140/90	88	104	FHaPW
12	44	39	162	69	+6	144/84	128/84	84	96	FGHaMNPa
13	43	35	162	106	+63	172/92		88		HHaTh
14	38	37	163	68	+5	116/80	122/86	72	80	Co
15	32	24	165	59	−12	100/60	100/72	68	88	FHILMN
16	49	17	174	76	+15	132/76	134/80	96	96	FLPTh
17	34	22	160	62	+6	134/88	122/86	80	76	HaMP
18	29	28	167	60	−12	100/66	96/80	60	80	FILHaSy
19	31	21	165	70	+4	104/62	98/68	84	100	FHaT
20	31	28	162	119	+88	132/72	120/90	80	116	FHa
21	44	26	170	63	−10	130/90	128/96	92	128	FHaPTlVo
22	30	26		81		154/96	144/96	96	104	FHaLP
23	46	30	164	76	+13	122/70		60		HHaLMNaP
24	33	25	158	86	+41	118/86	112/80	96	100	P
25	32	31	163	62	+3	110/80	120/80	96	96	HaNW
26	35	28		81		122/80	104/60	72	84	FP
27	65	64	151	71	+25	170/80	170/88	90	104	FG
28	24	21	162	68	+14	120/76	110/68	72	90	Dm
29	51	41	155	48	−19	140/88	132/92	68	76	Tl
30	59	46	157	65	+7	138/82	142/84	80	84	BHHaI
31	39	10	163	56	−7	90/50	84/60	88	108	HHaILZ
32	46	45	158	71	+25	136/82	134/86	92	104	Vo
33	45	33	162	48	−19	166/88	168/92	80	88	Ax
34	26	24	163	75	+15	132/82	132/80	84	104	
35	47	38	164	52	−22	102/68	90/60	100	120	FHHaLW megacolon
36	34	28	155	75	+27	162/68	160/74	108	108	RTh
37	32	27		75		130/72	124/80	84	92	FHaLMZ Crohn's
38	49	43	154	56	+2	150/86	126/78	88	92	HaNaW
39	29	25		62		106/84	108/84	72	82	
40	22	21	164	68	+1	130/80	128/84	76	84	H
41	28	26	170	70	0	130/86	114/84	72	112	HHaLMSY kinin high
42	48	45		58		152/92	122/82	76	80	FLQS kinin high
43	59	49	158	50	−18	142/70	122/70	100	104	CdHHa
44	35	30	166	98	+44	126/84	120/84	84	92	FHaMNaOSlTl
45	29	22	155	56	−5	124/68	106/90	84	130	FHLPV
46	43	31	170	64	−9	116/74	104/78	68	72	HaP
47	44	26	164	71	+18	110/80	84/70	72	100	FHHaIrMPaW
48	35	25	169	95	+38	136/76	130/86	84	104	P
49	25	24	162	64	−2	106/60	108/62	68	92	HM
50	20	18	158	54	−11	120/88	108/86	102	120	DmFRW
51	34	22	167	80	+18	106/68	100/68	84	88	P

Measured orthostatic changes						Therapy					
Urin Na	Urin osmol. (mOsm/kg)	Water excr. (%)	Change in leg volume a.m. to p.m. (ml)	Changes in balance study (kg)	Δ *Wt* intra diem (kg)	Δ *Wt* intra diem (kg)	Δ *Wt* a.m. (kg)	Drugs	Δ *Wt* intra diem (kg)	Δ *Wt* a.m. (kg)	Drug
5	297	56			1.6	0.4	−4	CES			
28	262	78	385	1.6	0.9	0.6	−9	L-Dopa			
30	320	—									
18	207	—			0.9	1.0	−10	D		−7	ECS
24	280					0.9	+1	D			
32	305	—			0.7						
13	201	109					−9	CS			
26	247	69									
12	182	—	450	1.3	0.8						
23	—	—									
6	293	—	320	1.2							
6	190	—			0.7	0.4	−2	DS			
12	259	72	355	1.4	0.6			Dopamine diuresis			
32	355	—				1.3	−1	CS			
29	—		456	1.8	2.0	1.3	−2	DS		0	S
21	290	76	261	1.6		0.2	−3	D			
28	246	—	642	1.6	1.0	0.5	−6	D			
22	—	86	348	1.7	0.9						
17	238		340	1.0	1.1	0.8	−2	D			
28	—						−2	ES			
32	267										
8	209	—			1.2	0.3	−4	D			
40	289	75	390	1.8	0.7	0.6	−5	D	0.2	−2	DS
33	—		390	1.7	1.4						
19	195										
25					0.8						
14	302		400	1.7	1.5	0.7	+1	D	0.8	−1	C
51	210	57	310	1.1							
13		95			1.7						
19	172	—	470	1.6	1.6	1.2	−6	DS	lost 6 kg in 3yr		
20	148	85	590	1.6			−4	D			
25	258	—		1.5	0.6	0.1	−4	CD			
14	—		346	1.7							
20	268	68									
22		—	490	2.6							
17					0.9	0.7	−1	PS	0.6	−1	S
23	214	—			1.2	0.5	−14	CES	lost 24 kg in 1yr		
22					0.7	0.4	−1	D			
15	224	—			1.1						
32	382										
33	302	88			2.7	2.1					
17		—		2.6	1.8		−1	D			
25	152	—	370	1.5	1.2	0.9	0	D	0.8	−1	C
42	285	65	450	2.4	1.1						
32	269	—	500	1.7	1.4	0.4	−1	D			
20		69	400	1.7	1.6						
24		100			1.6	0.4	−3	DSH	0.5	+2	SH
25	619	65					−25	Des			
29	504	87	320	0.6	0.8	0.6		E			
25	581	57	500	1.8	1.1	0.7	−3	D			
32	487	63	370	1.4	1.2						

(*continued*)

APPENDIX I. (*Continued*)

#	Age		Ht (cm)	Wt (kg)	Comp wt (%)	Blood pressure		Heart Rate		Symptoms
	When seen	Edema onset				Rec. (mm Hg)	Standing (mm Hg)	Rec. (per min)	Stand (per min)	
2. Orthostatic Sodium and Water Retainers										
52	42	27	160	81	+29	124/80	108/90	72	84	HLW
53	41	23	157	68	+11	106/70	96/68	88	100	FHP
54	50	50	169	105	+52	166/98	168/98	64	80	F
55	41	28		96		148/90	150/94	116	120	EFGQ
56	40	30	167	63	−7	128/98	126/98	72	84	HiVo
57	26	25	166	54	−21	110/70	104/82	80	92	FJLMPW
58	58	38	163	105	+62	192/108	166/102	80	84	V
59	33	31	154	79	+36	130/90	122/95	92	100	FHHaLPPaSw
60	30	27	168	65	+4	118/76	108/80	78	120	BMNTl
61	39	38	164	70	+4	124/74	112/80	84	92	FMSw
62	38	36	165	92	+37	148/86		88		H
63	39	22	162	57	−12	110/70	112/80	68	84	HaMNP
64	35	22	162	60	+1	110/68	108/78	76	88	HaMP
65	50	30	162	54	−10	106/58	112/64	92	94	PS
66	28	22	167	62	−9	116/76	112/82	84	96	HaJbL
67	46	22	163	110	+83	180/112	204/140	84	96	BFTl
68	52	50	161	87	+38	140/58	134/64	68	72	FL large sella
69	34	22	171	61	−14	128/70	128/82	88	96	FM
70	19	17	168	58	−16	120/80	120/108	84	92	Acute leg pain
71	45	40	171	59	−20	108/54	98/60	80	104	TlY
72	29	21	161	68	+6	128/60	130/78	72	100	HLMNQ
73	52	51	170	71	+1	120/70	120/90	92	120	CoN
74	38	34	174	124	+71	134/78		88		DF
75	42	22	172	79	+11	118/80	116/84	88	92	FlJbM
76	28	26	166	66	−3	118/80	116/84	72	98	HHaMN kinin+, AVP+
77	18	17	173	64	−11	98/64	84/80	68	120	FHHaLSSlW
78	20	13	161	61	−3	122/80	128/80	88	96	L
79	51	46	166	73	+7	160/90		88		HHaLTl
80	57	37	161	72	+23	122/76		76		DJTl
81	19	18	173	85	+18	128/80	122/96	84	112	HaDm
82	36	24	165	54	−19	124/74	114/72	76	84	FHHaIT purple legs
83	39	26	168	77	+12	122/76	116/70	108	120	FHHaMP
84	31	13	171	79	+11	102/74	100/84	88	96	Ha
85	73	63	152	92	+59	180/88	188/92	84	84	FJbTl
86	30	25	168	117	+71	166/104	142/90	88	94	DH adrenalex later
87	32	24	157	53	−13	132/84	112/84	78	102	HaM
88	42	40	165	99	+48	152/108	156/108	84	92	HaMPrxV
89	30	10	162	47	−23	84/72	68/64	80	108	DFSPs exercise tol.
90	30	27	165	69	+3	112/72	94/62	64	88	CoHa
91	46	34	163	54	−17	112/58	106/58	46	62	DLMP
92	19	18	167	62	−9	124/84	114/92	60	112	DHL
93	17	16	174	88	+21	126/74	122/88	92	104	FPrx TSH=7.2
94	48	47	165	54	−19	98/78	96/76	76	96	FL kinins high
95	19	17	165	91	+36	122/80	122/82	72	104	HPs+
96	24	22	173	83	+15	116/62	108/60	72	108	HPPs
97	50	49	166	62	−9	118/94	112/90	84	104	Vv
98	52	45	151	75	+32	160/92	160/92	96	100	DmHTl
99	35	27	166	65	−4	120/80	110/80	88	100	HJbLP
100	22	21	160	55	−13	150/60	138/74	84	90	J
101	40	39	165	61	−9	130/90	122/98	84	100	orth. nephroptosis

						Therapy					
Measured orthostatic changes											
Urin Na	Urin osmol. (mOsm/kg)	Water excr. (%)	Change in leg volume a.m. to p.m. (ml)	Changes in balance study (kg)	Δ *Wt* intra diem (kg)	Δ *Wt* intra diem (kg)	Δ *Wt* a.m. (kg)	Drugs	Δ *Wt* intra diem (kg)	Δ *Wt* a.m. (kg)	Drug
8	467	—	305	1.8							
14	444	—			2.1	0.5	−2	ESH			
10	475				1.8	0.7		ESH			
18	400	—									
11	292	11			0.9	0.5	−4				
23	540	—	333	1.5	1.3	0.5	−2	D			
17	460	—									
15	620										
13	438										
44	393	—	317	1.6	1.0	0.9	−4	D			
30	421				0.7	0.7	−4	D	0.7	+1	E
8	586										
22	448		630	1.4	2.0	0.5	−4	CD			
23	660	—	629	1.6	2.0	0.9		CD			
16	469	—	330	1.7		0.4	−3	C			
16	399				1.6						
3	600	32			0.8	0.7	−2	C			
6	654	42	468	1.8	2.0	0.8		Tenuate			
9	794	—			1.2	0.5	−4	D			
34	180	47			3.7	3.5	−1	Digitalis, L-thyroxine			
21	459				1.0	0.8	+1	D			
10	482				2.1	0.7	−1	D			
52	402	50	385	1.3			0	M captopril			
18	271	51			1.5	1.9	−3	FS			
20	157	54	470	1.5	2.6	0.7	−4	D	0.7	0	E
7		6			1.1	1.1	−4	E			
22	540	—	581	1.6	1.7	0.5	−1	D	0.4	−1	DS
21		17			0.6	0.5	−1	D	0.8	−1	DS
28	545	—	452	1.7	0.8	0.9	−4	DS			
19	157	29				0.5	−1	D	0.5	−1	F
21	198	13	290	0.8	1.9		+1	CM			
20	145	10	810	2.4	1.9	1.7	+1	DS captopril	1.9	+4	+M
33	244	52	448	1.9	1.7	1.0	−6	DS			
30	474	40			0.8	0.6	−5	DS			
19	720	49	404	1.4	1.5	1.5					
25	197	50									
28	685	45							lost 18 kg in 7 yr		
46	382	42	300	1.4	0.9	0.6	−3	ACD	0.5	−7	ACD
27	131	43							0.5	−4	D
45	196	41	275	0.7	1.3	0.7	−1	E	0.7	−1	DS
10	275	—	407	1.3	0.8	0.4	−6	D			
9	615	42	397	1.9			−5	diet			
31	610	51	325	2.2	1.2	0.7	−2	ESH			
23	657	11	478	1.7	0.7		−4	D			
20	331	29	285		1.4	1.0	−1	DDex	2.3	−3	DH
51	449	—	457	1.6	0.7	0.8	−1	D			
37	405	—	417	1.7	1.0	1.0	0	C			
15	607	52	268	1.9	1.6	0.9	−1	S			
19	403				0.4	0.4	−2	E			
14	387	—			0.5	0.4	0	D			

(*continued*)

APPENDIX I. (Continued)

#	Age: When seen	Age: Edema onset	Ht (cm)	Wt (kg)	Comp wt (%)	Blood pressure: Rec. (mm Hg)	Blood pressure: Standing (mm Hg)	Heart Rate: Rec. (per min)	Heart Rate: Stand (per min)	Symptoms
102	30	25	164	64	−4	120/80	110/80	84	110	H pregnancy edema
103	32	17	174	84	+15	126/80	128/96	82	96	HaP
104	35	33	160	133	+111	112/70		76		FHRW
3. Orthostatic Water Retainers										
105	55	45		57		108/68		92		Th
106	25	21	168	63	−9	114/72	120/80	56	72	BDTl
107	38	33	164	71	+6	90/78	90/70	80	108	Incomp. perforat. vv
108	36	30	168	73	+2	112/72	118/78	80	84	KS
109	32	28	162	54	−17	130/72	82/72	84	112	FHHal Pa toxemia
110	47	46	162	93	+43	150/76	130/82	84		Th
111	28	26	166	62	−9	118/82		88		M diuretic intolerance
112	32	22	170	80	+14	132/88	98/84	72	112	FH
113	42	31	165	72	+18	122/68		72		HaM
114	29	22	164	76	+13	110/56	110/56	80	84	HKLNSw
115	36	26	166	56	−18	110/76	106/86	72	80	FHHaSTh
116	29	22	164	91	+36	120/88	96/78	76	80	FHNaPZ
117	47	46	157	53	−13	114/70	116/76	52	60	LNPaT
118	41	37	172	110	+55	156/84	152/88	96	112	PTh
119	32	23	168	95	+38	140/90	126/98	96	140	D multip sclerosis
120	46	34	165	92	+37	122/80	118/72	76	90	HHaILP
121	52	42	163	60	−8	128/70	134/74	78	84	HMTl
122	32	22		45		112/76	104/78	80	96	F
123	42	25	154	91	+57	128/80	120/90	72	76	FHaMPU
124	27	10	154	46	−21	124/80	114/86	72	96	FJb kinins high
125	20	15	156	53	−5	122/78	118/82	66	86	
126	53	18	164	68	+1	118/84	110/88	92	96	HaMP
127	40	27	165	103	+54	114/66	106/70	68	84	FIMT ivc thrombosis
128	60	30	156	66	+18	148/68	128/60	80	80	S
129	20	18	168	62	−10	128/90	116/90	96	96	OTh+ regional ileitis
130	35	24	166	90	+32	140/86	130/96	120	136	ThVo
131	55	54	171	75	+6					FL
132	30	26		39		102/72	84/76	80	140	LQSwW
133	29	25	170	59	−16	106/72	100/72	72	82	F
134	43	33	161	72	+14	110/70	120/84	78	96	HaMU
135	32	30	156	57	+2	130/90		82		Ha
4. Nonorthostatic Edema										
136	42	32	165	59	−3	120/70	106/86	98	120	HaVo CHF, thalassemia
137	49	43	156	71	+20	150/80	144/72	76	80	MNTl
138	22	14	163	60	+8	110/84	108/90	76	104	NOT
139	21	19	164	57	−15	104/68	110/80	72	78	BF
140	57	23	156	54	−4	140/70	138/72	92		HHaP episodic edema
141	50	30	161	96	+52	180/94	152/100	96	124	HHaM adrex 10 yr ago
142	53	49	160	77	+22	138/90	146/92	92	100	CoFHNR
143	26	16	158	55	−4	118/78	106/80	104	120	DFNaT
144	16	13	156	78	+32	110/70	110/84	80	84	HHa
145	47	37	156	93	+41	180/112	164/114	68	80	T
146	43	22	159	60	−3	116/78	114/82	84	88	Pe
147	31	26	154	52	−12	118/78	104/78	52	60	HHaPZ EtOH aggravates

Measured orthostatic changes						Therapy					
Urin Na	Urin osmol. (mOsm/kg)	Water excr. (%)	Change in leg volume a.m. to p.m. (ml)	Changes in balance study (kg)	Δ *Wt* intra diem (kg)	Δ *Wt* intra diem (kg)	Δ *Wt* a.m. (kg)	Drugs	Δ *Wt* intra diem (kg)	Δ *Wt* a.m. (kg)	Drug
15	248	44			0.7						
5	396	—		0.8	1.0	1.0	−14	DH			
16	462	—			1.3		−19	CD			
65	620	8			0.7						
69	548				0.9	0.4	−3	T4			
74	316	41	308	1.4	2.6	0.4	−6	D			
37	574	18			1.9						
49	—	—			1.1	0.8	−1	S	0.6	−2	D
39	302	20									
38	134	52						Dopamine diuresis			
38		—			1.0	0.2	−3	D			
54		37									
55	504	31			0.9	0.6	+2	DES			
64	157	50	305								
47	539	25									
22	143	60 a.m. 45 p.m.			3.6	0.9	−2	SH		−3	D
48		23			1.5		0	E			
	154	33	585	1.8	1.3	1.4	−4	CDS	lost 16 kg in 1 yr		
37	281	37	395	2.0	1.5	1.0	−5	DS	lost 12 kg in 2.5 yr		
41	409	26									
72	294	27		0.9	0.9	0.6	−2				
	7				0.8	later TSH= 30 mIU/mL					
51	361	30	480	0.9	1.1	1.6	−1	CD	1.2	0	DH
58	162	36				0.2	0	D			
56	615	25			0.6	0.3	−2	C			
35	189	18	600	1.1	1.2	0.7	−2	D	lost 5kg in 3 yr		
62	232	42	571	1.8							
37		33									
54	420	27									
59	576	26			0.9						
57	675	—	340	1.1							
51		39		0.9							
66	275	37		2.3							
42	380	55									
40	161	—	249	1.1	0.1	0.2	−2	DS			
47		99						Thyroxine			
37		62									
39	203				0.5						
—	—	—			0.5						
97	232	—		0.4		0.2	−4	DS			
40	278	83			0.9	0.7	+1	H	0.4	0	DH
136	285	69			0.9	0.9	0	L-dopa			
46		—			0.5	0.6	−1	D	0.7	−1	DH
—		—			0.5	0.6	−7	D			
44	369	—	212	1.1	0.6			Dex			
180	151	80			0.4	0.1	−1	ES	0.5	+1	DS

(continued)

APPENDIX I. (*Continued*)

	Age					Blood pressure		Heart Rate		
#	When seen	Edema onset	Ht (cm)	Wt (kg)	Comp wt (%)	Rec. (mm Hg)	Standing (mm Hg)	Rec. (per min)	Stand (per min)	Symptoms
148	50	46	158	48	−16	88/50	96/60	60	84	F Lt nephroptosis
149	40	38	162	64	−2	110/76	106/76	88	100	DPeTl
150	37	35	160	85	+35	110/76	120/80	88	104	FHaZ
151	32	30	165	72	+7	138/86	122/84	76	76	HM
152	54	44	154	72	+24	158/90	160/96	80	84	FHaR
153	45	33	160	67	+6	132/84	120/84	80	96	DFHaM
154	34	20		88		138/78	132/114	88	92	B
155	59	54	155	68		100/70	110/80	100		Tl
156	35	28	165	85	+27	136/72		82		GHa
157	35	34	155	59	0	122/80	98/70		80	Worse sitting
158	48	35	174	74	−1	110/88	116/98	64	84	FHIr
159	35	16	150	50	−12	102/84	100/76	72 82	82	Co card. arrest, K = 5 mEq/L
160	42	40		54		112/76	120/86	64	68	Intermittent, face
161	49	29				154/90		112		FlSw T4, kinin nl
5. Other Patients										
162	44	12	161	54	−14	112/62	96/66	76	88	CoHa Heat sensitive
163	14	13	159	60	−3	114/76	108/80	76	110	DFHINaSl
164	37	30	157	78	+39	130/76	128/86	108	108	HLPSwSy
165	20	13	163	70	−8	146/68	132/100	80	92	BFWTl
166	33	24	170	65	−7	92/56	100/62	88	120	Co
167	39	38	165	57	−15	126/64		100		FGRTh Thyrotoxic
168	41	?	178	102	+38	140/70	106/58	56	64	none Male
169	48	42	182	98	+40	104/68	108/76	52	72	DIrSSw episodic Male

Measured orthostatic changes						Therapy					
Urin Na	Urin osmol. (mOsm/kg)	Water excr. (%)	Change in leg volume a.m. to p.m. (ml)	Changes in balance study (kg)	Δ *Wt* intra diem (kg)	Δ *Wt* intra diem (kg)	Δ *Wt* a.m. (kg)	Drugs	Δ *Wt* intra diem (kg)	Δ *Wt* a.m. (kg)	Drug
54	146	—		1.3							
32	564	50	140	1.0	0.3			Dex			
40	212	98			0.9	1.0	0	D			
36	276	74	130	1.2							
87	234	97	215	0.8	0.5	0.3	0	D			
50	318	—			0.5						
—		—			0.5	0.6	−1	D	1.1	−2	CS
48	200	97			1.7	2.2	−4	CD			
35	130	64			working:1.3	0.3	−4	ES 0.5	0.5	−3	D
36	255	79	235	1.6	1.3	0.9	−1	D			
49	163			0.8							
55	161	60									
—	—	—						Dexamyl diuresis			
69	229										
100	283	—	195	1.5	1.3	1.0	0	D			
57	(in heat)		285 (in heat)	1.8							
—	—	—			1.6	0.6	−6	D			
51	342	—	332	1.2	1.1						
41	319										
62	260				1.2		−2	DF Dopa dopamin. diuresis			
—	—		—	—	—	—	—				
37	—	—	207	0.6	1.0	0.7	−1	D			
	Male										
78		78									
	Male										

APPENDIX II

Clinical and Laboratory Data Obtained in 159 Patients with Orthostatic Blood Pressure Disorders

CLASSIFICATION

All patients had abnormalities in blood pressure in the upright posture and have been classified into five groups:

1. *Orthostatic diastolic hypotension:* Diastolic BP falls consistently by at least 10 mm Hg after standing for 3 min, either
   a. Associated with autonomic insufficiency manifested by subnormal standing plasma norepinephrine concentration (below 200 pg/ml) and/or orthostatic rise in heart rate of <10 beats/min, OR
   b. Associated with laboratory evidence of hypocortisolism, OR
   c. Idiopathic, associated with no evidence of subnormal orthostatic plasma norepinephrine concentration and with normal adrenal and cardiac function

2. *Orthostatic systolic hypotension:* Systolic BP alone falls by at least 20 mm Hg or to below 94 mm Hg after standing for 3 min,
   a. Associated with hypoaldosteronism, established by laboratory tests, OR
   b. Idiopathic

3. Orthostatic diastolic hypertension: Diastolic BP rises from <90 mm Hg in recumbency to at least 98 mm Hg after standing for 3 min.

4. *Orthostatic narrowing of pulse pressure* to 18 mm Hg or less:
   a. Associated with *hyperbradykininism,* established by finding blood bradykinin concentration above above 0.5 ng/ml and/or plasma bradykininase concentration below 0.4 μM/min per ml, OR
   b. Associated with plasma hypovolemia, OR
   c. Idiopathic

5. *Orthostatic tachycardia:* Heart rate rises by at least 28 beats/min and to above 108 beats/min after 3 min of standing:
   a. Associated with laboratory evidence of hypocortisolism, OR
   b. Associated with laboratory evidence of hyperbradykininism, OR
   c. Idiopathic

6. *Other:* Patients with recurrent orthostatic symptoms but normal blood pressure and heart rate changes in the upright posture.

KEY TO COLUMNS

#: patient number, followed by gender (Sex). Ages when first seen by us and when symptoms first occurred. Blood pressure and heart rate in recumbent (Rec.) and standing (Stand.) postures, after at least 3 min. Symptoms as follows: A: chest pain; Bv: blurred vision; C: cold intolerance; Dm: diabetes mellitus; E: facial flushes; Ed: edema present; F: fatigue; G: thyromegaly; H: headaches; Ha: aggravated by heat; I: impaired mental function in the upright posture; Im: impotence; In: urinary or fecal incontinence; Ir: irritability; J: joint pains; Jb: backache; K: hypoglycemic symptoms; L: lightheadedness; M: menstrual aggravation of symptoms; N: nocturia; Na: nausea; P: onset of symptoms during pregnancy; Pa: paresthesias; Pk: parkinsonism; Q: palpitations; R: heat intolerance; S: dyspnea; Sl: sleepiness; Sw: excessive sweating; Sy: syncope; Th: hyperthyroidism; T1: hypothyroidism; V: vomiting; W: weakness; Y: mitral valve prolapse documented by echocardiography; Z: mental depression.

Tests of Function: BP in G suit: blood pressure after standing for 3 min or more in an inflated G suit or MAST garment; Norepineph.: plasma concentrations of norepinephrine after reclining for 30 min (Rec.) and after standing for at least 5 min (Stand.), in pg/ml; Renin activity: plasma renin activity after furosemide (40 mg i.v.) and standing for 2 hr (in ng/ml per hr); Aldosterone: plasma aldosterone concentration (in ng/ml) after the same stimulation; Kinin: blood kinin concentration, recumbent or standing (NI = normal, not more than 0.5 ng/ml, by radioimmunoassay); ITT: insulin tolerance test with plasma response to hypoglycemia, expressed as cortisol/glucose slope (normal 0.20–0.66 μg/mg) (see Streeten *et al.*, 1984); ACTH test: maximal plasma cortisol (Cort) and aldosterone (Aldo) concentrations in 2- or 4-hourly blood sampling during infusion of cosyntropin (Cortosyn), 0.25 mg intravenously, over 8 hr; A-II: plasma aldosterone concentration before and at 1 or 2 hr after i.v. infusion of angiotensin, at a rate sufficient to raise diastolic BP by 20 mm Hg; Me and metyr: urinary 17-hydroxycorticosteroid excretion on day after metyrapone administration, 500 mg by mouth, every 2 hr, for 12 doses (normal: >10.5 mg) (see Streeten *et al.*, 1984).

THERAPY

Response in BP and heart rate (HR) after standing for 3 min, during treatment with the drugs indicated; FF: fludrocortisone (Florinef); Prop: propranolol; Co: hydrocortisone; Pheonx: pheonoxybenzamine; Spironz: spironolactone + hydrochlorothiazide, or other drugs, as indicated, in the doses shown (in mg). Jobst, waist high elastic garment (Jobst Co., Toledo, OH).

APPENDIX II

#	Sex	Ages		Blood pressure		Heart rate		Symptoms
		When seen	At onset	Rec. (mm Hg)	Stand. (mm Hg)	Rec. (per min)	Stand. (per min)	
1. Orthostatic Diastolic Hypotension								
a. With autonomic insufficiency								
1	M	59	57	134/88	70/52	116	116	EdImLPkSyW facial sweats, died
2	F	62	57	114/74	84/60	84	128	ABFLPkSSyVW
			later:	184/96	82/64	60	64	nursing home
3	M	74	72	192/104	54/40	64	64	BvHaImLSy no sweating
4	M	59	49	190/122	54/40	100	100	ImLPkSyW no sweating
5	M	56	56	156/76	104/60	56	56	DmLSy carcinoma lung
6	M	52	51	150/94	82/58	92	100	EdInLPkSy night sweats
7	M	82	81	140/84	80/60	72	84	EdL
8	M	63	62	142/68	84/42	56	56	ADmJbL myelopathy
9	M	63	62	184/116	66/56	80	92	InLN
10	M	69	66	144/74	42/18	76	80	LPkSy
11	M	52	45	188/106	72/48	76	76	EdImInSy no sweating
12	M	44	43	136/92	62/50	92	120	JbL laminectomy: L3–4 disc
			later:	214/108	142/98	88	104	
13	M	63	62	130/80	86/64	82	116	ALPk
14	M	72	68	194/88	54/40	60	56	LPkSy
15	F	45	44	106/72	60/20	120	120	DmL serum K = 8.2
16	M	71	64	132/64	54/36	72	80	ImLSy
			later:	158/82	66/42	60	72	BP v sensitive to AII
17	F	77	77	230/92	146/82	80	80	HLSy
18	F	49	48	178/80	108/68	84	96	DmLW
b. Adrenal Insufficiency								
19	F	41	22	112/66	68/50	104	140	HLNaW pigmented
20	F	57	57	90/48	70/40	96	104	FLNaW
21	F	51	50	136/80	80/50	72	102	FLNaSyW wt loss, pigmented
22	F	36	36	66/52	0/0	80	128	FLNaVW wt loss, pigmented
23	F	40	39	102/70	0/0	80	108	FLNaVW wt loss, pigmented
24	F	38	36	88/66	66/56	84	160	FLNaVW wt loss, pigmented
c. Idiopathic								
25	M	17	11	98/68	72/58	48	88	EHIIrLTZ behavior disorder
26	F	55	54	106/70	84/42	96	120	DmL ataxia
27	M	18	17	86/62	68/52	60	92	Weight loss
28	F	72		148/96	110/84	80	96	LSy
29	F	70	70	132/66	112/54	86	92	HLPaW
30	F	67	66	124/80	112/64	64	112	LSwW ct: adrenals enlarged, MIBG scan nl
31	F	74	73	170/92	104/76	90	108	L ataxia, wt loss
32	M	22	18	124/62	62/52	88	152	BvHL exercise aggravates

BP in G suit stand. (mm Hg)	Plasma concentrations of: Norepineph. Rec. (pg/ml)	Norepineph. Stand. (pg/ml)	Renin activ. (ng/ml per hr)	Aldosterone (ng/dl)	Kinin (ng/ml)	ITT cort./gluc. slope (μg/mg)	ACTH test: Cort. (μg/dl)	ACTH test: Aldo (ng/dl)	Therapy response: BP (mm Hg)	Therapy response: HR (per min)	Drug
	134	142				Nl			higher		FF 0.1
			10	30					Sl. better		FF 0.1
136/78	0				0.3, 0.6				94/66 64/40		Jobst Clonidine
						Nl	64	—			
							50	10			FF 0.1
102/62	0	279	9	34	1.1	Nl			Died, autopsy evidence of Parkinsonism only		
120/50											
						Nl			64/0		FF 0.2
	171	245							46/20		FF 0.6, died
							60	—	190/96		FF 0.1 + prednisolone
	105	245	2	60							
150/94			9				52		100/60		FF 0.2
	192	282									
			3								FF 0.5 G suit & Pitressin
60/44	167				0.8	low	82	18			
			0	3			43	8			
	117	260	1	7			48	15	118/72		Clonidine, 0.05
									106/74, 104		F + FF
											F + FF
							15		140/94, 76		F + FF
							3		118/70, 84		F + FF
						urine 17-OHCS= 1 mg/d			132/90, 80		F + FF
						urine 17-OHCS=0.7 mg/d			118/80, 80		F + FF
					0.5		40	21	96/64	84	FF 0.2
							120		116/80	116	FF 0.2, prop 40
104/68						Nl					FF 0.2 Died of ruptured aorta
						Nl			170/88	84	FF.2
			2	15			70	23			
							60				
							67		100/68	72	FF 0.1 Headache gone
									110/74	88	FF 0.1 + prop40

(*continued*)

APPENDIX II. (*Continued*)

#	Sex	Ages: When seen	Ages: At onset	Blood pressure: Rec. (mm Hg)	Blood pressure: Stand. (mm Hg)	Heart rate: Rec. (per min)	Heart rate: Stand. (per min)	Symptoms
33	M	18	17	148/84	152/70	64	84	BvHSw while playing football many PVC's standing
34	M	85	76	156/58	96/52	60	72	BvLW orth. seizures & aphasia
2. Orthostatic Systolic Hypotension								
a. With Hypoaldosteronism								
35	F	21	18	106/70	92/80	52	68	FHLSISy weight gain
36	M	61	59	122/80	88/62	72	90	EdL
37	F	36		114/66	88/84	56	80	Amenorrhea Prolactin = 54 ng/ml
38	F	11	11	104/40	84/40	96	120	LSy urticaria
39	F	64	61	130/86	60/50	88	112	LSy
b. With Hyperbradykininism								
40	M	27	20	100/66	86/60	52	84	HSY seizures, mother & sister (#61) affected
41	F	33	20	132/90	110/86			EFGHLQW legs blue
42	F	10	9	114/68	94/70	82	104	LW mother = #92
43	F	29	26	132/68	110/84	66	72	EHQSwW wt loss
44	F	35	16	102/60	88/68	60	72	FHJQW mother & daughter affected
45	F	48	33	170/110	130/110	56	88	FLQW
46	M	14	12	114/66	96/76	64	88	ELY can't stand still, son of #142
c. Idiopathic								
47	F	38	38	98/54	86/60	52	88	LQ
48	M	46	46	130/76	100/60	74	82	ALQRSSwW
				120/70	98/72	76	96	
49	M	43	42	146/84	126/84	68	100	BvHLY
50	M	27	26	108/60	88/66	86	120	BvDmFL
51	F	56	45	152/70	54/32	52	96	LSy Fabry's dis, legs & abdomen purple
			later:	222/114	194/120	72	108	
52	F	14	12	128/62	106/80	64	84	LSy
53	M	14	13	120/72	96/72	64	108	HL after running
54	M	35	22	120/72	102/78	80	88	ILNaQ SwSy, 6 yr later patient still asymptomatic
55	M	43	40	144/84	176/138	54		FGHaSw
56	M	64	63	100/66	86/64	56	80	LSy
57	F	26	25	104/74	88/68	64	88	FIrSI
58	F	79	74	138/64	84/60	80	112	BvHNaSwSyW wt loss

	Plasma concentrations of					ITT	ACTH test		Therapy response		
BP in G suit stand. (mm Hg)	Norepineph. Rec. (pg/ml)	Norepineph. Stand. (pg/ml)	Renin activ. (ng/ml per hr)	Aldosterone (ng/dl)	Kinin (ng/ml)	cort./gluc. slope (μg/mg)	Cort. (μg/dl)	Aldo (ng/dl)	BP (mm Hg)	HR (per min)	Drug
									PVC's & headache now gone		
142/64	146	417					36	24	154/88	72	FF 0.1 seizures now absent
			3	5							
			0.4	5			60	8	134/82	76	FF 0.2
						metyr: 36 A-II: aldo 0 to 4 ng/dl					
			4	7			70	24			FF 0.1
							43	9	116/72	96	FF 0.1
					metyr: 14						
			0.6	2			60	7	144/62	64	FF 0.1
						A-II: aldo 2 to 4 ng/dl					
112/60			2		4,1.5,.7		60	31	84/78	104	FF 0.1 + cyproheptadine
	165	537		22	1.2,.5		70	22			
					.1,.3 bradykininase low						
104/70			3	20	.6,.9		70	30			
						metyr: 11					
			1		2.6				134/86	60	nadolol
110/58			7	42	0.7, 1.1, 0.2, 1.1		100	39	84/70		ephedrine
						metyr: 26, aldo after A-II:48					
					can't stand still AII:aldo-48, metyr:26						
						metyr:20					
									98/72	96	FF 0.1
			2	19			51	34			
			9								
						metyr:22					
					0.1, 0.4						
						0.1			108/66	104	FF 0.1
							Nl		108/70	96	FF 0.1 + co
						0			126/78	80	prop 50
					bradykininase nl, metyr:26				asymptomatic 6 yr later		
94/70							92				
			2				40		108/74	88	FF 0.2 + prop 20
	208		3	16			44	41	100/64	88	FF 0.15
						metyr:11					
							Nl		136/88	84	FF.1

(continued)

APPENDIX II. (*Continued*)

#	Sex	Ages: When seen	Ages: At onset	Blood pressure: Rec. (mm Hg)	Blood pressure: Stand. (mm Hg)	Heart rate: Rec. (per min)	Heart rate: Stand. (per min)	Symptoms
3. Orthostatic Diastolic Hypertension								
59	F	16	15	124/84	112/106	76	88	FHISw
60	F	41	21	122/80	154/102	88	92	FHL adrenal CT normal
61	F	34	21	124/82	126/104	72	96	FLW sister of #40, 2 sons are affected
62	M	43	40	144/84	176/138	60	80	HLNaQSwSyW
63	M	50	23	140/90	136/100	66	90	no symptoms
64	F	45	35	138/88	120/112	84	120	FHLSy
65	M	14	13	136/78	128/98	80	100	no symptoms
66	M	41	36	150/90	148/100	88	110	no symptoms
67	M	14	14	132/58	124/98	76	86	BvHLW
68	F	50	32	172/80	192/100	64	68	LW
69	M	32	31	126/86	136/120	68	92	EQ
70	M	23	18	138/90	138/124	100	120	EFHHaQSwSy
71	M	30	?	126/86	124/102	76	100	no symptoms
72	F	64	?	152/86	158/104	60	68	no symptoms
73	M	47	37	138/80	130/106	60	96	FHLW
74	F	33	29	130/82	134/100	104	144	EFHLQ
75	M	57	39	152/82	126/106	64	92	FIIrLSw pl. histamine & VIP both normal
76	M	33	28	120/82	140/106	64	84	AHLW
77	F	57	55	128/82	126/106	72	80	H imbalance, legs blue standing
78	M	16	15	140/78	162/120	60	76	no symptoms
79	M	34	34	144/90	148/110	76	92	HQ
80	F	17	16	154/102	132/80	64	96	EdHL
81	M	36	22	120/68	104/98	80	112	EFLQW legs bluish
82	F	19	17	118/90		116	172	FILSyW
83	M	18	17	140/66	120/108	104	152	LNaQSwSy hypertensive spells
84	M	33	22	128/86	138/98	88	108	ELQ
4. Orthostatic Narrowing of Pulse Pressure								
a. With Hyperbradykininism								
85	F	30	24	102/68	104/92	52	68	EdHaLSy legs blue
86	F	20	18	112/80	78/76	96	180	AFHaLPQW legs blue, daughter of #41
87	F	30	18	112/72	84/80	88	128	AFHaLQSy legs blue, daughter affected
88	F	23	19	144/84	90/82	84	108	DmEdFLW legs blue
89	F	19	15	102/58	74/70	52	128	FLMSyW legs blue, better in pregnancy
90	M	14	11	104/62	104/98	72	108	HLNaSyW legs blue, fidgets, son of #92
91	F	11	10	126/68	96/82	80	120	FILW legs blue, daughter of 92
92	F	31	18	120/90	104/94	74	144	EdLQSyW legs blue, mother of #42, 90 and 91
93	F	51	50	126/88	138/132	84	120	FHILSwW mother of #142 and #143

BP in G suit stand. (mm Hg)	Plasma concentrations of: Norepineph. Rec. (pg/ml)	Norepineph. Stand. (pg/ml)	Renin activ. (ng/ml per hr)	Aldo-sterone (ng/dl)	Kinin (ng/ml)	ITT cort./gluc. slope (μg/mg)	ACTH test: Cort. (μg/dl)	ACTH test: Aldo (ng/dl)	Therapy response: BP (mm Hg)	Therapy response: HR (per min)	Drug
			14		18		NI				
			3		122	1.3, 0.3	72	25	144/106	60	prop 60
						0.8 (adrenal CT nl)			122/78	72	clonidine 0.2
122/84						0.6, 0.3					
144/98			15			3, 0.2	62	34	134/102	92	FF 0.2
						metyr: 15					
									140/112		prop 40
				phentolamine infusion:BP 134/98 std					164/126		phenoxyben30
156/102			11		103				130/92	72	prop 60
									118/80	78	+ FF.1
					NI						
						0.4, 0.3			140/70	88	FF 0.1
							3 yr later:		114/80	78	FF 0.1
			0.4		13			37			
						0.3					
						0.5			130/112	92	prop 60
									120/92	92	prop 40
						1.5, 1, 1.7	43		104/78	84	clonidine .3
						0.7, 0.3					
						0.2, 0, 0.2 plasma histamine, VIP normal					
									128/94	80	FF 0.1
148/86			6								
			3						140/102		spironz
									148/96		FF 0.1
						0.1, 0.2			140/90	96	prop 30
									120/82	80	prop 80
						0.3, 0.1			128/94	72	prop 120 much improved
			3				60		116/94	92	prop80+FF0.1
			9						134/118	72	FF 0.1 + prop 120
						0.9, 0.5, 0.1			132/96	84	Valium
					(bradykininase nl) NI						
						metyr:12					
126/70	169	459	4	30		0.7, 0.8, 1	70	41			
						0.9, 0.5, 0.4			112/92	84	prop 20
						(bradykininase 0.3, 0.4)					
						1.7, 2 (aldo sec rate 1910 μg/d on low Na)			84/78	104	FF 0.1 + cypro-heptadine
						(bradykininase 0.2, 0.3)					
						(bradykininase 0.3, 0.2)			124/90	84	prop 40
112/82									100/64	80	FF 0.1 + co
							metyr:15 aldo after A-II:48				
						1.2	60		122/98	80	prop 100
						metyr 24			124/86	84	FF 0.1 + prop60

(*continued*)

APPENDIX II. (*Continued*)

#	Sex	Ages		Blood pressure		Heart rate		Symptoms
		When seen	At onset	Rec. (mm Hg)	Stand. (mm Hg)	Rec. (per min)	Stand. (per min)	
94	F	38	29	120/60	102/94	68	80	EdFHILQW
95	F	36	26	120/86	112/106	88	132	EFHHaLNa legs blue, mother of #96
96	F	20	15	140/80	114/98	56	84	HLNa daughter of #95
97	F	23	21	114/62	100/88	80	120	HIrNaSw father and brother affected
98	F	22	18	86/72	0/0	92	112	FHaLNaQW
99	F	45	44	96/80	88/82	96	128	EdFHLS legs blue, wt change intra diem + 1.5kg
100	M	28	27	122/68	82/62	136	168	DmFLQTh weight loss
101	F	32	25	136/78	126/108	84	132	EdFLPaQS pulsus paradoxicus
102	M	16	14	126/84	100/84	60	124	EFHHaL mother also affected
103	F	36	35	108/74	98/88	72	116	FLQW mother of #102
104	F	35	29	116/76	102/88	72	84	BvW started after gastrectomy mother of #105 and 106
105	M	18	16	114/74	86/74	72	112	FL son of #104
106	F	16	15	116/58	82/68	88	132	EdFLSyY legs blue, daughter of #104
107	F	33	28	98/64	84/70	64	120	LSwW legs blue
108	F	58	57	118/78	102/88	112	136	IJLNaSIW legs blue, started after influenza
109	F	22	21	110/50	100/80	60	80	ALW panic attacks

b. With Plasma Hypovolemia

None studied

c. Idiopathic

#	Sex	When seen	At onset	Rec. (mm Hg)	Stand. (mm Hg)	Rec. (per min)	Stand. (per min)	Symptoms
110	F	23	13	114/56	94/80	84	108	HLSwSyY legs blue
111	F	28	23	110/82	98/80	76	92	EFLNa tremors
112	M	23	14	148/108	134/122	120	132	EQ
113	F	36	26	124/86	88/72	68	92	EHHaJNa mother of #114
114	M	17	13	98/60	96/82	44	68	AEHLY legs blue standing, son of #113, systemic mastocytosis
115	F	29	27	100/66	96/80	60	80	EEdLSy legs blue standing
116	F	40	35	96/64	100/84	76	100	EFQZ
117	F	42	34	112/82	90/86	100	136	EILW
118	M	44	43	112/60	86/70	64	104	FLRSw wt loss, PVC's standing
119	M	47	46	110/72	98/82	84	100	HIrL
120	F	21	20	116/60	88/70	80	120	BvL Raynauds, legs blue
121	F	42	42	108/66	108/90	60	64	BvEEdFL
122	F	28	12	94/62	74/68	68	120	BvFHHa legs blue, sister and son affected
123	F	39	13	116/66	66/64	56	112	AEdFHLSyW Acth increased freq/ of PVC's as serum K fell to 2.8

BP in G suit stand. (mm Hg)	Plasma concentrations of: Norepineph. Rec. (pg/ml)	Norepineph. Stand. (pg/ml)	Renin activ. (ng/ml per hr)	Aldo-sterone (ng/dl)	Kinin (ng/ml)	ITT cort./gluc. slope (μg/mg)	ACTH test: Cort. (μg/dl)	ACTH test: Aldo (ng/dl)	Therapy response: BP (mm Hg)	Therapy response: HR (per min)	Drug
			8		1,0	metyr:18	65				
					(bradykininase 0.3)		90		112/96	120	cyproheptadine
					(bradykininase 0.3, .4)						
									78/68	92	prop 120
			4	8	0.6, 1		48	16	96/90		FF 0.1 + prop160
					2, 3.3, 2.6, 4, 0.8, 1.8						
					(bradykininase 0.3, 0.3)	metyr:48	60		136/106	100	FF 0.1 + prop160
					(bradykininase 0.3, .4)	metyr:16	44		126/80	100	FF 0.1 + cyproheptadine
112/86					(bradykininase low)	metyr:12	55		112/80	116	FF 0.2
124/76	197	866	2.4		>4, 0.3		43	47			
					2,2				138/90,60		prop + cyproheptadine
					(bradykininase 0.2, 0.3)				98/78	80	FF 0.1
104/78	130	270			3.2, 0.5		48	32	84/80	100	FF 0.2 + prop 20
								later:	106/96	96	no therapy
			1	32	.5, 1 (bradykininase 0.2, 0.3)		72	22	felt much better		FF + Co
			2	65	0.4, 0.2, 0.4				98/68	60	FF 0.1 + atenolol 50
					0.04, 0.6						improved prop40
									128/104		prop 40
96/80					0.02, 0.3 (plasma histamine nl)						
					0.5 (plasma histamine nl)				82/66	92	H1 and H2 antagonists + FF
			6		0.2		112		140/100	90	FF 0.1 + prop30
									110/80	60	FF 0.2 much improved
					Nl						
							56				
118/78	125	493			0.3, 0.3		Nl		90/62	120	FF 0.1
				Nl			Nl				improved:prop100

(*continued*)

APPENDIX II. (*Continued*)

#	Sex	Ages: When seen	Ages: At onset	Blood pressure: Rec. (mm Hg)	Blood pressure: Stand. (mm Hg)	Heart rate: Rec. (per min)	Heart rate: Stand. (per min)	Symptoms
124	M	19	?	124/78	104/88	80	120	cannot gain weight
125	M	15	14	124/70	92/84	72	120	DmLNaTl,L worst after football
126	M	54	48	114/78	92/84	96	116	DmHaLSyW meals aggravate symps
127	F	23	21	150/94	110/104	88	164	HLSy
128	F	41	34	80/60	?72/70	80	132	LSSyW, has multiple sclerosis
129	F	32	29	104/78	88/86	92	152	HLQ, legs purple, migraine
130	F	15	14	114/64	100/88	72	120	HNa tremors
131	F	24	23	110/80	94/76	72	108	L
132	M	16	15	108/60	82/64	68	92	FLSlSyY, exhausted after basketball
133	F	28	20	112/60	94/76	76	128	HL legs blue, narcolepsy, daughter, mother, sister affected
134	F	53	48	122/80	94/88	84	114	FHLSyWY
5. Orthostatic Tachycardia								
a. With Hypocortisolism								
135	F	35	33	102/66	96/74	108	128	BvLNaW
136	M	14	13	120/40	90/58	84	120	BvHLSy
137	F	46	45	104/64	98/74	72	116	FHlQSwSyW, "spells"
138	F	32	?	110/70	82/70	84	142	HLW anorexia, wt loss
139	F	33	31	96/70	66/64	100	156	FLSlW
140	F	20	18	108/60	92/70	76	136	LW
b. With Hyperbradykininism								
141	F	38	21	102/70	98/76	92	128	ALQSy mother of #86
142	F	30	28	114/72	104/82	76	112	EFlLW daughter of #93, sister of #143, mother of #46
143	F	26	12	130/70	120/82	80	110	FLQSW daughter of #93
144	F	32	15	112/68	116/80	100	124	HaLSSwY legs blue, mother and daughter affected
145	F	39	37	108/68	106/74	90	132	EHLNaSy legs blue
146	F	16	14	142/78	136/86	76	120	HHaLSwThW thyrotoxic
c. Idiopathic								
147	F	42	?	140/80	138/92	96	120	FL multifocal ectopic beats with bigeminy when standing
148	F	37	35	132/84	118/88	96	120	L galactorrhea, hypertension
149	F	23	22	116/62	106/80	84	124	HHaLSwSy legs blue
150	F	31	30	106/72	98/70	72	104	BvFGHHaL

	Plasma concentrations of										
	Norepineph.					ITT	ACTH test		Therapy response		
BP in G suit stand. (mm Hg)	Rec. (pg/ml)	Stand. (pg/ml)	Renin activ. (ng/ml per hr)	Aldo-sterone (ng/dl)	Kinin (ng/ml)	cort./gluc. slope (μg/mg)	Cort. (μg/dl)	Aldo (ng/dl)	BP (mm Hg)	HR (per min)	Drug
						metyr:10.8					
									104/76	80	FF 0.2
								3yr later:	132/98	76	no treatment
96/70				0.3, 0.1			45		100/58	88	FF 0.1
140/118	224	547	4	39	0.3, 0.4, 0						
									94/84	88	prop 100
108/70				172	0 (plasma aldo after IV NaCl 2 L: 28 ng/dl)				106/78	92	FF 0.1 + prop
			50	151	(ITT: NI, metyr:24)		100		104/84	88	FF 0.1
					4, 0.5, 0.2				86/48	80	FF 0.1 + prop40
96/64			13		0.3, 0.2, 0.7				102/66 88/66	88 112	FF 0.1 pacemaker
			7	13	0.3, 0, .2		68	37			FF 0.1
						(pl aldo during AII infusion: 7.4 to 18.9 ng/dl)					
				40		NI metyr:8	8	62			improved on Co
					0.5						
				mean plasma co:4.7μg/dl, metyr:12		0.05	34		98/74	116	on triamcinolone
						metyr:9			132/90	104	FF.1 + Co
						NI	metyr:3		108/80	68	FF.1 + Co
						NI metyr:9			128/78,	108	FF.1 + Co
104/82	550	900			0.5, 0.7						
						metyr:14			114/84	88	FF 0.05 + prop 60
									124/90	84	FF 0.1 + prop 60
114/70	92	612			1.7, 1.6 0.9, 1.3						
122/90	417	1460			2, 3, 1.5	70 metyr:19		25			no response to FF, prop, midodr
					2.2	NI					
							84		108/74	100	FF 0.1 + Co

(continued)

APPENDIX II. (*Continued*)

#	Sex	Ages: When seen	Ages: At onset	Blood pressure: Rec. (mm Hg)	Blood pressure: Stand. (mm Hg)	Heart rate: Rec. (per min)	Heart rate: Stand. (per min)	Symptoms
151	F	17	17	106/60	96/70	76	112	Sy legs blue
152	F	61	60	112/70	98/68	132	164	InLW Brown-Sequard lesion from metastatic carcinoma
153	F	25	24	128/74	106/72	88	128	HILSyY
154	F	20	19	102/50	80/45	68	132	LSY
155	F	34	29	132/90	118/84	84	112	LNaW vomiting
6. Other								
156	F	43	40	150/80	136/86	100	110	EEdHLQW G suit: improved ataxia
157	F	41	31	106/74	98/78	68	88	FIrIY very sleepy
158	F	21	?	122/70	106/84	56	88	BvHIL
159	F	26	23	172/86	156/90	80	92	AFHILTIS/W

BP in G suit stand. (mm Hg)	Plasma concentrations of: Norepineph. Rec. (pg/ml)	Norepineph. Stand. (pg/ml)	Renin activ. (ng/ml per hr)	Aldo-sterone (ng/dl)	Kinin (ng/ml)	ITT cort./gluc. slope (μg/mg)	ACTH test Cort. (μg/dl)	ACTH test Aldo (ng/dl)	Therapy response BP (mm Hg)	Therapy response HR (per min)	Drug
							NI				
							96				FF .1 + prop60
							NI				
					0.1						
			2								FF 0.2
						(clinically improved in G suit)					
				15	0.2, 0.6, 0.4 0.5, 0.5		38 metyr:30	38	15		FF 0.2 little better
							bradykininase 0.3, 0.3, 0.4				
					0.2, 0.5, 0.4		NI				

References

Abate G, Polimeni RM, Cuccurrullo F, et al: Effect of indomethacin on postural hypotension in Parkinsonism. *Br Med J* 2:1466–1468, 1979.

Abboud FM, Eckberg DL, Johannsen UJ, et al: Carotid and cardiopulmonary baroreceptor control of splanchnic and forearm vascular resistance during venous pooling in man. *J. Physiol (Lond)* 286:173–184, 1979.

Adamski SW, Svensjö E, Kay S, et al: Effects of captopril and propranolol on bradykinin-induced changes in vascular pressures, lymph total protein concentration, and weight in canine forelimbs. *Microvasc Res* 25:307–321, 1983.

Ahlquist RP: A study of the adrenotropic receptors. *Am J Physiol* 153:586–600, 1948.

Åkesson S: Über Veränderungen des Elektrokardiogramms bei orthostatischer Zirkulationsstörung. *Ups Lakareforens forhandl* 41:381, 1936.

Åkesson S: On arterial orthostatic anemia in cases of essential hypertonia. (A contribution to the question of the genesis of orthostatic electrocardiographic changes.) *Acta Med Scand (Suppl)* 170:324–347, 1946.

Alexander K, Teusen R, Mitzkay HJ: Measurement of the integrated capillary pressure in reactive hyperaemic phase in diabetics and normal subjects. *Bibl Anat* 9:516–519, 1967.

Alexander RS: The influence of constrictor drugs on the distensibility of the splanchnic venous system, analyzed on the basis of an aortic model. *Circ Res* 2:140–147, 1954.

Alexander RW, Gill JR Jr, Yamabe H, et al: Effects of dietary sodium and of acute saline infusion on the interrelationship between dopamine excretion and adrenergic activity in man. *J Clin Invest* 54:194–200, 1974.

Al-Khader AA, Aber GM: The relationship between the ''idiopathic oedema syndrome'' and subclinical hypothyroidism. *Clin Endocrinol* 10:271–279, 1979.

Allen SC, Taylor CL, Hall VE: A study of orthostatic insufficiency by the tiltboard method. *Am J Physiol* 143:11–20, 1945.

Altura BM: Evaluation of neurohumoral substances in local regulation of blood flow. *Am J Physiol* 212:1447–1454, 1967.

Altura BM: Chemical and humoral regulation of blood flow through the precapillary sphincter. *Microvasc Res* 3:361–384, 1971.

Altura BM: Pharmacology of venular smooth muscle: new insights. *Microvasc Res* 16:91–117, 1978*a*.

Altura BM: Humoral, hormonal and myogenic mechanisms in microcirculatory regulation, including some comparative pharmacologic aspects of microvessels. In Kaley G, Altura BM (eds): *Microcirculation*. Vol. 2. University Park Press, Baltimore, 1978*b*, pp. 431–502.

Anderson GH Jr, Dalakos TG, Elias A, et al: Diuretic therapy and response of essential hypertension to saralasin. *Ann Intern Med* 87:183–187, 1977.

Appenzeller O: *The Autonomic Nervous System.* 3rd ed. Elsevier, Amsterdam, 1982.

Asmussen E: The distribution of the blood between the lower extremities and the rest of the body. *Acta Physiol Scand* 5:31–38, 1943.

Asmussen E, Christensen EH, Nielsen M: Über die Kreislaufinsufficienz in stehender Stellung bei normalem arteriellem Druck und herabgesetztem Minutenvolumen. *Scand Arch Physiol* 81:214–224, 1939.

Atkinson JP, Waldmann TA, Stein SF, et al: Systemic capillary leak syndrome and monoclonal IgG gammopathy. *Medicine (Baltimore)* 56:225–239, 1977.

Atzler E, Herbst R: Die Schwankungen des Fussvolumens und deren Beeinflussing. *Z Ges Exp Med* 38:137–152, 1923.

Auchincloss JH, Streeten DHP, Gilbert R, et al: Dyspnea in patients with hyperbradykininism and excessive venous pooling. *Am J Med* 1986, in press.

August JT, Nelson DH, Thorn GW: Response of normal subjects to large amounts of aldosterone. *J Clin Invest* 37:1549–1555, 1958.

Aull JC, McCord WM: Effects of posture and activity on the major fractions of serum protein. *Am J Clin Pathol* 27:52–55, 1957.

Bachman DM, Youmans WB: Effects of posture on renal excretion of sodium and chloride in orthostatic hypotension. *Circulation* 7:413–421, 1953.

Balikian HM, Brodie AH, Dale SL, et al: Effect of posture on the metabolic clearance rate, plasma concentration and blood production rate of aldosterone in man. *J Clin Endocrinol Metab* 28:1630–1640, 1968.

Bannister R: Degeneration of the autonomic nervous system. *Lancet* 2:175–179, 1971.

Bannister R: Clinical features of progressive autonomic failure. In Bannister R (ed): *Autonomic Failure: A Textbook of Clinical Disorders of the Autonomic Nervous System.* Oxford University Press, Oxford, 1983, pp 67–73.

Bannister R, Ardill L, Fentem P: Defective autonomic control of blood vessels in idiopathic orthostatic hypotension. *Brain* 90:725–746, 1967.

Bannister R, Ardill L, Fentem P: An assessment of various methods of treatment of idiopathic orthostatic hypotension. *Q J Med* 38:377–395, 1969.

Bannister R, Sever P, Gross M: Cardiovascular reflexes and biochemical responses in progressive autonomic failure. *Brain* 100:327–344, 1977.

Bannister R, Davies B, Holly E, et al: Defective cardiovascular reflexes and supersensitivity to sympathomimetic drugs in autonomic failure. *Brain* 102:163–176, 1979.

Bansi HW, Olsen JM: Water retention in obesity. *Acta Endocrinol (Copenh)* 32:113–122, 1959.

Barcroft H, Swan HJC: *Sympathetic Control of Human Blood Vessels.* Arnold, London, 1953.

Barger AC, Berlin RD, Tulenko JF: Infusion of aldosterone, 9-α-fluorohydrocortisone and antidiuretic hormone into the renal artery of normal and adrenalectomized unanesthetized dogs. Effect on electrolyte and water excretion. *Endocrinology* 62:804–815, 1958.

Barraclough MA, Sharpey-Shafer EP: Hypotension from absent circulatory reflexes. Effects of alcohol, barbiturates, psychotherapeutic drugs, and other mechanisms. *Lancet* 1:1121–1126, 1963.

Bartter FC, Schwartz WB: The syndrome of inappropriate secretion of antidiuretic hormone. *Am J Med* 42:790–806, 1967.

Behar A, Tournoux A, Baillet J, Lagrue G: Untersuchungen zer Bestimmung der kapillaren Durchlässigkeit mit markiertem menschlichem Albumin. *Nucl Med* 15:214–216, 1976.

Benowitz NL, Byrd R, Schambelan M, et al: Dihydroergotamine treatment for orthostatic hypotension from vacor rodenticide. *Ann Intern Med* 92:387–388, 1970.

Beretta-Piccoli C, Weidmann P: Metoclopramide alone or combined with flurbiprofen in the treatment of orthostatic hypotension associated with diabetes mellitus. *Klin Wochenschr* 60:863–865, 1982.

Berry MR: Influence of the position of arm and body on blood pressure determined by auscultation. *Mayo Clin Proc* 16:29–32, 1941.

Best JB, Bett JHN, Coghlan JP, et al: Circulating angiotensin-II and aldosterone levels during dietary sodium restriction. *Lancet* 2:1353–1354, 1971.

Biglieri EG: Hypokalemic alkalosis and edema with increased desoxycorticosterone excretion. *J Clin Endocrinol Metab* 25:884–894, 1965.

Bjure A, Laurell H: Abnormal static circulatory phenomena and their symptoms. Arterial orthostatic anemia, a neglected clinical picture. *Ups Lakaref Forh* 33:1–23, 1927.

Boblin RP, Guth PS: Venoconstrictive action of bradykinin. *J Pharmacol Exp Ther* 160:11–21, 1968.

Bohr DF, Bonaccorsi A, Greenberg S: Mechanisms of action of vasoactive agents. In Kiley G, Altura BM (eds): *Microcirculation.* Vol. II. University Park Press, Baltimore, 1978, pp 311–348.

Borst C, Wieling W, van Brederode JFM, et al: Mechanisms of initial heart rate response to postural change. *Am J Physiol* 243:H676–681, 1982.

Borst C, van Brederode JFM, Wieling W, et al: Mechanisms of initial blood pressure response to postural change. *Clin Sci* 67:321–327, 1984.

Boucher R, Veyrat R, DeChamplain J, et al: New procedures for measurement of human plasma angiotensin and renin activity levels. *Can Med Assoc J* 90:194–201, 1964.

Boyd GW, Adamson AR, Arnold M, et al: The role of angiotensin II in the control of aldosterone in man. *Clin Sci* 42:91–104, 1972.

Bradbury S, Eggleston C: Postural hypotension; report of three cases. *Am Heart J* 1:73–86, 1925.

Bravo EL, Tarazi RC, Gifford RW, et al: Circulating and urinary catecholamines in pheochromocytoma. Diagnostic and pathophysiologic implications. *N Engl J Med* 301:682–686, 1979.

Bravo EL, Tarazi RC, Fouad FM, et al: Clonidine suppression test: A useful aid in the diagnosis of pheochromocytoma. *N Engl J Med* 305:623–626, 1981.

Brehm H: Der orthostatische Symptomenkomplex und seine Therapie. *Z Kreislaufforsch* 44:471–483, 1955.

Brennan LA Jr, Malvin RL, Jochim KE, et al: Influence of right and left atrial receptors on plasma concentrations of ADH and renin. *Am J Physiol* 221:273–278, 1971.

Brun C, Knudsen EOE, Raaschou F: The influence of posture on the kidney function. I. The fall of the diuresis in the erect posture. *Acta Med Scand* 122:315–331, 1945.

Burns A, Brown TM, Semple P: Clinical reports. Extreme metabolic alkalosis with fludrocortisone therapy. *Postgrad Med J* 59:506–507, 1983.

Burns CR, McGiff JC: Mechanism of the natriuretic action of dopamine. *Circulation* 35–36 (Suppl 2):ii–79, 1967.

Burnstock G, Chamley JH, Campbell GR: The innervation of arteries. In Schwartz CJ, Werthessen NT, Wolf S (eds): *Structure and Function of the Circulation.* Vol. 1. Plenum, New York, 1981, pp 729–767.

Caird FI, Andrews GR, Kennedy RD: Effect of posture on blood pressure in the elderly. *Br Heart J* 35:527–530, 1973.

Campbell IW, Ewing DJ, Clarke BF: Therapeutic experience with fludrocortisone in diabetic postural hypotension. *Br Med J* 1:872–874, 1976.

Campese VM, Romoff M, DeQuattro V, et al: Relationship between plasma catecholamines, plasma renin activity, aldosterone and arterial pressure during postural stress in normal subjects. *J Lab Clin Med* 95:927–933, 1980.

Cannon WB, Rosenblueth A: *The Supersensitivity of Denervated Structures. A Law of Denervation.* Macmillan, New York, 1949, p 1.

Cantwell DP: *The Hyperactive Child: Diagnosis, Management and Current Research*. Spectrum Publications, New York, 1975.

Carmichael SM, Eagleton L, Ayers CR, et al: Orthostatic hypotension during vincristine therapy. *Arch Intern Med* 126:290–293, 1970.

Catt KJ, Zimmet PZ Cain MD, et al: Angiotensin II blood-levels in human hypertension. *Lancet* 1:459–463, 1971.

Chambers R, Zweifach BW: Topography and function of the mesenteric capillary circulation. *Am J Anat* 75:173–205, 1944.

Chapman EM, Maloof F: Bizarre clinical manifestations of hyperthyroidism. *N Engl J Med* 254:1–5, 1956.

Cherrick GR, Kerr DNS, Read AE, et al: Colloid osmotic pressure and hydrostatic pressure relationships in the formation of ascites in hepatic cirrhosis. *Clin Sci* 19:361–375, 1960.

Chobanian AV, Volicer L, Liang CS, et al: Use of propranolol in the treatment of orthostatic hypotension. *Trans Assoc Am Physicians* 90:324–334, 1977.

Chobanian AV, Volicer L, Tifft CP, et al: Mineralocorticoid-induced hypertension in patients with orthostatic hypotension. *N Engl J Med* 301:68–73, 1979.

Chokroverty S, Barron KD, Katz FH, et al: The syndrome of primary orthostatic hypotension. *Brain* 92:743–768, 1969.

Clarke BF, Ewing DJ: Resting heart rate and diabetic autonomic neuropathy. *NY J Med* 82:908–913, 1982.

Clarkson B, Thompson D, Horwith M, et al: Cyclical edema and shock due to increased capillary permeability. *Am J Med* 1:193–206, 1960.

Clements IP, Offord KP, Baron DW, et al: Cardiovascular hemodynamics of bicycle and handgrip exercise in normal subjects before and after administration of propranolol. *Mayo Clin Proc* 59:604–611, 1984.

Clift GV, Schletter FE, Speller PJ, et al: Studies on the pathogenesis of idiopathic edema. *Clin Res* 13:235A, 1965.

Clorius JH, Kjelle-Schweigler M, Ostertag H, et al: 131-I-Hippuran renography in the detection of orthostatic hypertension. *J Nucl Med* 19:343–347, 1978.

Cody RJ, Franklin KW, Laragh JH: Postural hypotension during tilt with chronic captopril and diuretic therapy of severe congestive heart failure. *Am Heart J* 103:480–484, 1982.

Cohen EL, Rovner DR, Conn JW: Postural augmentation of plasma renin activity. Importance in diagnosis of renovascular hypertension. *JAMA* 197:973–978, 1966.

Cohen ME, Badal DW, Kilpatrick A, et al: The high familial prevalence of neurocirculatory asthenia (anxiety neurosis, effort syndrome). *Am J Hum Genet* 3:126–158, 1951.

Coleman M, Horwith M, Brown JL: Idiopathic edema. Studies demonstrating protein-losing angiopathy. *Am J Med* 49:106–113, 1970.

Coleridge HM, Coleridge JCG, Kidd C: Cardiac receptors in the dog with particular reference to two types of afferent ending in the ventricular wall. *J Physiol (Lond)* 174:323–339, 1964.

Coleridge JCG, Kidd C: Reflex effects of stimulating baroreceptors in the pulmonary artery. *J Physiol (Lond)* 166:197–210, 1963.

Collier JG, Nachev C, Robinson BF: Effect of catecholamines and other vasoactive substances on superficial hand veins in man. *Clin Sci* 43:455–467, 1972.

Conn JW, Fajans SS: The prediabetic state. A concept of dynamic resistance to a genetic diabetogenic influence. *Am J Med* 31:839–850, 1961.

Conway N, Seymour J, Gelson A: Cardiac failure in patients with valvular heart disease after use of propranolol to control atrial fibrillation. *Br Med J* 2:213–214, 1968.

Cooper KE: Functional aspects of the venous system. In Schwartz CJ, Werthessen NT, Wolf S (eds): *Structure and Function of the Circulation*. Vol. 2. Plenum, New York, 1981, pp 457–485.

Corcoran JC, Browning JS, Page IH: Renal hemodynamics in orthostatic hypotension. Effects of angiotonin and head-up bed. *JAMA* 119:793–794, 1942.
Crabbé J: Stimulation of active sodium transport by the isolated toad bladder with aldosterone in vitro. *J Clin Invest* 40:2103–2110, 1961.
Crane MG, Harris JJ: Suppression of plasma aldosterone by partial immersion. *Metabolism* 23:359–368, 1974.
Crane MG, Harris JJ, Shankel S: Case report. Tetany related to postural diuresis. *Am J Med Sci* 265:153–165, 1973.
Cranston WI, Brown W: Diurnal variation in plasma volume in normal and hypertensive subjects. *Clin Sci* 25:107–114, 1963.
Cryer PE: Mechanisms and management of postural hypotension. *Spec Top Endocrinol Metab* 1:79–91, 1979.
Cryer PE, Weiss S: Reduced plasma norepinephrine response to standing in autonomic dysfunction. *Arch Neurol (Chicago)* 33:275–277, 1976.
Cryer PE, Santiago JV, Shah S: Measurement of norepinephrine and epinephrine in small volumes of blood by a single isotope derivative method: Response to the upright posture. *J Clin Endocrinol Metab* 39:1025–1029, 1974.
Cuche JL, Kuchel O, Barbeau A, et al: Relationship between the adrenergic nervous system and renin during adaptation to upright posture: A possible role for 3,4-dihydroxyphenethylamine (dopamine). *Clin Sci* 43:481–491, 1972.
Currens JH: A comparison of the blood pressure in the lying and standing positions: A study of 500 men and 500 women. *Am Heart J* 35:646–654, 1948.
Da Costa JM: On irritable heart; a clinical study of a form of functional cardiac disorder and its consequences. *Am J Med Sci* 61:17–52, 1871.
Davies B, Bannister R, Sever P: Pressor amines and amine-oxidase inhibitors for treatment of postural hypotension in autonomic failure. Limitations and hazards. *Lancet* 1:172–175, 1978.
Davies B, Bannister R, Mathias C, et al: Pindolol in postural hypotension: The case for caution. *Lancet* 2:982–983, 1981.
Davies B, Sudera D, Sagnella G, et al: Increased numbers of alpha receptors in sympathetic denervation supersensitivity in man. *J Clin Invest* 69:779–784, 1982.
Davis JO, Myers CR, Carpenter CCJ: Renal origin of an aldosterone-stimulating hormone in dogs with thoracic caval constriction and in sodium depleted dogs. *J Clin Invest* 40:1466–1474, 1961.
de Bold AJ, Borenstein HB, Veress AT, et al: A rapid and potent natriuretic response to intravenous injection of atrial myocardial extract in rats. *Life Sci* 28:89–94, 1981.
Deitrick JE, Whedon GD: The effects of bed rest and immobilization upon some aspects of calcium metabolism and circulation in normal men: their modification by the use of the oscillating bed. *J Clin Invest* 25:915, 1946 (abs).
DeMey JG, Vanhoutte PM: Differences in pharmacological properties of postjunctional alpha-adrenergic receptors among arteries and veins. *Arch Int Pharmacodyn Ther* 244:328–329, 1980.
Dent RG, Edwards OM: Idiopathic oedema: A study of the effects of bromocriptine. *Clin Endocrinol* 11:75–80, 1979*a*.
Dent RG, Edwards OM: Bromocriptine-responsive form of idiopathic oedema. *Lancet* 2:355–356, 1979*b*.
Depace N, Segal BL, Fischl SJ, et al: Mitral valve prolapse and orthostatic hypotension. *Pract Cardiol* 7:160–162, 1981.
Devine CE: Vascular smooth muscle morphology and ultrastructure. In Kaley J, Altura BM (eds): *Microcirculation*. Vol. II. University Park Press, Baltimore, 1978, pp 1–39.
De Wardener HE: Idiopathic edema: Role of diuretic abuse. *Kidney Int* 19:881–892, 1981.

Diamond MA, Murray RH, Schmid PG: Idiopathic postural hypotension: physiologic observations and report of a new mode of therapy. *J Clin Invest* 49:1341–1343, 1970.

Dietlen H: Über die klinische Bedeutung der Veränderungen am Zirkulationsapparate, insbesondere der wechseln den Herzgrösse, bei verschiedener Körperstellung (Liegen und Stehen). *Dtsch Arch Klin Med* 97:132–164, 1909.

Docci D, Turci F, Salvi G: Therapeutic response of idiopathic edema to captopril. *Nephron* 34:198–200, 1983.

Dzau VJ: Vascular wall renin-angiotensin pathway in control of the circulation: A hypothesis. *Am J Med* 77(4A):31–36, 1984*a*.

Dzau VJ: Vascular renin-angiotensin: A possible autocrine or paracrine system in control of vascular function. *J Cardiovasc Pharmacol* 6:S377–S382, 1984*b*.

Ead HW, Green JH, Neil E: A comparison of the effects of pulsatile and non-pulsatile blood flow through the carotid sinus on the reflexogenic activity of the sinus baroreceptors in the cat. *J Physiol (Lond)* 118:509–519, 1952.

Eckstein JW, Hamilton WK: The pressure–volume responses of human forearm veins during epinephrine and norepinephrine infusions. *J Clin Invest* 36:1663–1671, 1957.

Edmonds ME, Archer AG, Watkins PJ: Ephedrine: A new treatment for diabetic neuropathic oedema. *Lancet* 1:548–551, 1983.

Edwards OM, Bayliss RIS: Postural fluid retention in patients with idiopathic oedema: Lack of relationship to the phase of the menstrual cycle. *Clin Sci* 48:331–333, 1975.

Edwards OM, Bayliss RIS: Idiopathic oedema of women. A clinical and investigative study. *Q J Med* 45:125–144, 1976.

Edwards CRW, Besser GM, Thorner MO: Bromocriptine-responsive forms of idiopathic oedema. *Lancet* 2:94, 1979.

Ehinger B, Falck B, Sporrong B: Adrenergic fibres to the heart and to peripheral vessels. *Bibl Anat* 8:35–45, 1967.

Eide I, Campese V, Stein D, et al: Clinical assessment of sympathetic tone: Orthostatic blood pressure responses in borderline primary hypertension. *Clin Exp Hypertension* 1:51–65, 1978.

Eisenhofer G, Lambie DG, Johnson RH, et al: Deficient catecholamine release as the basis of orthostatic hypotension in pernicious anaemia. *J Neurol Neurosurg Psychiatry* 45:1053–1055, 1982.

Ellis LB, Haynes PW: Postural hypotension with particular reference to its occurrence in disease of the central nervous sytem. *Arch Intern Med* 58:773–798, 1936.

Emerson K Jr, Armstrong SH Jr: High protein edema due to diffuse abnormality of capillary permeability. *Trans Am Clin Climatol Assoc* 67:59–72, 1955.

Epstein FH, Goodyer AVN, Lawrason FD, et al: Studies of the antidiuresis of quiet standing: The importance of changes in plasma volume and glomerular filtration rate. *J Clin Invest* 30:63–72, 1951.

Epstein M, Saruta T: Effect of water immersion on renin-aldosterone and renal sodium handling in normal man. *J Appl Physiol* 31:368–374, 1971.

Erlanger J, Hooker DR: An experimental study of blood-pressure and of pulse-pressure in man, including a consideration (a) of blood-pressure and pulse-pressure under various physiological conditions, (b) of the effect of blood-pressure and pulse-pressure upon the secretion of urine, and (c) of the relation between blood-pressure and pulse-pressure and the output of albumin in a case of orthostatic albuminuria. *Johns Hopkins Hosp Rep* 12:147–376, 1905.

Evered DC, Horrobin DF, Vice PA, et al: Idiopathic oedema and prolactin. *Proc R Soc Med* 69:427–428, 1976.

Ewing DJ, Campbell IW, Clarke BF: The natural history of diabetic autonomic neuropathy. *Q J Med* 49:95–108, 1980.

Ewing DJ, Martyn CN, Young RJ, et al: The value of cardiovascular autonomic function tests: 10 year's experience in diabetes. *Diabetes Care* 8:491–498, 1985.

Farhi LE, Nisarajah MS, Olszowka AJ, et al: Cardiac output determination by simple one-step rebreathing technique. *Respir Physiol* 28:141–159, 1976.

Fasola AF, Martz BL: Peripheral venous renin activity during 70° tilt and lower body negative pressure. *Aerospace Med* 43:713–715, 1972.

Faucheux B, Buu NT, Kuchel O: Effects of saline and albumin on plasma and urinary catecholamines in dogs. *Am J Physiol* 232:F123–F127, 1977.

Favre H, Mach RS: Etude du "facteur natriurétique" chez des malades atteints d'oedèmes idiopathiques. *Schweiz Med Wochenschr* 110:1107–1111, 1980.

Fawcett JK, Wynn V: Effects of posture on plasma volume and some blood constituents. *J Clin Pathol* 13:304–310, 1960.

Ferrer MI: The sick sinus syndrome. *Hosp Pract* 79–89, Nov 1980.

Fisher DA, Morris MD: Idiopathic edema and hyperaldosteronuria: Postural venous plasma pooling. *Pediatrics* 35:413–424, 1965.

Folkow B: Cardiovascular structural adaptation; its role in the initiation and maintenance of primary hypertension. *Clin Sci Mol Med* 55:3S–22S, 1978.

Food and Drug Administration: Amphetamines: Drugs for human use; drug efficacy study implementation; amendment of previous notice and opportunity for hearing. *U.S. Federal Register* 44:41552–41571, 1979.

Fritz I, Levine R: Action of adrenal cortical steroids and norepinephrine on vascular responses of stress in adrenalectomized rats. *Am J Physiol* 165:456–465, 1951.

Frohlich ED, Tarazi RC, Ulrych M, et al: Tilt test for investigating a neural component in hypertension. Its correlation with clinical characteristics. *Circulation* 36:387–393, 1967.

Furness JB: Arrangement of blood vessels and their relation with adrenergic nerves in the rat mesentery. *J Anat* 115:347–364, 1973.

Gabbay KH, Merola LO, Field RA: Sorbitol pathway: Presence in nerve and cord with substrate accumulation in diabetes. *Science* 151:209–210, 1966.

Gauer OH: Die Wechselbeziehungen zwischen Herz- und Venensystem. *Verh Dtsch Ges Herz Kreislaufforsch* 22:61–78, 1956.

Gauer OH, Henry JP: Circulatory basis of fluid volume control. *Physiol Rev* 43:423–481, 1963.

Gauer OH, Thron HL: Properties of veins in vivo: Integrated effects of their smooth muscle. *Physiol Rev* 42 (Suppl 5):283–303, 1962.

Gauer OH, Thron HL: Postural changes in the circulation. In Hamilton WF and Dow P (eds): *Handbook of Physiology. Circulation.* Sect. 2, Vol. III. American Physiological Society, Washington, DC, 1965, pp 2409–2439.

Gavras H, Ribeiro AB, Gavras I, et al: Reciprocal relation between renin dependency and sodium dependency in essential hypertension. *N Engl J Med* 295:1278–1283, 1976.

Gill JR Jr: The role of the sympathetic nervous system in the regulation of sodium excretion by the kidney. In Ganong WF, Martini L (eds): *Frontiers in Neuroendocrinology.* Oxford University Press, New York, 1969, pp 289–305.

Gill JR Jr, Mason DT, Bartter FC: "Idiopathic" edema resulting from occult cardiomyopathy. *Am J Med* 38:475–480, 1965.

Gill JR Jr, Cox J, Delea CS, et al: Idiopathic edema. II: Pathogenesis of edema in patients with hypoalbuminemia. *Am J Med* 52:452–456, 1972*a*.

Gill JR Jr, Waldmann TA, Bartter FC: Idiopathic edema. I. The occurrence of hypoalbuminemia and abnormal albumin metabolism in women with unexplained edema. *Am J Med* 52:444–451, 1972*b*.

Glezer GA, Moskalenko NP: The physiological and pathological haemodynamic changes in orthostasis in subjects with a normal arterial pressure. *Cor Vasa* 14:265–277, 1972.

Glover WE, Greenfield ADM, Kidd BSL, et al: The reactions of the capacity blood vessels of the human hand and forearm to vasoactive substances infused intraarterially. *J Physiol (Lond)* 140:113–121, 1958.

Goetz RH, Warren JV, Gauer OH, et al: Circulation of the giraffe. *Circ Res* 8:1049–1058, 1960.

Gordon ES, Graham DT: Metabolic edema. *J Lab Clin Med* 54:818–819, 1959.

Gordon RD, Wolfe LK, Island DP, et al: A diurnal rhythm in plasma renin activity in man. *J Clin Invest* 45:1587–1592, 1966.

Gordon RD, Kuchel O, Liddle GW, et al: Role of the sympathetic nervous system in regulating renin and aldosterone production in man. *J Clin Invest* 46:599–605, 1967.

Gowenlock AH, Mills JN, Thomas S: Acute postural changes in aldosterone and electrolyte excretion in man. *J Physiol (Lond)* 146:133–141, 1959.

Graham JG, Oppenheimer DR: Orthostatic hypotension and nicotine sensitivity in a case of multiple system atrophy. *J Neurol Neurosurg Psychiatry* 32:28–34, 1969.

Green DM, Metheny D: The estimation of acute blood loss by the tilt test. *Surg Gynecol Obstet* 84:1045–1050, 1947.

Green RS, Iglauer A, McGuire J: Alterations of radial or brachial intra-arterial blood pressure and of the electrocardiogram induced by tilting. *J Lab Clin Med* 33:951–960, 1948.

Greenough WB, Sonnenblick EH, Januszewicz V, et al: Correction of hyperaldosteronism of massive fluid retention of unknown cause by sympathomimetic agents. *Am J Med* 33:603–614, 1962.

Gregory R: Treatment of orthostatic hypotension with particular reference to use of desoxycorticosterone. *Am Heart J* 29:246–252, 1945.

Grill C: Investigations into the displacements in the blood mass due to changes in the body positions, and the resultant changes in the work of the heart, in the blood pressure and in the volume of the extremities under physiological conditions and in certain pathological conditions; and a contribution to the pathogenesis of so-called arterial orthostatic anaemia. *Acta Med Scand* 92:267–307, 1937.

Gross M: The effects of posture on subjects with cerebrovascular disease. *Q J Med* 39:485–491, 1970.

Gullbring B, Holmgren A, Sjostrand T, et al: The effect of blood volume variations on the pulse rate in supine and upright positions and during exercise. *Acta Physiol Scand* 50:62–71, 1960.

Guy WA: The effect produced upon the pulse by change of posture. Being part of a paper read before the physical society of Guy's Hospital in the month of October 1837. *Guys Hosp Rep* 3:92–110, 1838.

Guyton AC, Lindsey AW, Kaufman BN, et al: Effect of blood transfusion and hemorrhage on cardiac output and on the venous return curve. *Am J Physiol* 194:263–267, 1958.

Guyton AC, Abernathy B, Langston JB, et al: Relative importance of venous and arterial resistances in controlling venous return and cardiac output. *Am J Physiol.* 196:1008–1014, 1959.

Haddy FJ, Scott JB: Active hyperemia, reactive hyperemia, and autoregulation of blood flow. In Kaley G, Altura BM (eds): *Microcirculation.* Vol. 3. University Park Press, Baltimore, 1978, pp 531–544.

Haddy FJ, Molnar JI, Borden CW, et al: Comparison of direct effects of angiotensin and other vasoactive agents on small and large blood vessels in several vascular beds. *Circulation* 25:239–246, 1962.

Hammarström S: Arterial hypertension. I. Variability of blood pressure. II. Neurosurgical treatment, indications and results. *Acta Med Scand (Suppl)* 192:1–301, 1947.

Hatton R, Clough DP, Adigun SA, et al: Functional interaction between angiotensin and sympathetic reflexes in cats. *Clin Sci* 62:51–56, 1982.

Helgeland A: Treatment of mild hypertension: A five-year controlled drug trial. The Oslo study. *Am J Med* 69:725–732, 1980.

Heymans C, Neil E: *Reflexogenic Areas of the Cardiovascular System*. Little, Brown, Boston, 1958, pp 23–25, 78–82.

Hickler RB: Orthostatic hypotension and syncope. Editorial. *N Engl J Med* 296:336–337, 1977.

Hickler RB, Thompson GR, Fox LM, et al: Successful treatment of orthostatic hypotension with 9-alpha-fluorohydrocortisone. *N Engl J Med* 261:788–791, 1959*a*.

Hickler RB, Wells RE, Tyler HR, et al: Plasma catecholamine and electroencephalographic responses to acute postural change. *Am J Med* 26:410–423, 1959*b*.

Hickler RB, Hoskins RG, Hamlin JT III: The clinical evaluation of faulty orthostatic mechanisms. *Med Clin North Am* 44:1237–1250, 1960.

Hill L: The influence of the force of gravity on the circulation of the blood. *J Physiol (Lond)* 18:15–53, 1895.

Hill L, Barnard H: The influence of the force of gravity on the circulation. Part II, Section I. The action of the respiratory pump. Section II. The escape of the heart from vagal arrest. Section III. The mean pressure of the vascular system. *J Physiol (Lond)* 21:323–352, 1897.

Hill SR Jr, Hood WG Jr, Farmer TA Jr, et al: Idiopathic edema: Report of a case with orthostatic edema and hyperaldosteronism. *N Engl J Med* 263:1342–1345, 1960.

Hjemdahl P, Eliasson K: Sympatho-adrenal and cardiovascular response to mental stress and orthostatic provocation in latent hypertension. *Clin Sci* 57:189s–191s, 1979.

Holland OB, Nixon JV, Kuhnert L: Diuretic-induced ventricular ectopic activity. *Am J Med* 70:762–768, 1981.

Holmes LB, Fields JP, Zabriskie JB: Hereditary late-onset lymphedema. *Pediatrics* 61:575–579, 1978.

Holmgren A, Ovenfors CO: Heart volume at rest and during muscular work in the supine and in the sitting position. *Acta Med Scand* 167:267–277, 1960.

Horwith M, Hagstrom JWC, Riggins RCK, et al: Hypovolemic shock and edema due to increased capillary permeability. *JAMA* 200:101–104, 1967.

Hughes RO, Cartlidge NEF, Millac P: Primary neurogenic orthostatic hypotension. *J Neurol Neurosurg Psychiatry* 33:363–371, 1970.

Hull DH, Wolthuis RA, Cortese T, et al: Borderline hypertension versus normotension: Differential response to orthostatic stress. *Am Heart J* 94:414–420, 1977.

Hypertension Detection and Follow-up Program Cooperative Group: *Circ Res* Suppl I:106–109, 1977.

Ibrahim MM, Tarazi RC, Dustan HP: Orthostatic hypotension: Mechanisms and management. *Am Heart J* 90:513–520, 1975.

Ingle DJ: The relationship of the diabetogenic effect of diethylstilbestrol to the adrenal cortex in the rat. *Am J Physiol* 138:579–581, 1942–1943.

Ingle DJ: Permissive action of hormones. *J Clin Endocrinol Metab* 14:1272–1274, 1954*a*.

Ingle DJ: Permissibility of hormone action: A review. *Acta Endocrinol (Copenh)* 17:172–186, 1954*b*.

Itskovitz HD, Wartenburg A: Combined phenylephrine and tranylcypromine for postural hypotension. *Am Heart J* 106:598–599, 1983.

Jacox R, Waterhouse C, Tobin R: Periodic disease associated with muscle destruction. *Am J Med* 55:105–110, 1973.

Jennings G, Esler M, Holmes R: Treatment of orthostatic hypotension with dihydroergotamine. *Br Med J* 2:307, 1979.

Johnson JA, Moore WW, Segar WE: Small changes in left atrial pressure and plasma antidiuretic hormone titers in dogs. *Am J Physiol* 217:210–214, 1969.

Johnson JM, Rowell LB, Niederberger M, et al: Human splanchnic and forearm vasoconstrictor responses to reductions of right atrial and aortic pressures. *Circ Res* 34:515–524, 1974.

Johnson RH, Smith AC, Spalding JMK, et al: Effect of posture on blood pressure in elderly patients. *Lancet* 1:731–733, 1965.

Joint National Committee on Detection, Evaluation and Treatment of High Blood Pressure: 1980 Report. *Arch Intern Med* 140:1280–1285, 1980.

Joint National Committee on Detection, Evaluation and Treatment of High Blood Pressure: 1984 Report. *Hypertension* 7:457–468, 1985.

Jones NF: Sodium homeostasis in patients with ''idiopathic oedema.'' *Heilkunst* 86:158–162, 1973.

Kaley G: Microcirculatory–endocrine interactions. Role of the prostaglandins. In Kaley G, Altura BM (eds): *Microcirculation.* Vol. 2. University Park Press, Baltimore, 1978, pp 503–529.

Kangawa K, Matsuo H: Purification and complete amino-acid sequence of alpha-human atrial natriuretic polypeptide (a-hANP). *Biochem Biophys Res Commun* 118:131–139, 1984.

Kaplan AP; Angioedema (Editorial). *N Engl J Med* 310:1662–1664, 1984.

Kaplan NM: *Clinical Hypertension.* 3rd ed. Williams & Wilkins, Baltimore, 1982, pp 103–107.

Kapoor WN, Karpf M, Wieand S, et al: A prospective evaluation and follow-up of patients with syncope. *N Engl J Med* 309:197–204, 1983.

Kappagoda CT, Linden RJ, Snow HM: The effect of stretching the superior vena caval-right atrial junction on right atrial receptors in the dog. *J Physiol (Lond)* 227:875–887, 1972.

Katz, FH: Diurnal variation of plasma renin activity, aldosterone and cortisol in idiopathic edema. *J Clin Endocrinol Metab* 45:419–424, 1977.

Kirkendall WM, Feinleib M, Freis ED, et al: AHA Committee Report. Recommendations for human blood pressure determination by sphygmomanometers. Subcommittee of the AHA Postgraduate Education Committee. *Circulation* 62:1145A–1155A, 1980.

Kirsch KA, Röcker L, Gauer OH, et al: Venous pressure in man during weightlessness. *Science* 225:218–219, 1984.

Knox R: On the relation between the time of day and various functions of the human body; and the manner in which the pulsations of the heart and arteries are affected by muscular exertion. *Edinburgh Med J* 11:52–65, 1815.

Knox R: Physiological observations on the pulsations of the heart, and on its diurnal revolution and excitability. *Edinburgh Med Surg J* 47:358–377, 1837.

Kochar MS, Itskowitz HD: Treatment of idiopathic orthostatic hypotension (Shy-Drager syndrome) with indomethacin. *Lancet* 1:1011–1014, 1978.

Kopin IJ, Polinsky RJ, Oliver JA, et al: Urinary catecholamine metabolites distinguish different types of sympathetic neuronal dysfunction in patients with orthostatic hypotension. *J Clin Endocrinol Metab* 57:632–637, 1983.

Kristinsson A: Programmed atrial pacing for orthostatic hypotension. *Acta Med Scand* 214:79–83, 1983.

Krogh A, Landis EM, Turner AH: The movement of fluid through the human capillary wall in relation to venous pressure and to the colloid osmotic pressure of the blood. *J Clin Invest* 11:63–95, 1932.

Kuchel O, Horky SD, Gregorova I, et al: Inappropriate response to upright posture: A precipitating factor in the pathogenesis of idiopathic edema. *Ann Intern Med* 73:245–252, 1970.

Kuchel O, Cuche JL, Buu NT, et al: Catecholamine excretion in ''idiopathic'' edema; decreased dopamine excretion a pathogenic factor? *J Clin Endocrinol Metab* 44:639–646, 1977.

Kuchel O, Buu NT, Gutkowska J: Treatment of severe orthostatic hypotension by metoclopramide. *Ann Intern Med* 93:841–843, 1980.

Lake CR, Ziegler MG, Kopin IJ: Use of plasma norepinephrine for evaluation of sympathetic neuronal function in man. *Life Sci* 18:1315–1326, 1976.

Landgren S, Neil E: Chemoreceptor impulse activity following haemorrhage. *Acta Physiol Scand* 23:158–167, 1951.

Landis EM, Gibbon JH Jr: The effects of temperature and of tissue pressure on the movement of fluid through the human capillary wall. *J Clin Invest* 12:105–138, 1933.

Langer SZ: Presynaptic regulation of the release of catecholamines. *Pharmacol Rev* 32:337–362, 1981.

Laragh JH, Angers M, Kelly WG, et al: Hypotensive agents and pressor substances. The effect of epinephrine, norepinephrine, angiotensin II and others on the secretory rate of aldosterone in man. *JAMA* 174:234–240, 1960.

Laurell H: Die "orthostatische arteriele Anämie," ein gewöhnliches, aber oft fehlgedeutetes Krankheitsbild. *Fortschr Geb Roentgenstrahl* 53:501–519, 1936.

Ledsome JR, Linden RJ: Reflex increase in heart rate from distention of the pulmonary-vein–atrial junctions. *J Physiol (Lond)* 170:456–473, 1964.

Ledsome JR, Linden RJ: The effect of distending a pouch of the left atrium on the heart rate. *J Physiol (Lond)* 193:121–129, 1967.

Levin JM, Ravenna P, Weiss M: Idiopathic orthostatic hypotension. Treatment with a commercially available counter pressure suit. *Arch Intern Med* 114:145–148, 1964.

Lewis RK, Hazelrig CG, Fricke FJ, et al: Therapy of idiopathic orthostatic hypotension. *Arch Intern Med* 129:943–949, 1972.

Lewis T: Report on neurocirculatory asthenia and its management. *Milit Surg* 42:409–426, 1918.

Lewis T: *The Soldier's Heart and the Effort Syndrome*. Shaw & Sons, London, 1919 and Hoeber, New York, 1920.

Liddle GW: Sodium diuresis induced by steroidal antagonists of aldosterone. *Science* 126:1016–1018, 1957.

Linden RJ: Function of cardiac receptors (George E Brown Memorial Lecture). *Circulation* 48:463–480, 1973.

Looke H: Über die Volumenänderungen der unteren extremitäten unter verschiedenen Bedingungen. *Arbeitsphysiol* 9:496–504, 1937.

Luetscher JA, Lieberman AH: Idiopathic edema with increased aldosterone output. *Trans Assoc Am Physicians* 70:158–166, 1957.

Luetscher JA, Dowdy AJ, Arnstein AR, et al: Idiopathic edema and increased aldosterone excretion. In Baulieu EE, Robel PFA (eds): *Aldosterone: A Symposium*. FA Davis, Philadelphia, 1964, p 487.

Luft R, von Euler US: Two cases of postural hypotension showing a deficiency in release of norepinephrine and epinephrine. *J Clin Invest* 32:1065–1069, 1953.

MacGregor GA, de Wardener HE: Idiopathic oedema. *Lancet* 2:355, 1979.

MacGregor GA, Tasker PRW, de Wardener HE: Diuretic-induced oedema. *Lancet* 1:489–492, 1975.

MacGregor GA, Roulston JE, Markandu ND, et al: Is "idiopathic oedema" idiopathic? *Lancet* 1:397–400, 1979.

Mach RS, Fabre J, Muller AF, et al: Oedèmes par rétention de chlorure de sodium avec hyper-aldostéronurie. *Schweiz Med Wochenschr* 85:1229–1234, 1955*a*.

Mach RS, Fabre J, Muller AF, et al: Oedème idiopathique par rétention sodique avec hyper-aldostéronurie. *Bull Mem Soc Med Hop Paris* 19/20:726–732, 1955*b*.

MacLean AR, Allen EV: Orthostatic hypotension and orthostatic tachycardia. Treatment with the "head-up" bed. *JAMA* 115:2162–2167, 1940.

MacLean AR, Allen EV, Magath TB: Orthostatic tachycardia and orthostatic hypotension: Defects in return of venous blood to the heart. *Am Heart J* 27:145–163, 1944.

Magrini F, Ibrahim MM, Tarazi RC: Abnormalities of supine hemodynamics in idiopathic orthostatic hypotension. *Cardiology* 61(Suppl 1):125–135, 1976.

Malcolm AD, Broughner DR, Kostuk WJ, et al: Clinical features and investigative findings in presence of mitral leaflet prolapse. Study of 85 consecutive patients. *Br Heart J* 38:244–256, 1976.

Management Committee: The Australian therapeutic trial in mild hypertension. *Lancet* 1:1261–1267, 1980.

Man in 't Veld AJ, Schalekamp MADH: Pindolol acts as beta-adrenoceptor agonist in orthostatic hypotension. Therapeutic implications. *Br Med J* 282:929–931, 1981.

Man in 't Veld AJ, Boomsma F, Schalekamp MADH: Effects of β-adrenoceptor agonists and antagonists in patients with peripheral autonomic neuropathy. *Br J Clin Pharmacol* 13:367S–374S, 1982.

Mann S, Altman DG, Rafferty EB, et al: Circadian variation of blood pressure in autonomic failure. *Circulation* 68:477–483, 1983.

Marieb NJ, Mulrow PJ: Failure to escape: A mechanism in idiopathic edema. *J Clin Invest* 43:1279, 1964 (abs).

Mark AL, Kerber RE: Augmentation of cardiopulmonary baroreflex control of forearm vascular resistance in borderline hypertension. *Hypertension* 4:39–46, 1982.

Matalon SV, Farhi LE: Cardiopulmonary readjustments in passive tilt. *J Appl Physiol* 47:503–507, 1979.

McCann WS, Romansky MJ: Orthostatic hypertension: The effect of nephroptosis on the renal blood flow. *JAMA* 115:573–578, 1940.

McCuskey RS: A dynamic and static study of hepatic arterioles and hepatic sphincters. *Am J Anat* 119:455–471, 1966.

McDonald RH Jr, Goldberg LI, McNay JL, et al: Effects of dopamine in man: augmentation of sodium excretion, glomerular filtration rate and renal plasma flow. *J Clin Invest* 43:1116–1124, 1964.

Meyer JS, Leiderman H, Denny-Brown D: Electroencephalographic study of insufficiency of the basilar and carotid arteries in man. *Neurology (NY)* 6:455–477, 1956.

Miles DW, Hayter CJ: The effect of intravenous insulin on the circulatory responses to tilting in normal and diabetic subjects with special reference to baroreceptor reflex block and atypical hypoglycaemic reactions. *Clin Sci* 34:419–430, 1968.

Mimran A, Targhetta R: Captopril treatment of idiopathic edema. *N Engl J Med* 301:1289–1290, 1979.

Molzahn M, Dissman TL, Halim S, et al: Orthostatic changes of haemodynamics, renal function, plasma catecholamines and plasma renin concentration in normal and hypertensive man. *Clin Sci* 42:209–222, 1972.

Moritz F: Methodisches und Technisches zur Orthodiagraphie. *Dtsch Arch Klin Med* 81:1–33, 1904.

Moss AJ, Glazer W, Topol E: Atrial tachypacing in the treatment of a patient with primary orthostatic hypotension. *N Engl J Med* 302:1456–1457, 1980.

Muller AF, Manning EL, Riondel AM: Diurnal variation of aldosterone related to position and activity in normal subjects and patients with pituitary insufficiency. In Muller AF, O'Connor CM (eds): *An International Symposium on Aldosterone*. Little, Brown, Boston, 1958*a*, pp 111–142.

Muller AF, Manning EL, Riondel AM: Influence of position and activity on the secretion of aldosterone. *Lancet* 1:711–713, 1958*b*.

Naimark A, Wasserman K: The effect of posture on pulmonary capillary blood flow in man. *J Clin Invest* 41:949–954, 1962.

Nanda RN, Johnson RH, Keogh HJ: Treatment of neurogenic orthostatic hypotension with a monoamine oxidase inhibitor and tyramine. *Lancet* 2:1164–1167, 1976.

Neil E: Chemoreceptor areas and chemoreceptor circulatory reflexes. *Acta Physiol Scand* 22:54–65, 1951.

Neil E, cited by Heymans C, Neil E: *Reflexogenic Areas of the Cardiovascular System*, Little, Brown, Boston, 1958, p 81.

Norbiato G, Bevilacqua M, Raggi U, et al: Effect of metoclopramide, a dopaminergic inhibitor, on renin and aldosterone in idiopathic edema: Possible therapeutic approach with Levodopa and Carbidopa. *J Clin Endocrinol Metab* 48:37–42, 1979.

Nordenfelt O: Über funktionelle Veränderungen der P- und T-Zacken im Elektrokardiogramm. *Acta Med Scand (Suppl)* 119:1–186, 1941.

Nylin G, Levander M: Studies of the circulation with the aid of tagged erythrocytes in a case (orthostatic hypotension. *Ann Intern Med* 28:723–746, 1948.

Obeid AI, Streeten DHP, Eich RH, et al: Cardiac function in idiopathic edema. *Arch Intern Med* 134:253–258, 1974.

Oelkers W, Marsen M, Molzahn M, et al: Spontaneous changes in weight, leg volume, renin, aldosterone and sex hormones in patients with cyclical oedema. *Klin Wochenschr* 53:509–517, 1975.

Oelkers W, Rawer C, Wiederholt M, et al: Katamnesen und endokrinologische Befunde bei Frauen mit idiopathischem Ödem. *Klin Wochenschr* 55:495–502, 1977.

Oliver JA, Sciacca RR: Local generation of angiotensin I as a mechanism of regulation of peripheral vascular tone in the rat. *J Clin Invest* 74:1247–1251, 1984.

Oppenheimer BS, Levine SA, Morison RA, et al: Report on neurocirculatory asthenia and its management (foreword by T Lewis). *Milit Surg* 42:409–426, 1918*a*.

Oppenheimer BS, Levine SA, Morison RA, et al: Illustrative cases of neurocirculatory asthenia. *Milit Surg* 42:711–719, 1918*b*.

Ota K, Kimura T, Matsui K, et al: The effects of postural changes on ADH release and the renal handling of sodium and water in patients with idiopathic edema. *Endocrinol Jpn* 31:459–469, 1984.

Overstall PW, Exton-Smith AN, Imms FJ, et al: Falls in the elderly related to postural imbalance. *Br Med J* 1:261–264, 1977.

Page EB, Hickam JB, Sieker HO, et al: Reflex venomotor activity in normal persons and in patients with postural hypotension. *Circulation* 11:262–270, 1955.

Page MM, Watkins PJ: Provocation of postural hypotension by insulin in diabetic autonomic neuropathy. *Diabetes* 25:90–95, 1976.

Parving H-H, Hansen JM, Nielsen SL, et al: Mechanisms of edema formation in myxedema: increased protein extravasation and relatively slow lymphatic drainage. *N Engl J Med* 301:460–465, 1979.

Payen DM, Safar ME, Levenson JA, et al: Prospective study of predictive factors determining borderline hypertensive individuals who develop sustained hypertension: prognostic value of increased diastolic orthostatic blood pressure tilt-test response and subsequent weight gain. *Am Heart J* 103:379–383, 1982.

Pearce ML, Newman EV: Some postural adjustments of salt and water excretion. *J Clin Invest* 33:1089–1094, 1954.

Pelletier CL, Edis AJ, Shepherd JT: Circulatory reflex from vagal afferents in response to hemorrhage in the dog. *Circ Res* 29:626–634, 1971.

Pelletier CL, Shepherd JT: Circulatory reflexes from mechanoreceptors in the cardio-aortic area. *Circ Res* 33:131–138, 1973.

Pfeiffer MA, Weinberg CR, Cook DL, et al: Autonomic neural dysfunction in recently diagnosed diabetic subjects. *Diabetes Care* 7:447–453, 1984.

Phalen GS: Reflections of 21 years' experience with the carpal tunnel syndrome. *JAMA* 212:1365–1367, 1970.

Pinals RS, Dalakos TG, Streeten DHP: Idiopathic edema as a cause of non-articular rheumatism. *Arthritis Rheumatism* 22:396–399, 1979.

Polinsky RJ, Kopin IJ, Ebert MH, et al: Pharmacologic distinction of different orthostatic hypotension syndromes. *Neurology (Minneapolis)* 31:1–7, 1981.

Polinsky RJ, Samaras GM, Kopin IJ: Sympathetic neural prosthesis for managing orthostatic hypotension. *Lancet* 1:901–904, 1983.

Porter JM, Lindell TD, Lakin PC: Leg edema following femoropopliteal autogenous vein bypass. *Arch Surg* 105:883–888, 1972.

Preston GM, Rees JR, Spathis GS: A man with cyclical oedema. *Guys Hosp Rep* 111:69–79, 1962.

Rapoport JL, Buchsbaum MS, Zahn TP, et al: Dextroamphetamine: Cognitive and behavioral effects in normal prepubertal boys. *Science* 199:560–562, 1978.

Reid AC, Matheson MS, Teasdale G: Volume of the ventricles in benign intracranial hypertension. *Lancet* 2:7–8, 1980.

Reilly FD, McCuskey RS, Cilento EV: Hepatic microvascular regulatory mechanisms. I. Adrenergic mechanisms. *Microvasc Res* 21:103–116, 1981.

Richards AM, Nicholls MG, Ikram H, et al: Syncope in aortic valvular stenosis. *Lancet* 2:1113–1116, 1984.

Riley CM, Day RL, Greeley DM, et al: Central autonomic dysfunction with defective lacrimation. I. Report of 5 cases. *Pediatrics* 3:468–478, 1949.

Riley CM, Moore RH: Familial dysautonomia differentiated from related disorders: Case reports and discussions of current concepts. *Pediatrics* 37:435–446, 1966.

Riley TL, Friedman JM: Stroke, orthostatic hypotension and focal seizures. *JAMA* 245:1243–1244, 1981.

Roberts LJ: Recurrent syncope due to systemic mastocytosis. Clinical Conference. *Hypertension* 6:285–294, 1984.

Roberts LJ II, Fields JP, Oates JA: Mastocytosis without uticaria pigmentosa: A frequently unrecognized cause of recurrent syncope. *Trans Assoc Am Physicians* 95:36–41, 1982.

Robertson D, Johnson GA, Robertson RM, et al: Comparative assessment of stimuli that release neuronal and adrenomedullary catecholamines in man. *Circulation* 59:637–643, 1979.

Robertson D, Goldberg MR, Hollister AS, et al: Clonidine raises blood pressure in severe idiopathic orthostatic hypotension. *Am J Med* 74:193–200, 1983.

Robinson S: Physiological adjustments to heat. In Newburgh LH (ed): *Physiology of Heat Regulation and the Science of Clothing*. WB Saunders, Philadelphia, 1949, p 205.

Robson D: Pindolol in postural hypotension. *Lancet* 2:1280, 1981.

Rosa RM, Silva P, Young JB, et al: Adrenergic modulation of extrarenal potassium disposal. *N Engl J Med* 302:431–434, 1980.

Roscher AA, Manganiello VC, Jelsema CL, et al: Autoregulation of bradykinin receptors and bradykinin-induced prostacyclin formation in human fibroblasts. *J Clin Invest* 74:552–558, 1984.

Rose JC, Kot PA, Cohn JN, et al: Comparison of effects of angiotensin and norepinephrine on pulmonary circulation, systemic arteries and veins and systemic vascular capacity in the dog. *Circulation* 25:247–253, 1962.

Rosen SG, Cryer PE: Postural tachycardia syndrome. Reversal of sympathetic hyperresponsiveness and clinical improvement during sodium loading. *Am J Med* 72:847–850, 1982.

Rosenhamer G, Thorstrand C: Effect of G-suit in treatment of postural hypotension. *Acta Med Scand* 193:277–280, 1973.

Rosenthal T, Birch M, Osikowska B, et al: Changes in plasma noradrenaline concentration following sympathetic stimulation by gradual tilting. *Cardiovasc Res* 12:144–147, 1978.

Ross EJ, Crabbé J, Renold AE, et al: A case of massive edema in association with an aldosterone-secreting adrenocortical adenoma. *Am J Med* 25:278–292, 1958.

Rovner DR: The enigma of idiopathic cyclic edema. *Hosp Pract* 103–110, 1972.

Rowell LB,Wyso CR, Brengelmann GL: Sustained human skin and muscle vasoconstriction with reduced baroreceptor activity. *J Appl Physiol* 34:639–643, 1973.

Rubini ME, Kleeman CR, Lamdin E: Studies on alcohol diuresis. II. The effect of ethyl alcohol ingestion on water, electrolyte and acid–base metabolism. *J Clin Invest* 34:439–447, 1955.

Safar ME, Weiss YA, Levenson JA, et al: Hemodynamic study of 85 patients with borderline hypertension. *Am J Cardiol* 31:315–319, 1973.

Santos AD, Puthenpurakal KM, Hilal A, Wallace WA: Orthostatic hypotension: A commonly unrecognized cause of symptoms in mitral valve prolapse. *Am J Med* 71:746–750, 1981.

Sapru RP, Sleight P, Anand IS, et al: Orthostatic hypertension. *Am J Med* 66:177–182, 1979.

Schatz, IJ: Orthostatic hypotension: Diagnosis and treatment. *Hosp Pract* 59–69, April 1984.

Schatz IJ, Podolsky S, Frame B: Idiopathic orthostatic hypotension: Diagnosis and treatment. *JAMA* 186:537–540, 1963.

Schirger A, Hines EA Jr, Molnar GD, et al: Idiopathic orthostatic hypotension. *JAMA* 181:822–826, 1962.

Schirger A, Thomas JE: Idiopathic orthostatic hypotension: Clinical spectrum and prognosis. *Cardiology* 61(Suppl 1):144–149, 1976.

Schirger A, Sheps SG, Thomas JE, et al: Midodrine, a new agent in the management of idiopathic orthostatic hypotension and Shy-Drager syndrome. *Mayo Clin Proc* 56:429–433, 1981.

Schmid PG, Eckstein JW, Abboud FM: Effect of 9-alpha-fluorohydrocortisone on forearm vascular responses to norepinephrine. *Circulation* 34:620–626, 1966.

Schneider EC, Truesdell D: A statistical study of the pulse rate and the arterial blood pressures in recumbency, standing and after a standard exercise. *Am J Physiol* 61:429–474, 1922.

Schneider PB: Orthostatic hypotension. Observations on the effect of levarterenol and Hypertensin. II. *Arch Intern Med* 110:240–248, 1962.

Schuster DS: Erythema of legs on standing. *JAMA* 202:670–671, 1967.

Seller RH: Idiopathic orthostatic hypotension. Report of successful treatment with a new form of therapy. *Am J Cardiol* 23:838–844, 1969.

Sever PS: Plasma noradrenalin in autonomic failure. In Bannister R (ed): *Autonomic Failure. A Textbook of Clinical Disorders of the Autonomic Nervous System.* Oxford University Press, Oxford, 1983, pp 155–173.

Sewall H: On the clinical significance of postural changes in the blood pressure and the secondary waves of arterial blood pressure. *Am J Med Sci* 158:786–816, 1919.

Shadle OW, Zukof M, Diana J: Translocation of blood from the isolated dog's hindlimb during levarterenol infusion and sciatic nerve stimulation. *Circ Res* 6:326–333, 1958.

Sharpey-Schafer EP: Venous tone. *Br Med J* 2:1589–1595, 1961.

Sharpey-Schafer EP: Venous tone: Effects of reflex changes, humoral agents and exercise. *Br Med Bull* 19:145–148, 1963.

Sharpey-Schafer EP, Taylor PJ: Absent circulatory reflexes in diabetic neuritis. *Lancet* 1:559–562, 1960.

Shear L: Renal function and sodium metabolism in idiopathic orthostatic hypotension. *N Engl J Med* 268:347–352, 1963.

Sheps SG: Use of an elastic garment in the treatment of orthostatic hypotension. *Cardiology* 6(Suppl 1):271–279, 1976.

Shy GM, Drager GA: A neurological syndrome associated with orthostatic hypotension. *Arch Neurol (Chicago)* 3:511–527, 1960.

Sieker HO, Burnum JF, Hickam JB, et al: Treatment of postural hypotension with counterpressure garment. *JAMA* 161:132–135, 1956.

Sims EAH, Mackay BR, Shirai T: The relation of capillary angiopathy and diabetes mellitus to idiopathic edema. *Ann Intern Med* 63:972–987, 1965.

Slaton PE Jr, Biglieri EG: Reduced aldosterone excretion in patients with autonomic insufficiency. *J Clin Endocrinol Metab* 27:37–45, 1967.

Smith AA, Dancis J: Catecholamine release in familial dysautonomia. *N Engl J Med* 277:61–64, 1967.

Smithwick RH, Greer WER, Robertson CW, et al: Pheochromocytoma. A discussion of symptoms, signs and procedures of diagnostic value. *N Engl J Med* 242:252–257, 1950.

Sowers JR, Beck FW, Berg G: Altered dopaminergic modulation of 18-hydroxycorticosterone secretion in idiopathic edema: Therapeutic effects of bromocriptine. *J Clin Endocrinol Metab* 55:749–756, 1982*a*.

Sowers JR, Catania R, Paris J, et al: Effects of bromocriptine on renin, aldosterone and prolactin responses to posture and metoclopramide in idiopathic edema: Possible therapeutic approach. *J Clin Endocrinol Metab* 54:510–516, 1982*b*.

Speller PJ, Streeten DHP: Mechanism of the diuretic action of D-amphetamine. *Metabolism* 13:453–465, 1964.

Spingarn CL, Hitzig WM: Orthostatic circulatory insufficiency. Its occurrence in tabes dorsalis and Addison's disease. *Arch Intern Med* 69:23–40, 1942.

Stead EA Jr, Ebert RV: Postural hypotension: A disease of the sympathetic nervous system. *Arch Intern Med* 67:546–562, 1941.

Steiner JA, Low PA, Huang CY, et al: L-dopa and the Shy-Drager syndrome. *Med J Aust* 2:133–136, 1974.

Streeten DHP: The use of aldosterone antagonists in idiopathic edema. In Bartter FC (ed): *The Clinical Use of Aldosterone Antagonists.* Charles C Thomas, Springfield, IL, 1960*a*, pp 738–745.

Streeten DHP: Primary and secondary aldosteronism: Definition and diagnosis. In Moyer JH, Fuchs M (eds): *Hahnemann Symposium on Edema.* WB Saunders, Philadelphia, 1960*b*, pp 121–132.

Streeten DHP: Symposium on the experimental pharmacology and clinical use of antimetabolites. VII. The spirolactones. *Clin Pharmacol Ther* 2:359–373, 1961.

Streeten DHP: Effects of epinephrine and norepinephrine infusions on aldosterone excretion in man. In discussion of Ganong WF, Biglieri EG, Mulrow PJ: Mechanisms regulating adrenocortical secretion of aldosterone and glucocorticoids. *Rec Prog Horm Res* 22:381–430, 1966.

Streeten DHP: Hyperbradykininism. *Univ Mich Med Cent J* 42:16–21, 1976.

Streeten DHP: Idiopathic edema: Pathogenesis, clinical features and treatment. *Metabolism* 27:353–383, 1978.

Streeten DHP: Idiopathic oedema (Letter). *Lancet* 1:775–776, 1979.

Streeten DHP, Conn JW: Studies on the pathogenesis of idiopathic edema. *J Lab Clin Med* 54:949–950, 1959.

Streeten DHP, Conn JW: Observations on the pathogenesis of idiopathic edema. Advanced abstracts of short communications. *First International Congress of Endocrinology, Copenhagen, 1960.*

Streeten DHP, Speller PJ: The role of aldosterone and vasopressin in the postural changes in renal excretion in normal subjects and patients with idiopathic edema. *Metabolism* 15:53–64, 1966.

Streeten DHP, Hirschowitz BI, Henley KS, et al: Effects of adrenocortical steroids on the propulsive motility of small intestine. *Am J Physiol* 189:108–112, 1957.

Streeten DHP, Conn JW, Louis LH, et al: Secondary aldosteronism. The metabolic and adrenocortical responses of normal man to high environmental temperatures. *Metabolism* 9:1071–1092, 1960*a*.

Streeten DHP, Louis LH, Conn JW: Secondary aldosteronism in idiopathic edema. *Trans Assoc Am Physicians* 73:227–239, 1960*b*.

Streeten DHP, Schletter FE, Clift GV, et al: Studies of the renin-angiotensin-aldosterone system in patients with hypertension and in normal subjects. *Am J Med* 46:844–861, 1969*a*.

Streeten DHP, Stevenson CT, Dalakos TG, et al: The diagnosis of hypercortisolism. Biochemical criteria differentiating patients from lean and obese normal subjects and from females on oral contraceptives. *J Clin Endocrinol Metab* 29:1191–1211, 1969*b*.

Streeten DHP, Kerr LP, Kerr CB, et al: Hyperbradykininism: A new orthostatic syndrome. *Lancet* 2:1048–1053, 1972.

Streeten DHP, Dalakos TG, Souma M, et al: Studies of the pathogenesis of idiopathic oedema. *Clin Sci Mol Med* 45:347–373, 1973.

Streeten DHP, Anderson GH Jr, Dalakos TG, et al: Normal and abnormal function of the hypothalamic–pituitary–adrenocortical system in man. *Endocr Rev* 5:371–394, 1984.

Streeten DHP, Auchincloss JH Jr, Anderson GH Jr, et al: Orthostatic hypertension. Pathogenetic studies. *Hypertension* 7:196–203, 1985.

Strong CG, Bohr DF: Effects of prostaglandins E1, E2, A1 and F1α on isolated vascular smooth muscle. *Am J Physiol* 213:725–733, 1967.

Su PC, Rosen AD, Peress NS: Orthostatic hypotension of central neurogenic origin. *NY J Med* 77:1960–1963, 1977.

Sundin T: The influence of body position on the urinary excretion of adrenaline and noradrenaline. *Acta Med Scand (Suppl)* 313:1–57, 1956.

Surtshin A, White HL: Postural effects on renal tubular activity. *J Clin Invest* 35:267–271, 1956.

Takada Y, Shimizu H, Kazatani Y, et al: Orthostatic hypertension with nephroptosis and aortitis disease. *Arch Intern Med* 144:152–154, 1984.

Tanz RD: Studies on the inotropic action of aldosterone on isolated cardiac tissue preparations; including the effects of pH, ouabain and SC-8109. *J Pharmacol Exp Ther* 135:71–78, 1962.

Taylor C, Allen SC: Unpublished report to National Research Council 1941. Cited by Allen *et al.*: A study of orthostatic insufficiency by the tiltboard method. *Am J Physiol* 143:11–20, 1945.

Thibonnier MJ, Marchetti JP, Corvol PL, et al: Abnormal regulation of antidiuretic hormone in idiopathic edema. *Am J Med* 67:67–73, 1979.

Thibonnier MJ, Marchetti JP, Corvol PL, et al: Influence of previous diuretic intake on the humoral and hormonal profile of idiopathic oedema. *Eur J Clin Invest* 11:9–24, 1981.

Thomas S: Some effects of change of posture on water and electrolyte excretion by the human kidney. *J Physiol (Lond)* 139:337–352, 1957.

Thomas JE, Schirger A: Idiopathic orthostatic hypotension: A study of its natural history in 57 neurologically affected patients. *Arch Neurol (Chicago)* 22:289–293, 1970.

Thomas JE, Schirger A, Fealey RD, et al: Orthostatic hypotension. *Mayo Clin Proc* 56:117–125, 1981.

Thompson WO, Thompson PK, Dailey ME: The effect of posture upon the composition and volume of the blood in man. *J Clin Invest* 5:573–604, 1928.

Thorn GW: Cyclical edema. *Am J Med* 23:507–509, 1957.

Thorn GW: Approach to the patient with "idiopathic edema" or "periodic swelling." *JAMA* 206:333–338, 1968.

Thorn GW: *Idiopathic Edema*. Searle & Co, San Juan, Puerto Rico, 1972.

Thulesius O: Pathophysiological classification and diagnosis of orthostatic hypotension. *Cardiology* 61(Suppl 1):180–190, 1976.

Tifft CP, Chobanian AV: A case of chronic orthostatic hypotension: Evaluation and therapy. *Med Grand Rounds* 1:296–306, 1982.

Tobian L, Branden M, Maney J: The effect of unilateral renal denervation on the secretion of renin. *Fed Proc* 24:405, 1965.

Tohmeh JF, Shah SD, Cryer PE: The pathogenesis of hyperadrenergic postural hypotension in diabetic patients. *Am J Med* 67:772–778, 1979.

Tooke JE: A capillary pressure disturbance in young diabetics. *Diabetes* 29:815–819, 1980.

Turk J, Oates JA, Roberts LJ II: Intervention with epinephrine in hypotension associated with mastocytosis. *J Allergy Clin Immunol* 71:189–192, 1983.

Vander AJ: Effects of catecholamines and the renal nerves on renin secretion in anesthetized dogs. *Am J Physiol* 209:659–662, 1965.
Vanhoutte PM: Heterogeneity in vascular smooth muscle. In Kaley G, Altura BM (eds): *Microcirculation*. Vol. 2. University Park Press, Baltimore, 1978, pp 181–309.
Veress AT, Milojevic S, Sonnenberg H: Characterization of the natriuretic activity in the plasma of hypervolaemic rats. *Clin Sci* 59:183–189, 1980.
Veterans Administration Cooperative Study Group on Antihypertensive Agents: Effects of treatment on morbidity in hypertension. II. Results in patients with diastolic blood pressure averaging 90 through 114 mm Hg. *JAMA* 213:1143–1152, 1970.
Veyrat R: Les oedèmes idiopathiques avec hyperaldostéronisme (secondaire). Définition, historique, pathogénie. *J Urol Nephrol* 76:969–976, 1970.
Veyrat R, Robert M, Mach RS: Etude de la rénine dans les oedèmes idiopathiques avec hyperaldostéronisme secondaire. *Schweiz Med Wochenschr* 98:1499–1507, 1968.
von Euler US, Franksson C, Hellstrom J: Adrenaline and noradrenaline output in urine after unilateral and bilateral adrenalectomy in man. *Acta Physiol Scand* 31:1–5, 1954.
Wagner E: Fortgesetzte Untersuchungen über den Einfluss der Schwere auf den Kreislauf. *Arch Ges Physiol* 39:371, 1886.
Wagner HN Jr: Influence of autonomic vasoregulatory reflexes on rate of sodium and water excretion in man. *J Clin Invest* 36:1319–1327, 1957.
Wagner HN Jr: Orthostatic hypotension. *Bull Johns Hopkins Hosp* 105:322–359, 1959.
Wagner HN Jr, Braunwald E: The pressor effect of the antidiuretic principle of the posterior pituitary in orthostatic hypotension. *J Clin Invest* 35:1412–1418, 1956.
Wald H, Guernsey M, Scott FH: Some effects of alteration of posture on arterial blood pressure. *Am Heart J* 14:319–330, 1937.
Waldmann TA: Gastrointestinal protein loss demonstrated by ^{51}Cr-labelled albumin. *Lancet* 2:121–123, 1961.
Waterfield RL: The effect of posture on the volume of the leg. *J Physiol (Lond)* 72:121–131, 1931*a*.
Waterfield RL: The effects of posture on the circulating blood volume. *J Physiol (Lond)* 72:110–120, 1931*b*.
Watkins PJ: Facial swelling after food: A new sign of diabetic autonomic neuropathy. *Br Med J* 1:583–587, 1973.
Weidinger P, Kaindl F, Kroiss A, et al: Zur Beurteilung der Orthostasereaktion mit der Venenverschlussrheographie. *Cardiology* 61(Suppl 1):191–198, 1976.
Weinbren I: Spontaneous periodic oedema. *Lancet* 2:544–546, 1963.
Weissler AM, McCraw BW, Warren JV: Pulmonary blood volume determined by a radioactive tracer technique. *J Appl Physiol* 14:531–534, 1959.
Wells HS, Youmans JB, Miller DG Jr: Tissue pressure (intracutaneous, subcutaneous and intramuscular) as related to venous pressure, capillary filtration and other factors. *J Clin Invest* 17:489–499, 1938.
Werning C, Baumann K, Gysling E, et al: Renin und Aldosterone bei idiopathischen Ödemen. *Klin Wochenschr* 47:1256–1263, 1969.
Wesson LG Jr: Glomerular and tubular factors in the renal excretion of sodium chloride. *Medicine (Baltimore)* 36:281–396, 1957.
Wiggins RC, Basar I, Slater JDH, et al: Vasovagal hypotension and vasopressin release. *Clin Endocrinol (Oxf)* 6:387–393, 1977.
Wilcox CS, Aminoff MJ, Slater JDH: Sodium homeostasis in patients with autonomic failure. *Clin Sci Mol Med* 53:321–328, 1977.
Wilcox CS, Puritz R, Lightman SL, et al: Plasma volume regulation in patients with progressive autonomic failure during changes in salt intake or posture. *J Lab Clin Med* 104:331–339, 1984.
Williams GH, Cain JP, Dluhy RG, et al: Studies of the control of plasma aldosterone concentration in

normal man. I. Response to posture, acute and chronic volume depletion and sodium loading. *J Clin Invest* 51:1731–1742, 1972.

Winkle RA, Lopes MG, Popp RL, et al: Life-threatening arrhythmias in the mitral valve prolapse syndrome. *Am J Med* 60:961–967, 1976.

Wolfe LK, Gordon RD, Island DP, et al: An analysis of factors determining the circadian pattern of aldosterone excretion. *J Clin Endocrinol Metab* 26:1261–1266, 1966.

Wong PY, Talamo RC, Williams GH, et al: Response of the kallikrein-kinin and renin-angiotensin systems to saline infusion and upright posture. *J Clin Invest* 55:691–698, 1975.

Wood JE, Eckstein JW: A tandem forearm plethysmograph for study of the acute responses of the peripheral veins of man: The effect of environmental and local temperature change, and the effect of pooling blood in the extremities. *J Clin Invest* 37:41–50, 1958.

Youmans JB, Akeroyd JH Jr, Frank H: Changes in the blood and circulation with changes in posture. The effect of exercise and vasodilatation. *J Clin Invest* 14:739–753, 1935.

Zerbe RL, Henry DP, Robertson GL: Vasopressin response to orthostatic hypotension. Etiologic and clinical implications. *Am J Med* 74:265–271, 1983.

Ziegler MG, Lake CR, Kopin IJ: Deficient sympathetic nervous response in familial dysautonomia. *N Engl J Med* 294:630–633, 1976.

Ziegler MG, Lake CR, Kopin IJ: The sympathetic nervous defect in primary orthostatic hypotension. *N Engl J Med* 296:293–297, 1977.

Zimmerman BG: Actions of angiotensin on adrenergic nerve endings. *Fed Proc* 37:199–202, 1978.

Zoller RP, Mark AL, Abboud FM, et al: The role of low pressure baroreceptors in reflex vasoconstrictive responses in man. *J Clin Invest* 51:2967–2972, 1972.

Zweifach BW: Microcirculation. *Annu Rev Physiol* 35:117–150, 1973.

Zweifach BW, Shorr E, Black MM: The influence of the adrenal cortex on behavior of terminal vascular bed. *Ann NY Acad Sci* 56:626–633, 1952–1954.

Index

GPSR Compliance

The European Union's (EU) General Product Safety Regulation (GPSR) is a set of rules that requires consumer products to be safe and our obligations to ensure this.

If you have any concerns about our products, you can contact us on ProductSafety@springernature.com

In case Publisher is established outside the EU, the EU authorized representative is:

Springer Nature Customer Service Center GmbH
Europaplatz 3
69115 Heidelberg, Germany

Batch number: 10620163

Printed by Printforce, the Netherlands